Also by Angela Scriven:

Alliances in Health Promotion: Theory and Practice*

Health Promotion: Professional Perspectives*

*Also published by Palgrave Macmillan

Promoting Health

Global Perspectives

edited by

Angela Scriven and Sebastian Garman

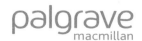

palgrave
macmillan

First published 2005 by
PALGRAVE MACMILLAN
Houndmills, Basingstoke, Hampshire RG21 6XS and
175 Fifth Avenue, New York, N.Y. 10010
Companies and representatives throughout the world.

PALGRAVE MACMILLAN is the global academic imprint of the Palgrave
Macmillan division of St. Martin's Press, LLC and of Palgrave Macmillan Ltd.
Macmillan® is a registered trademark in the United States, United Kingdom
and other countries. Palgrave is a registered trademark in the European
Union and other countries.

ISBN-13: 978-1-4039-2136-9 hardback
ISBN-10: 1-4039-2136-9 hardback
ISBN-13: 978-1-4039-2137-6 paperback
ISBN-10: 1-4039-2137-7 paperback

This book is printed on paper suitable for recycling and made from fully
managed and sustained forest sources.

A catalogue record for this book is available from the British Library.

10 9 8 7 6 5 4 3 2 1
14 13 12 11 10 09 08 07 06 05

Printed in China.

Contents

List of Figures and Tables

Figures

Tables

Foreword

Ilona Kickbusch

In order to understand the key challenges facing health promotion at this point in time we need to situate it within the new dynamics of the 21st century. There is of course an extensive literature that aims to identify the key driving forces of change. For health promotion in a global perspective two defining elements of modernity, globalisation and individualisation, are of particular importance.

These factors are not only a 'new' context or a new set of determinants of health but they change the very nature of health promotion and public health, its focus and its key strategies. This new quality is reflected in the two central themes of the present debate on global health: the understanding of health as a global public good (which addresses the collective dimension of health) and the understanding of health as a human right (which addresses the individual dimension of health). Both themes address the extreme inequalities in access to health and indicate new approaches on how they should be addressed. The data speak a stark language of global inequality: 1.2 billion people live on less than US $1 a day and the gap between the richest fifth and the poorest fifth is growing. Additionally we need to take into account that about 70 per cent of the world's poor are women and children and that no country treats its women as well as its men.

Health as global public good: the macro dimension

While there is a significant and controversial debate whether health can be a global public good, it does address the fact that we need to move beyond seeing health only in terms of national challenges. Public health, and health promotion, have emerged historically as a key element of the modern nation state, as part and parcel of the state responsibility for the security and safety of its citizens and its economic development. Globalisation has clearly shifted this 'national' premise. Kaul et al. (1999) define global public goods as outcomes (or intermediary products) that tend towards universality in the sense that they benefit all countries, population groups and generations. '....Its benefits extend to more than one group of countries and do not discriminate against any population group or any set of generations, present or future.' In a borderless world the health of one part of the world depends on the health of another and from that emerges a new conceptualisation of health as a new form of global politics. In health promotion terms this gives a totally new meaning to what we define as healthy public policy. Health is now part of foreign policy, security policy, trade and economic policy and geopolitics. Increasingly therefore in macro terms health is seen as being 'at the core of human development.'

Health as an individual right: the micro dimension

There has also been a whole new development discourse starting from a new view of the individual. The concept of human capabilities, as expressed in the work of Amartya Sen and Martha Nussbaum, reflects much of what we have considered to be a health promotion perspective with a focus on empowerment. Martha Nussbaum's studies on sex and social justice are a central contribution to the debate around a new global ethics based on gender equity. She underlines that a person's human rights derives just from the fact of being human; human rights she says, are in effect 'justified claims to basic capabilities and opportunities.' Nussbaum has developed a basic set of central human functional capabilities which all citizens (women and men) should have and which should be the goal of public policies that aim to reach gender equality – and I would add, health.

The most recent campaign against stigma by the UNAIDS programme reinforces this approach: AIDS is not presented as a disease but through a sea of faces of individuals identifying some of the most painful symptoms of HIV/ AIDS as shame, stigma, ignorance and injustice. Health and disease in many variations have become a defining factor of increasing areas of personal and social life and an increasing number of everyday behaviours and deviations, compulsions and addictions are defined in health terms and regulated through the health system. An important part of this development is the creation of a self, an identity. Again HIV/AIDS is the obvious example, the identity is one of a person living with HIV or AIDS and the politics are related to this identity, fighting for oneself and others with the same disease related identity.

Just as in the global arena health has entered multiple policy arenas in the context of everyday life; health is now indivisible from the discourse on sexuality, violence, gender and beauty to name but a few. Increasingly therefore health is seen as being at the core of human development also in micro terms.

Linking globalisation, individualisation and health promotion

Health is created in the context of everyday life. Health promotion can contribute to a differentiated view of how globalisation and its dynamics affects not only economies, the state, nations and institutions but also personal lives and experiences. Globalisation brings with it the pressure of being forced to live a more flexible and reflexive life towards an open future, a process which can be liberating for some and carries great costs, burdens and fears for others.

This interface between the macro and the micro dimensions of public health and health promotion will be central for its development in the twenty-first century. The five action areas of the Ottawa Charter take on new meaning and we are challenged to reframe them with a global perspective in mind.

Global health opens great opportunities, as outlined in this book, to understand and reposition health promotion as a global strategy.

Ilona Kickbusch
Professor and Head of the Division of Global Health
Department of Epidemiology and Public Health
Yale University School of Medicine

References

Giddens, A. (1990) *The Consequences of Modernity*. London: Polity Press.

Kickbusch, I. (2003) Global Health Governance: some new theoretical considerations on the new political space. In Lee, K. (ed) *Globalization and Health*. London: Palgrave 2003, pp. 192–203.

Kaul, I., Grunberg, I. and Stern, M.A. (1999) (eds) *Global Public Goods. International Cooperation in the 21st Century*. New York: UNDP.

Nussbaum, M. (1999) *Sex and Social Justice*. Oxford: Oxford University Press 1999.

Sen, A. (1999) *Development as Freedom*. New York: Anchor.

Singer, P. (2002) *One World. The ethics of Globalization*. New Haven: Yale University Press.

Notes on Contributors

Peter Aggleton is Professor in Education and Director of the Thomas Coram Research Unit at the Institute of Education, University of London, UK. The author and editor of over 30 books on the social aspects of HIV/AIDS, and the editor of the journal *Culture, Health and Sexuality* (Published by Taylor and Francis), Professor Aggleton is a senior advisor to UNAIDS, UNESCO, UNICEF, WHO and a wide range of other international agencies.

Laurie Anderson is a health scientist at the US Centers for Disease Control and Prevention (CDC) where she works with the Task Force on Community Preventive Services conducting systematic reviews of public health programmes to synthesise research on intervention effectiveness. Her work focuses on public health nutrition programs and policies, and on broad socio-cultural determinants of health, such as housing, education and employment. Prior to joining the Community Guide she worked in chronic disease prevention and health promotion with CDC's Behavioural Risk Factor Surveillance System and the Division of Cancer Prevention and Control.

Hiram Arroyo is Professor and Chair of the Department of Social Sciences, School of Public Health, Medical Sciences Campus, University of Puerto Rico. He has been teaching and researching in the fields of Health Promotion and Health Education for over 20 years. He is a Regional Director of the International Union on Health Promotion and Health Education for the Latin America Region. He is co-author and editor of three books: *Desde Uncinariasis hasta Estilos de Vida- Crónicas de la Educación para la Salud en Puerto Rico (1994), La Promoción de la Salud y la Educación para la Salud en América Latina- Un Análisis Sectorial (1997) and Formación de Recursos Humanos en Promoción de la Salud y Educación para la Salud en América Latina-Modelos y Prácticas en las Américas (2001).*

Samira Asma is the Associate Director for Global Tobacco Control at the Office on Smoking and Health, National Center for Chronic Disease Prevention and Health Promotion, US Centers for Disease Control and Prevention.

Robert Beaglehole trained in medicine in New Zealand and in epidemiology and public health in England and the USA. He is now Director, Office of the Assistant Director-General, Evidence and Information for Policy Cluster, WHO, Geneva. His responsibilities include being Editor-in-Chief of World Health Reports. He has published over 200 scientific papers, several books on epidemiology and public health, and is co-editor of the *Oxford Textbook of Public Health*, Fourth Edition.

Chris Brown is a health promotion and development specialist working in the WHO/European Office for Investment for Health and Development. She has been working with international agencies for over 10 years and has been responsible for the design management and evaluation of many cross-sectoral development programmes in Europe and internationally. Since 1997, she has been working with countries across the European region to undertake reviews of their population health promotion policy, capacity and infrastructures, with a view to strengthening systems and practice to address the social and economic determinants of health.

Martin Caraher is Reader in Food and Health policy at City University, London, UK. He originally trained as an environmental health officer, subsequently moving in to health promotion and community development. He has written extensively on issues related to cooking skills, local sustainable food supplies, the role of markets and cooperatives in promoting health, farmers' markets, food access and poverty, retail concentration and globalisation of the food chain. Current research includes the role of local food projects in promoting health and the relationship between the state and local/regional funded food projects in England.

Sophia Chan is currently Head of Department of Nursing Studies of the University of Hong Kong. Over the years, she had developed her professional and academic career as a clinical nurse, nurse educator and nurse researcher. She has designed and implemented a number of pioneering programmes in Hong Kong including the smoking cessation counselling training programme for nurses and social workers. Her research expertise is in the evaluation of tobacco dependency treatment interventions and outcomes, health promotion and education, nursing education and gerontology.

John Coveney has worked in clinical, community and public health nutrition settings in UK, Papua New Guinea and Australia. He is currently coordinator of the Postgraduate Programme in Primary Health Care at Flinders University, Adelaide, Australia. He is the author of two books, *Good Vegetarian Food for Children*, co-author Rhonda Mooney, and *Food, Morals and Meaning*, and has publications in the fields of health promotion and food policy.

Basiro Davey is Senior Lecturer in Health Sciences, Department of Biological Sciences at The Open University, UK. Her writing on a wide range of topics, including HIV/AIDS, asthma and emerging infectious diseases, takes a multidisciplinary approach to public health issues. She is a major contributor to and Series Editor for the nine books in the *Health and Disease* series, Open University Press/McGraw Hill. Her ethnographic research on acute surgical wards focuses on interactions between health professionals, patients and carers in contested situations, such as decisions not to attempt resuscitation.

Sebastian Garman is Senior Tutor to the Department of Health and Social Care at Brunel University, London, UK. He is leader for a postgraduate module on Global Perspectives in Public Health and Health Promotion and has helped design, teach and publish for health related courses for 30 years. He is a sociologist with a research interest in collective memory and the role of the mass media. He is on the Advisory Council of the *Association for the Study of Ethnicity and Nationalism* and on the editorial committee of its journal, *Nations and Nationalism.*

Joana Godinho is a medical Doctor with a specialism in public health and communication. She is a Senior Health Specialist at the World Bank, where she has been working on human development, environment and infrastructure. For the last 10 years, she has been assisting Governments of the Former Soviet Union and other stakeholders carrying out analytical work. This work has involved preparing and implementing investment operations on reproductive health, water and sanitation, TB and HIV/AIDS control, and health sector reforms, including establishment of health promotion and primary healthcare.

Prakash Gupta is a Senior Research Scientist at the Tata Institute of Fundamental Research, and Honorary Consultant at the Tata Memorial Centre, Mumbai, India. He is the Vice President of Action Council against Tobacco, India and is connected with numerous NGOs working on cancer control and tobacco control. He has a longstanding interest in tobacco control research for over 30 years, published numerous research papers and has received several honours and awards including Luther Terry Award from the American Cancer Society for Exemplary Leadership in Tobacco Control in the category of Outstanding Research Contribution.

Spencer Hagard is a senior lecturer in health promotion at the London School of Hygiene and Tropical Medicine where he organised the MSc Health Promotion Sciences course until 2003. His main research and consultancy work is in national systems and infrastructures for effective health promotion policy making and practice. He was previously chief executive of the former Health Education Authority for England, and from 1996 to 2001 was President of the International Union for Health Promotion and Education.

Corinna Hawkes is currently working on the development of a long-term strategy for noncommunicable disease prevention at the World Health Organization. Previously she was a New York City based freelance consultant working on food policy issues both at the international and community level. She also taught at the Department of Nutrition, Food Studies and Public Health at New York University, and is now an honorary research fellow in the Department of Health Management and Food Policy at City University, London.

Shane Hearn is the first Aboriginal Lecturer to be appointed permanently to the School of Public Health at the University of Sydney, Australia. He is also a Director of the Australian Centre for Health Promotion and chairs the Australian Indigenous Health Promotion Network. He lecturers in public policy and Aboriginal health and convenes the Graduate Diploma in Indigenous Health Promotion at the University of Sydney. His research and consultancy work has been in the area of education, evaluation, policy and capacity building in Indigenous communities in Australian.

John Hubley is Principal Lecturer in Health Promotion at Leeds Metropolitan University in the UK. He has been involved in training, consultancy and research activities in more than 25 countries in Africa, Caribbean, Asia, Europe and the Pacific. He is the author of *Communicating Health* and *The AIDS Handbook* both published by Macmillan and co-author of *Public Health in Developing Countries* published by Oxford University Press. His main research interests focus on the maintenance of the Leeds Health Education Database of evidence-based health promotion in developing countries.

Tim Lang is Professor of Food Policy at City University's Institute of Health Sciences in London, UK, following nine years as Director of the Centre for Food Policy at Thames Valley University, London. He has worked widely across food and public health, as an academic, in the voluntary sector and as a consultant to local, national and international bodies. He was the Director of the London Food Commission, from 1984 to 1990 and the Director of Parents for Safe Food, 1990–94.

Gabriel Leung is a public health medicine specialist. He currently has a joint appointment as Clinical Assistant Professor at the University of Hong Kong School of Public Health and as Associate Consultant in Family Medicine at Queen Mary Hospital. His research expertise spans the areas of epidemiology, health services research and health policy and economics, with over 60 scientific papers. As a Fulbright Scholar, he trained in public health and health policy and management at Harvard University. He is a medical graduate of the University of Western Ontario and completed his specialty training in family medicine at the University of Toronto.

Debra Lightsey is the Acting Associate Director for Planning, Evaluation and Legislation of the National Center for Chronic Disease Prevention and Health Promotion (NCCDPHP), at the Centers for Disease Control and Prevention (CDC) in Atlanta, Georgia, USA. As such, she is responsible for the policy agenda of the Center. Prior to joining CDC, she was the Chief Policy Advisor at the Delaware Department of Health and Social Services, directing policy activities including the agency's legislative agenda and regulatory initiatives. Prior to her work in Delaware, Ms Lightsey was on the faculty of Georgetown University, where she directed the Healthy Start National Resource Center, a national infant mortality reduction initiative.

David McDaid is Research Fellow in Health Economics and Health Policy at the London School of Economics and Political Science and also at the European Observatory on Health Care Systems. He is a director of the Health Equity Network, coordinator of the Mental Health Economics European

Network and editor of Eurohealth. Current research interests include tackling inequalities related to mental health and methods of incorporating economic evaluation into complex interventions including those for health promotion.

David McQueen is a Senior Biomedical Research Scientist and Associate Director for Global Health Promotion at the National Center for Chronic Disease Prevention and Health Promotion (NCCDPHP), at the Centers for Disease Control and Prevention (CDC) in Atlanta, Georgia, USA. Prior to joining the Office of the Director he was Director of the Division of Adult and Community Health at NCCDPHP and Director of the Office of Surveillance and Analysis at NCCDPHP. Prior to joining CDC he was Professor and Director of the Research Unit in Health and Behavioural Change at the University of Edinburgh, Scotland (1983–92), and prior to that Associate Professor of Behavioural Sciences at the Johns Hopkins University School of Hygiene and Public Health in Baltimore. He has served as Director of WHO Collaborating Centers as well as a technical consultant with the World Bank.

Hine Martin is the Director of a Public Health Workforce Development Company based in Northland, New Zealand. She has been involved in public health for 18 years with particular interest in health promotion and Māori health. At the time of writing she is completing a PhD at the University of Auckland on obesity and health service utilisation for Māori women.

Maurice Mittelmark earned his PhD in psychology in 1978 at the University of Houston. He conducted behavioural epidemiology research at the University of Minnesota from 1978 to 1987. While at Wake Forest University from 1987 until 1995, he directed the Center for Human Services Research. There, community studies were mounted on health and health services related to vulnerable population sub-groups. Since 1995, he has held a Chair in Health Promotion at the University of Bergen, Norway. Professor Mittelmark is President of the International Union for Health Promotion and Education.

David Nyamwaya holds a doctoral degree in medical anthropology from the University of Cambridge, UK. He is currently Regional Adviser, Health promotion, WHO Office for Africa, Brazzaville. He was director of Health Behaviour and Education Department of the African Medical and Research Foundation, Nairobi, 1986–99. He has taught health promotion at various universities in Africa and coordinated a course on International Health at the Kaloniska Institute, Sweden. He has undertaken numerous research projects in health and development and published on a wide range of subjects, including three editorials for *Health Promotion International*. He is a member of the IUHPE for which he has served as a member of the Board of Trustees since 1991.

Adam Oliver is Research Fellow and Lecturer in Health Economics and Health Policy at the London School of Economics and Political Science. He is Co-Founder and Chair of the Health Equity Network, Co-Founder and

Co-ordinator of the Preference Elicitation Group, a former Co-ordinator of the European Health Policy Group, and Founding Co-Editor of *Health Economics, Policy and Law*.

Michel O'Neill is a Professor in the School of Nursing at Laval University in Quebec City, Canada. He obtained his doctorate in sociology from Boston University and has been involved in community health for about 30 years as a community health worker, professor, researcher, consultant and activist. His long-standing teaching and research interests pertain to the political and policy dimensions of health promotion. He is co-editor of several books including *Health Promotion in Canada*, has authored and co-authored several dozen chapters and articles and has presented more than 100 papers in various scientific and professional meetings.

Ann Pederson is the Manager of Research and Policy at the British Columbia Centre of Excellence for Women's Health in Vancouver, Canada. She has co-authored several pieces on the evolution of health promotion in Canada with her colleagues, Irving Rootman and Michel O'Neill, beginning with their edited collection, *Health Promotion in Canada: Provincial, National and International Perspectives* in 1994. She has a substantial track record in women's health research and policy and is currently studying health sector reform and its implications for girls and women in Canada.

Irving Rootman is a Professor and Michael Smith Foundation for Health Research Distinguished Scholar at the University of Victoria, Canada. He has been a researcher and research manager for more than 25 years for the Canadian Federal Government, the World Health Organization, University of Calgary, and the University of Toronto before joining the University of Victoria in 2002. He has co-edited several books including *Health Promotion in Canada, Settings for Health Promotion* and *Evaluation in Health Promotion* as well as co-authored *People-Centred Health Promotion*. His current research is centred on the study of literacy and health and the impact of the school environment on health.

Angela Scriven is the Course Leader for the MSc in Health Promotion and Public Health at Brunel University in London, UK. She has been teaching and researching in the field of health promotion for over 20 years and has published widely including the two edited books *Health Promotion Alliances: Theory and Practice* and *Health Promotion: Professional Perspectives*. Her research is centred on the relationship between health promotion policy and practice within specific contexts.

Louise Signal is a Senior Lecturer in Health Promotion in the Department of Public Health at the Wellington School of Medicine and Health Sciences, Otago University. She has been involved in health promotion for over 15 years as a practitioner, teacher and researcher. Her current research interests include tackling inequalities in health, health promotion in primary care and health impact assessment.

Charles Warren is a Distinguished Consultant and leads the global tobacco surveillance effort for the Office on Smoking and Health, National Center for Chronic Disease Prevention and Health Promotion, US Centers for Disease Control and Prevention. Dr. Warren has led the development and implementation of the largest youth surveillance system, Global Youth Tobacco Survey.

Paul Wilkinson is an environmental epidemiologist and Head of the Public and Environmental Health Research Unit, London School of Hygiene and Tropical Medicine. He trained in clinical medicine and then epidemiology and public health in the UK, and has research interests in the health impacts of environmental pollution and climate change.

Marilyn Wise is the Executive Director of the Australian Centre for Health Promotion and a Senior Lecturer in the School of Public Health at the University of Sydney. She has more than 20 years' experience in health promotion practice, research, teaching and policy. Her current areas of interest include Indigenous health promotion, evidence-based health promotion, public health workforce planning, social exclusion/inclusion, and community/organisational capacity for health promotion. She is the Vice President for Advocacy in the International Union for Health Promotion and Education.

Derek Yach has over the past two decades initiated, managed and implemented several epidemiological and policy related programmes in priority public health areas at the national and international levels. Major areas of activity have included conducting a critical assessment of the successes and failures of the Health for All strategy that led a new HFA policy adopted by the World Health Assembly in May 1998; directing the development of WHO's first international treaty, the Framework Convention on Tobacco Control, adopted in May 2003, and directing development of a Global Strategy for diet, physical activity and health.

Erio Ziglio is the head of the recently established WHO European Office for Investment for Health and Development, based in Venice, Italy. He has been working for the last ten years with the European Office of the World Health Organization with main responsibility for health promotion and the social and economic determinants of population health. Prior to his work at the WHO, Dr Ziglio has worked as a lecturer and researcher in several universities in Europe, University of Edinburgh, and North America, Toronto and Carleton, Ottawa and Yale, USA. He has published extensively in the fields of health promotion, evaluation research and health policy.

Acknowledgements

We would like to thank all the contributors for their enthusiasm and cooperation in supporting this book and all those who have helped with the development of ideas in individual chapters. Particular thanks go to Bethan Rylance for her excellent secretarial skills and assistance in finalising the manuscript and to Helen Chalmers, Elaine Chase, Kim Rivers, Paul Tyrer, Ian Warwick and Kate Wood, all of the Thomas Coram Research Unit, Institute of Education, University of London for their contribution to earlier papers around which elements of Chapter 17 were developed.

CHAPTER 1

Promoting Health: A Global Context and Rationale

ANGELA SCRIVEN

We live in an interconnected world, where spatial, temporal and cognitive boundaries (Lee et al., 2002) separating us as individuals and societies are becoming rapidly eroded. The global health implications of this inter-connectedness are serious, wide ranging and multifaceted and are coming under increasing scrutiny. What this scrutiny reveals is that national health profiles are largely determined by socioeconomic factors outside the con-trol of individual population groups and that a number of anti-health forces are compromising the fundamental prerequisites for health. There are approaches that can be taken to improve health at a global level and whilst complex, these are affordable given international commitment. The first action programmes are underway (see Kickbusch, 1997) but there is much to be achieved, as this volume will demonstrate. The purpose of this opening chapter is to provide the general context and rationale for focusing on the promotion of global health, to review the book's contents and to discuss the terms and concepts that are used and that are central to developing a global perspective.

There are a number of reasons why a global view on health has become nec-essary. The first relates to the interconnectedness mentioned above and is con-cerned with the way the health profiles of countries and regions interact. Commenting on the global health challenges faced by the World Health Organisation (WHO) for the next decade, Dare (2003) challenges the WHO to be more cognisant of the way the health of every nation depends on the health of others. To reinforce his point he asserts that if Africa's ill health and its vicious relation to poverty and poor socioeconomic development is not addressed it will have significant repercussions for global health. Dare's use of the situation in sub-Saharan Africa presents a rather pessimistic picture. On certain indicators world health appears to be improving, with figures suggest-ing that there has been an increase in life expectancy in all countries over the past 50 years and some are forecasting this will continue (for a further discus-sion of these predictions see Lomborg, 2002; WHO, 2003 and in this text Part I, Chapters 2 and 3).

Notwithstanding some positive indicators, many authors would agree with Dare's suppositions. Stephens (2003a), to take one example, points to increasing

1

inequalities between countries creating huge global asymmetries that may reverse earlier positive health gains, a position also taken up in Chapters 2 and 3 of this text. Moreover, some (such as Buve et al., 2002; Sanders and Chopra, 2003) predict that the rapid spread of HIV and AIDS will impact dramatically on life expectancy in sub-Saharan Africa, which is amongst those regions where improvements have been made (see Chapter 9 by Aggleton in this text for a critical analysis of the global impact of HIV/AIDS). Whilst HIV/AIDS is seen as the first widespread emergent infection of our globally interconnected era (Berkley, 2002), the transmission of infectious diseases generally is a critical issue for global health in the twenty-first century and an obvious example of the health interaction between countries, regardless of their geospatial boundaries. The SARS virus discussed in Part III, Chapter 14 manifestly demonstrates that geographical boundaries are highly permeable to communicable diseases, helped in part by the increase in international travel and the effects of global climate change. Such examples illustrate that the nature of health problems have become globalised, with the need for a global view and a global approach to public health imperative.

A second equally important reason for taking a global perspective is that there are emerging and significant threats to health that require global action if they are to be tackled effectively. These include environmental degradation (Cole et al., 1999; MacArthur, 2002; Wilkinson, Chapter 10 in this text) social, economic and health inequalities inflated by a neoliberal economic orthodoxy that promotes global free trade and unregulated markets (Labonte, 1998; Leon and Walt, 2000; McDaid and Oliver, Chapter 3 in this text) and a related growth in noncommunicable diseases (WHO, 1997; see also Chapters 6 and 7 of this text) and international conflict and terrorism (Lee et al., 2002). These are matters of serious global concern, creating challenges for those promoting health within and across national boundaries.

Finally, a global perspective is required because evidence-based decision making about how to deal with the set of universal problems outlined above can only be done in the global arena. This will avoid duplication of effort, but more importantly will allow the development of global strategies involving political, economic and policy initiatives that directly address the complexity of health determinants that have to be confronted. The expansion of global information systems and networks that support those working to promote health within countries are clearly needed, to provide synergy and to facilitate the accomplishment of intercountry public health goals. As Malaspina (1998) so cogently argues, it is only by perceiving health promotion as a global challenge requiring global cooperation and partnerships at all levels that we will be able to work toward a safer and healthier world.

Hence the fundamental motivation in producing this volume is to add to the discourse about global health by reviewing national and international priorities, critically examining the diverse global health issues and challenges, postulating on future trends and disseminating some of the strategies that are being used in addressing global health impediments.

Examining global health

Recent additions to the research and literature on global health emerge from a range of disciplinary starting points, such as the excellent contributions from Lee et al. (2002) from an international relations standpoint, with its specific focus on the impact of globalisation on health and Beaglehole (2003) from a public health perspective. The promotion of health is a multi-professional field of activity with those involved coming from a range of disciplinary backgrounds. This book is different from others because it presents a comprehensive overview of global health issues, challenges and strategies that reflects this multidisciplinary base, drawing on theoretical positions from sociology, social policy, epidemiology, public health medicine, public health nutrition, food policy, health and environmental sciences, health economics, psychology, anthropology, gender studies and education.

The authors examine many of the central issues associated with the promotion of health at a global level, some of which are alluded to elsewhere in this opening chapter. Transcending the orthodoxies of traditional public health they offer a critique of where things are at, where they seem to be going and provide a future orientation for current practice. Insights are provided into the key determinants of health between and within countries, the significant health challenges to be faced in the twenty-first century are signalled and assessments are made of how effective the methodologies of health promotion and public health are in achieving health gain at a global level. The text endeavours to present a critical discourse on the issues, dilemmas and diverse perspectives relating to promoting health within and across countries and regions and to make recommendations for the future.

Contributors of chapters consist of a highly distinguished group drawn internationally and covering the disciplines noted above. Amongst them are representatives from health promotion and public health academic and research communities across the world (Aggleton, Caraher Arroyo, Coveney, Chan, Davey, Haggard, Hearn, Hubley, Lang, Martin, McDaid, Mittlemark, Oliver, O'Neill, Pederson, Rootman, Signal, Wilkinson, Wise and Scriven and Garman the editors of the book), the World Health Organisation (Beaglehole, Brown, Hawkes, Nyamwaya, Ziglio, Yach), the International Union of Health Promotion and Education (IUHPE) (Mittlemark, Wise), the US Centers for Disease Control and Prevention (Anderson, Asma, Lightsey, McQueen, Sheldon, Warren), the World Bank (Godhino) and Non Governmental Organisations (NGOs) (Gupta). Most of the authors have influence and experience that go beyond one setting and one country. Aggleton, for example, is an eminent academic and researcher, who also acts as a senior advisor to global organisations such as UNAIDS, UNESCO, UNICEF, WHO, whilst Mittlemark holds both a professorial post in health promotion and the presidency of the global professional association, the IUHPE.

Together, the contributors comprise an internationally recognised group of specialists in health promotion, public health and health related policy, and the contents and scope of this book reflect this wide range of experience and expertise. Whilst there are no chapters devoted to an examination of the role of the key international and national agencies that promote health, such as the WHO and the different divisions of the UN, their activities are integral to the content and their roles and functions are delineated throughout the text.

The approach taken by the authors is intended to challenge current thinking and to stimulate debate. The range of chapters covered are illustrative of the current pressing problems in relation to global health and of some of the strategies that are being employed across the world to tackle these.

The volume is constructed around three main areas of analysis, namely *issues, challenges and strategies*, each forming a distinct section but together creating the framework to the text in which the chapters are located. The parts are introduced by a brief overview that identifies some of the themes addressed in the chapters and makes links where appropriate. The ordering of the sections reflects the principle of moving from the analysis of generic health *issues* in Part I that establish the foundation and context for the critical exami-nation of a set of specific health *challenges* that need to be confronted at a global level in Part II. These first two sections then provide the backdrop for an assessment of the national and regional *strategies* that are being employed to promote health in Part III.

Part I begins by establishing the key health issues to be confronted at a global level. Davey (Chapter 2) and MacDaid and Oliver (Chapter 3) offer a detailed epidemiological review of the global patterns of disease and disability, their determinants and the nature of inequalities both within and between countries. Mittlemark (Chapter 4) and Garman (Chapter 5) follow this by considering critically the strategies for promoting health and the barriers that might confound efforts. There is confirmation in each chapter that promoting individual, population and global health is a complex process, that there are numerous anti-health forces to be overcome and that the rising health inequal-ities gap between and within countries is a significant obstacle to global health.

Part II focuses on particular topics that have emerged as global public health *challenges* in the twenty-first century. Each of the five chapters forming this second part of the book will provide a detailed examination of a specific health related topic and an assessment of comprehensive health promoting approaches that might be employed in addressing the issues that emerge. The five topics, *noncommunicable diseases, food and diet, tobacco, HIV/AIDS, envi-ronment*, have been chosen because of their global significance and are presented by key researchers in the field. What is interesting and at the same time disturbing about this section is the global complexity that is inherent in the discussion of the specific health problem, clearly demonstrating that local action is insufficient on its own to deal with these health challenges and that national and global solutions that include stronger health governance are required.

Part III concentrates on a critical review of *strategies* in place in a number of countries and regions. The chapters take the form of case studies that offer clear insights into the complexity of having to address the *issues* and the *challenges* set out in Parts I and II in a national or regional context. It would be difficult to cover all regions and countries adequately, so a selection has been made on the basis of geographical spread, areas of high population and a balance between low income, middle income, and high income countries and regions of the world. Included are chapters on Africa, Latin America, the Greater China Region, the Former Soviet Union, Europe, Australia and New Zealand, Canada, the USA and a more generic chapter that considers the achievements and challenges for the future in a range of low and middle income countries, including India.

Terminology used in discussing global health

There are key terms that are used throughout this volume and it is important at the outset to establish how they are being employed, as they are not defined beyond this opening chapter. There are three areas of particular importance: the classification of countries and the use of the terms globalisation and health promotion.

Categorisation of countries and regions

There are numerous ways of categorising the countries and regions of the world. Groupings are usually done on the basis of economic or geographical classification so that global comparisons can be undertaken, as is the case in this text. However, all classifications are problematic, often simplistic and fail to group countries in a precise manner. One problem is that the categories are generally too broad, usually amounting to just two divisions such as *developed* and *developing, first world* and *third world*. This broad approach results in difficulties of assignment, with a large number of countries being placed in the same category but often having little in common. This can be misleading. Countries assigned the developed label for example, can be very different in terms of their economic and industrial maturity and global standing. *Developing* as an idiom can also be misleading as it implies advances are taking place and that a country is moving toward a more finite point called *developed*, when little or no improvement is taking place. Equally, those classifications based on geography such as north and south are generally erroneous because, as Gray (2001) argues, the differences between countries in these two broad regions are often more important than their similarities. The type of terminology used to identify and categorise countries is also frequently value laden, hierarchical in character with a condescending resonance that can be demeaning to the populations who are grouped in this way. The term developing, for example, implies under development or lack of maturity and the term third world carries the connotation of a lower order or class than first or second world.

In order to ensure linguistic consistency contributors to this book are using the following three categories proposed by Gray (2001), which assigns countries according to whether national income per person is low, middle or high:

Low income: sub-Saharan Africa and Central and East and South Asia
Middle income: Eastern Europe, Central and South America, the Middle East and North Africa
High income: Western Europe, North America, Japan, Australia and New Zealand.

The advantage of using the Gray classification is that it is in line with the World Bank national statistics and avoids some of the problems associated with the other types of terminology discussed earlier.

Whilst these categories will be used throughout this text to facilitate comparative debate, their limitations are recognised. Some of these limitations have already been discussed and relate to the significant differences between the countries within the bands of high, middle and low income. These differences create problems for any classification. Of perhaps more significance is that the high, middle and low categories as others, fail to indicate the differences between groups *within* countries and can inadvertently disguise these variations, particularly those linked to national inequalities and resource distribution. Caraher et al., Part II, Chapter 7 and McDaid and Oliver, Part I, Chapter 3 expands this discussion when examining specific issues linked to relative and absolute levels of income within countries.

It is acknowledged therefore that in the countries and regions clustered in these three broad bands there will be differences in population groups within countries and that countries differ significantly in terms of their histories, cultures, geographical and population sizes, politics and global influences. All of these factors will impact on the health of populations and will therefore feature significantly as themes throughout the book.

Globalisation

Towards the end of the twentieth century, Potter (1997) articulated what many already knew, that the world was in the midst of a global revolution in trade, politics, finances, communications, research, technology and the movement of people. The term globalisation, introduced to describe this revolution, is used to mark the increasing economic and social interdependence between countries. Whilst the term is still relatively novel, some argue the globalisation process is not a new phenomenon. One theory discussed by Farrar (2004) suggests that globalisation is a recurring process that dates back at least 2000 years to the Roman Empire, when the integration of people, culture, technology and ideas was on an unprecedented scale. However, modern globalisation as referred to in many of the chapters in this text is a much faster and more complex process and is linked to changes to the world economy, particularly capitalism in the latter part of the twentieth century.

The exact meaning of the term globalisation is contested, but there is general agreement that the discourses, practices and technologies relating to globalisation have powerful influences on and are in turn influenced by governments, economies, the media and cultural identity (see Schirato and Webb, 2003 for a further discussion). The exact impact of globalisation on health is also contested, with it being viewed as both a threat and a benefit. On the one hand, Stevens (2003b) asks the question whether globalisation is good or bad for health, in an article the title of which, *Globalisation is killing us*, offers a frank answer. The World Bank, on the other hand, asserts that globalisation will bring benefits for all. Neither argument is entirely accurate, but there is evidence that the liberalisation of trade and capital flows is increasing inequality both between and within countries (Sanders and Chopra, 2003) undermining public health protection, weakening public healthcare services and destroying the global eco system (Stephens, 2003b).

Perhaps the adverse impact of globalisation is most evident when it comes to food. Pretty (2003) refers to what he calls extraordinary times in his review of the new book of Millestone and Lang (2003) *The Atlas of Food: Who eats what, where and why.* He points to the paradox of 800 million hungry people in the world whilst in high income countries health problems associated with people who eat too much have resulted in obesity being regarded as one of the key public health concerns of the twenty-first century. Chapter 7 in Part II of this book pursues this debate further by exploring the irony of nutritional transition (Popkin, 1998) brought on by world trade processes associated with globalisation and the growing problem of obesity in low and middle income countries. Clearly there has been a major failing in dealing with such problems, both through national and international policies and through the institutions that have responsibilities to protect public health at a global level. There are those who gain and those who lose as a result of globalisation, and this is reflected in the diverse global health profiles, examined in Chapters 2 and 3 of this book. Lee et al. (2002) makes a strong case for globalisation being more inclusive and equitable if the true roots of so many global health risks are to be tackled, a theme explored in many of the following chapters.

Health promotion

Health promotion is a late twentieth-century idiom, used for the first time in the mid-1970s (Lalonde, 1974) although it is acknowledged that the existence of the concept predates the explicit use of the expression (MacDonald, 1998; Webster and French, 2002). An early and frequently cited influence on the thinking in relation to health promotion was the McKinlay (1979) analogy that advocated the need for upstream, preventative action. The idea of refocusing resources upstream proved to be a powerful and persuasive argument, articulating the need for more preventative approaches to be adopted in targeting the general population.

Whilst preventative goals continue to dominate practice in some countries, as reflected in Part III of this book, the definition and scope of health promotion has been a source of polemic that has engaged health professionals and others for the last three decades. It is not the intention here to reproduce these long and often impassioned debates; it is sufficient to record that the term is now universally perceived as referring to an holistic field of overlapping activity at primary, secondary and tertiary levels encompassing health education, lifestyle and preventative approaches alongside the policy, environmental, legal and fiscal measures designed to advance health (for further discussion on this issue see, for example, Jones, 2000; Scriven and Orme, 2001; Bell, 2003). Globally, people in statutory and non-statutory settings and multidisciplinary areas of practice and expertise draw on a range of disciplines and methodologies to undertake health promotion activities at these three levels (Bunton and MacDonald, 2002; Webster and French, 2002).

More recently the polemic around health promotion has been shifting to focus on the relationship between health promotion and public health. This debate is ongoing, but it is worth noting as pointed out by Bunton and MacDonald (2002) that few would challenge the centrality of health promotion in public health practice or its contribution to the development of thought and theory in an evolving social model of health. This latter point is crucial to understanding the health promotion practice discussed in this book, which has distinctive methodologies drawn from community development and primary healthcare programmes (Green and Frankish, 2002).

Because of its centrality to public health, some countries have established a specialised form of health promotion provision with an emphasis on the wider determinants of health. This mirrors current thinking in health promotion, which prioritises sustainable interventions and the building of social systems for health with integrated and strategic investment (see Mittlemark, Chapter 4 for analysis of health promotion and the case studies in Part III for practice examples). The WHO policies and charters relating to the promotion of health, one of which is discussed next, have directed health promotion strategies and have resulted in health promotion being perceived by many as a key global investment and an essential element of social and economic development.

Policy focus

Many diverse international and national policies are referred to throughout this text but there are two in particular, the Millennium Development Goals (http://www.develpmentgoals.org/) and the Ottawa Charter (WHO, 1986) that receive frequent attention, so an introductory overview is presented here.

Millennium Development Goals

The Millennium Development Goals (MDGs) were produced by the Organisation for Economic Cooperation and Development (OECD) and are used by the international community as a normative framework to guide its policies and programmes. They emerged from the Millennium Declaration signed by 189 countries, including 147 Heads of State in September 2000. The goals and targets are interrelated and together they represent a commitment to create an environment at national and global levels that is conducive to development and to the elimination of poverty. Given the vital link between health and development (see Kickbusch, 1997) these goals have a direct relevance to those working to promote global health.

The indicators for the Millennium Development Goals have been reviewed and finalised by an expert panel drawn from the secretariats of the UN system, the International Monetary Fund (IMF), the OECD and the World Bank. The 8 goals, 18 targets, and 48 indicators for monitoring progress are highly relevant to health as they focus on the eradication of extreme poverty and hunger, the empowerment of women, the advance of both primary and female education, the reduction in child mortality and the improvement in maternal health, the combating of HIV/AIDS, malaria and other diseases, the promotion of environmental sustainability and finally the establishment of a global partnership for development. These are commendable targets that would suggest a determination by the international community to reduce health inequalities. Authors in this text and elsewhere (see Dare, 2003), however, are pessimistic about the likely success in achieving the goals, with some stating categorically that they are unattainable. Chapter 3 for example is instructive in this respect, with a forceful argument by McDaid and Oliver that only two of the MDGs are likely to be met in the 15-year timescale set. These views are shared outside this book, with Dare (2003) pointing to a World Bank analysis when suggesting that no African country will achieve any of the mid-decade goals. These are disappointing assessments given the importance of the MDGs to global health. It will be essential to monitor the progress against the indicators in the next decade.

Ottawa Charter

The Ottawa Charter is generally regarded as having heralded the new public health (Kickbusch and Payne, 2003) and it has significantly informed other international and national policies and continues to have a strong global influence on health promotion practice (Sindall, 2001). The charter endorsed the process of enabling people to increase control over and improve their health, but also made a strong link to structural adjustment through political, economic and social change that is so relevant to tackling some of the issues and challenges in global health. There was also affirmation that the attainment of global health is not just the business of those professionals who work within the health and social services, but that significant measures to improve health must be taken outside these sectors and are the responsibility of politicians and planners at a national and international level.

In line with this, the charter embraced the social model of health and the targeting of the wider determinants, particularly health inequalities. Those actively engaged in health promoting roles were encouraged to act as *advocates*, ensuring that the conditions favourable to health are in place, as *enablers* to facilitate population groups to achieve their fullest health potential and to overcome health inequalities and finally as *mediators*, to arbitrate between differing interests in society for the pursuit of health. These remain important ideas and roles in relation to some of the political and economic challenges facing the promotion of global health, and are reflected in the recommendation for action made in the chapters that follow.

In addition to the above, five approaches, in italics below, were advocated and have permeated both the philosophy and practice in the promotion of health and accordingly are reflected throughout this book. *Healthy public policies* are crucial for global health, forming the framework for coordinated action to foster greater equity, which many authors advocate (see Part I for recommendations that relate to these approaches and III for examples of these in action). The *creating of supportive environments* emphasises a socio-ecological approach to health in the form of reciprocal maintenance. This involves everyone taking responsibility for the protection of the natural and built environments and the conservation of natural resources, a key challenge for global health (see Wilkinson, Part II, Chapter 10 for a detailed examination of this theme) and is linked to *Strengthening community action* and the empowerment of communities, their ownership and control of their own endeavours and destinies (see Part III for examples of this approach, particularly Chapter 11 by Hubley). *Developing personal skills* involves education for health and enhancing life skills. Action here is advocated in multiple settings including schools, homes, workplaces and communities and is regarded as crucial for increasing the options available to people to exercise more control over their own health and to make choices conducive to health (see Part III, but also Part II, Chapter 9 by Aggleton with its specific focus on HIV/AID interventions). Finally, *reorienting health services* has repositioned the healthcare sector beyond its responsibility for providing clinical and curative services to one that contributes to the pursuit of health. This changing mandate has resulted in collaborative partnerships across sectors, and a refocusing on the individual as a whole person who participates in health decisions. A number of chapters in the book advocate the need for new, innovatory collaborative partnerships (see for example, Part I, Mittelmark, Chapter 4).

Other WHO conference declarations such as the Jakarta Declaration on Health Promotion (WHO, 1997) have affirmed and advanced Ottawa, with priorities for the twenty-first century around increased investment, expansion of partnerships, social responsibility, sustainability, community capacity and empowerment and the securing of an infrastructure for the promotion of health. These declarations have not been without their critics, such as Jones (2000) who argues that they create catchphrase frameworks and all-encompassing agendas for the promotion of health in which the priorities are unclear. Generally however, the Ottawa guiding principles are seen as seminal as testified by the frequent references to them in this book, illustrating that the Charter continues to have a strong influence on the strategies, methodologies, and the thinking employed in the promotion of global health. Worthy of additional note is a recent assessment of the effectiveness of health promotion where Baum (2002) suggests that comprehensive strategies that use all five Ottawa approaches are the most effective.

By the time the book is published, we will have almost reached the twentieth anniversary of the publication of the Ottawa Charter. Many believe that the values, principles and strategies outlined in the Charter are as relevant today as they were when it was first published. Indeed, some arguments relating to the promotion of global health in the twenty-first century closely reflect these principles. Notably, what is needed to improve health globally, is a collectivist, participatory and interdisciplinary approach, which requires power *with* rather than power *over* populations and groups (Green and Frankish, 2002). Social and economic justice (Germain, 2003), combined international resolve and concerted health governance are essential in addressing the key public health targets, including a reduction of poverty and health inequalities both within and between countries. These guiding principles are the basis for a global perspective in promoting health and form the essence of what follows.

References

Baum, F. (2002) *The New Public Health: An Australian Perspective* (2nd edn). Oxford: Oxford University Press.

Beaglehole, R. (2003) *Global Public Health – A New Era*. Oxford: Oxford University Press.

Bell, S. (2003) Health promotion and the role of the health promotion specialist. In Watson, A. (ed.) *Public Health in Practice*. Basingstoke: Palgrave.

Berkley, S.F. (2002) The outlook for eradicating AIDS. In Koop, E.C., Pearson, C.E. and Schwatz, M.R. (eds) *Critical Issues in Global Health*. San Francisco: Jossey-Bass.

Bunton, R. and MacDonald, G. (eds) (2002) *Health Promotion: Disciplines or Diversity* (2nd edn). London: Routledge.

Buve, A., Bishokwabo-Nsarhaza, K. and Mutangadurs, G. (2002) The spread and effects of HIV-1 infection in sub-Saharan Africa. *Lancet*, **359**: 2011–17.

Cole, D.C., Eyles, J., Gibson, B.L. and Ross, N. (1999) Links between humans and ecosystems: the implication for framing for health promotion strategies. *Health Promotion International*, **14** (1): 65–72.

Dare, L. (2003) WHO and the challenges of the next decade. *Lancet*, **361**: 170–71.

Farrar, S. (2004) Sorry, Mr Bush, the Romans got there before you. *The Times Higher Education Supplement*, 2 January 2004.

Germain, A. (2003) Addressing inequalities: the role for the new WHO Director General. *Lancet*, **361**: 171-72.

Gray, A. (2001) *World Health and Disease* (3rd edn). Buckingham: the Open University Press.

Green, L.W. and Frankish, C.J. (2002) Health promotion, Health education, and disease prevention. In Koop, E.C., Pearson, C.E. and Schwatz, M.R. (eds) *Critical Issues in Global Health*. San Francisco: Jossey-Bass.

Jones, L. (2000) Promoting health: everybody's business? In Katz, J., Peberdy, A. and Douglas, J. (eds) *Promoting Health: Knowledge and Practice (2nd edn)*. Basingstoke: Palgrave.

Kickbusch, I. (1997) Think health: what makes the difference? *Health Promotion International*, **12** (4): 265–72.

Kickbusch, I. and Payne, L. (2003) Twenty-first century health promotion: the public health revolution meets the wellness revolution. *Health Promotion International*, **18** (4): 275–78.

Labonte, R. (1998) Healthy public policy and the World Trade Organization: a proposal for an international health presence in future world trade/investments talks. *Health Promotion International*, **13** (3): 245–56.

Lalonde, M. (1974) *A New Perspective on the Health of Canadians*. Ottowa: Information Canada.

Lee, K., Kent, B. and Fustukian, S. (eds) (2002) *Health Policy in a Globalising World*. Cambridge: Cambridge University Press.

Leon, D. and Walt, G. (2000) Poverty, inequality and health in international perspective. In Leon, D. and Walt, G. (eds) *Poverty, Inequality and Health – An International Perspective*. Oxford: Oxford University Press.

Lomborg, B. (2002) How healthy is the world? *British Medical Journal*, **325**: 1461–64.

MacArthur, I. (2002) Fresh in our minds. *Health Matters*, **50**: 18–19.

MacDonald, T.H. (1998) *Rethinking Health Promotion: A Global Approach*. London: Routledge.

McKinlay, J.B. (1979) A case for refocusing upstream: the political economy of health. In Javco, E.G. (ed.) *Patients, Physicians and Illness*. Basingstoke: Macmillan.

Malaspina, A. (1998) Global partnerships for a safer, healthier world- the work of the International Life Sciences Institute. *Health Promotion International*, **13** (3): 187–89.

Millstone, E. and Lang, T. (2003) *The Penguin Atlas of Food: Who Eats What, Where and Way*. New York: Penguin Books.

Popkin, B. (1998) The nutrition transition and its health implications in lower-income countries. *Public Health Nutrition*, **1** (1): 5–21.

Potter, I. (1997) Looking back, looking ahead– health promotion: a global challenge. *Health Promotion International*, **12** (4): 273–7.

Pretty, J. (2003) Staple diet of inequity and hypocrisy. *The Times Higher*, 31 October: 29.

Sanders, D. and Chopra, M. (2003) Two key issues for the WHO leadership. *Lancet*, **361**: 172–73.

Schirato, T. and Webb, J. (2003) *Understanding Globalization*. London: Sage.

Scriven, A. and Orme, J. (2001) *Health Promotion: Professional Perspectives* (2nd edn). London: Palgrave.

Sindall, C. (2001) Health promotion and chronic disease: building on the Ottawa Charter, not betraying it? *Health Promotion International*, **16** (3): 215–17.

Stephens, C. (2003a) We must not go on like this. *Health Matters*, **50**: 12–15.

Stephens, C. (2003b) "La globalisation nos matan"– globalisation is killing us. *Health Matters*, **41**: 6–8.

Webster, C. and French, J. (2002) The cycle of conflict: the history of the public health promotion movements. In Adams, L., Amos, M. and Munro, J. (eds) *Promoting Health: Politics and Practice*. London: Sage.

World Health Organisation (WHO) (1986) *Ottawa Charter for Health Promotion*. Geneva: WHO.

World Health Organisation (WHO) (1997) *The Jakarta Declaration on Health*. Geneva: WHO.

World Health Organisation (WHO) (2003) *The World Health Report 2003 – Shaping the Future*. Geneva: WHO.

PART I

GLOBAL ISSUES IN PROMOTING HEALTH: AN OVERVIEW

Angela Scriven

This first part of the book critically examines a range of issues that are central to informing the promotion of health in the global arena and as such, creates the context for what follows in the remaining parts.

The opening chapter presents the global patterns of disease and Disability Adjusted Life Years (DALYs) and raises highly pertinent considerations for those responsible for promoting health. There is a richness of detail in the assessment of the global health figures, with critical problems identified. One crucial issue highlighted is the process of risk transition, which is creating a double jeopardy for low income countries confronted by degenerative diseases brought on by open market-induced lifestyle changes, alongside the causes of mortality and morbidity that dominated their health profiles in the past (see part II for further examination of risk transition, particularly Chapters 6 and 7). Those promoting health are called on not to be complacent about the continuing impact of infectious and parasite-mediated diseases for the twenty-first century, but there is the clear identification of emerging key global health concerns. Two are given particular attention. First, the predicted global mortality and DALYs in relation to traffic accidents and second the level of mental health problems globally, with five mental illness categories appearing in the top ten causes of DALYs worldwide. The latter is particularly important, as mental health promotion has not always received the attention it deserves and this analysis might advance the position of mental health on global agendas. A valuable assessment is provided of the interconnection of the fundamental causes of ill health and there is a positive affirmation that health promotion initiatives can intervene effectively at many different points in the mesh of interacting causes.

This opening chapter is followed in Chapter 2 by a focus on what many consider to be the key public issue to be addressed at a global level, inequalities in health. The normative concept of equity and the empirical concept of inequality are debated and the distinction is made between inequitable health disparties and those caused by poor lifestyle choices or by unavoidable biological factors. Questions emerge from this discussion that reflect the complexity that those promoting health have to overcome if they are to enable populations to achieve a minimum standard in health and to reduce global health inequalities.

The actions of the international community in addressing adult, child and gender related health inequalities are critically assessed and the Millennium Development Goals in particular are seen as ineffectual. Important recommendations emerge from this chapter. Of particular note is that the development and the health development communities work more closely and that the cost effectiveness of health promotion interventions is made overt in terms of its potential impact on economic development and reducing health service costs.

A lively discourse in Chapter 4 centres on the challenges for health promotion of the global health determinants discussed in Chapters 2 and 3. As in the preceding chapters there is an impassioned call for a joining up of resources with health promoters encouraged to form new alliances with social progress movements and the business sector. Two areas receive particular attention, the notion of health promoters as social activists and the contention that health promotion is too insular. Health promotion is seen as sufficiently robust to meet current and future public health challenges, but it is suggested that it needs invigorating by the inclusion of other academic disciplines, particularly community psychology and by establishing new partnerships with the corporate social responsibility, environmental and human rights movements. Some interesting insights are offered about the conceptual variations in health promotion in different parts of the world that will underpin the chapters in Part III. A rallying call to health promoters to keep developing and advancing their discipline and alliance base to ensure they do not become complacent or stagnate ends this discussion.

The debate is advanced, however in the final chapter by an analysis of the dialectics that provide the creative tensions that move health promotion forward, with a gap identified between rhetoric and practice. A number of global conundrums are presented that those promoting health must overcome, including the negative health impacts of economic globalisation and disrupted social fabric and war. There are important discussions on the contradictory role that mass communication plays and a critique of research in underpinning the evidence base for promoting health.

Through the examination of these fundamental issues, the chapters in this section represent an important conceptual and epidemiological foundation for the rest of the book. The authors move beyond simply identifying what the global health problems are to making recommendations based on their assessment of current and future trends.

Concluding remarks

The issues debated in these first chapters will be examined further in other parts of the book, but there are clear conclusions that can be drawn from this opening section.

Those professionals with a responsibility to promote health are undoubtedly facing challenges that are global in nature. Confronting these challenges will require concerted efforts and innovatory and outward-looking, rather than insular, ways of working. This must include effective collaborative long-term planning and the combining of resources between different statutory and non-statutory agencies. This is crucial if health inequalities and other public health problems are to be successfully addressed at a global level. These global health partnerships should be wide-ranging and include environmental, developmental, human rights and private sector industry and business organisations (see both Mittelmark and McDaid and Oliver on this issue) in committed and focused alliances with the health sector. It is clear from these early Chapters that these partnerships are necessary because progress in tacking global public health problems will only be achieved through the wider context of social reforms and national and international investment. To offer just one example, there is little point in health promoters encouraging the use of condoms to prevent the spread of HIV and AIDS in sub-Saharan Africa if, as Davey points out in Chapter 2, there is an estimated annual shortage of 13 billion condoms. International investment through private and public finding is required, therefore, not simply to resolve income inequalities, but to adequately fund health promotion activities so that they have maximum impact.

The overriding conclusion is that there is much to be done in tackling significant problems in global health. This must involve, as Garman argues in Chapter 4, moving beyond the rhetoric of upstream political, public policy and legislative reforms, to action that ensures delivery on these strategies. There is no room for complacency. These are serious issues that need to be addressed, requiring the mediation of power relations connected to both the alliances mentioned earlier and to the control of the negative impact of communications, media and multinational industries. These are daunting challenges that require enhanced workforce capacity and capability, but as a starting point, a high degree of political resolve at an international level.

CHAPTER 2

Key Global Health Concerns for the Twenty-first Century

BASIRO DAVEY

The central purpose of this chapter is to identify the key patterns of disease and disability among the global population of just over six billion at the start of the twenty-first century, emphasising differences in the major health problems affecting different age groups. This review forms the background to analyses in later chapters in this book of the underlying causes of disease patterns and trends in the context of local, national and internationally directed health promotion strategies and the challenges faced by the individuals, organisations and governments involved in their implementation.

As the new millennium began, the gap in health status between the poorest nations and those in middle income and wealthier countries was becoming wider. The rate of premature mortality was accelerating in sub-Saharan Africa, parts of Eastern Europe and in war-torn countries such as Afghanistan, Iraq and Sudan, in stark contrast to the gains being made elsewhere. Within populations, the causes of illness, disability and death remained sharply divided along gradients of gender, ethnicity, education and material circumstances (as Chapter 3 in this part of the book demonstrates). Although there are signs of progress, for example the near eradication of polio and the continuing decline in deaths from diarrhoeal diseases, key indicators of health status such as life expectancy at birth testify that in areas of high HIV prevalence the steady gains of previous decades are being rapidly eroded.

Several chapters in this book are concerned primarily with health promotion aimed at reducing noncommunicable diseases (NCDs), particularly heart disease, stroke, and food and tobacco related disorders (see Chapters 6, 7 and 8 among others). This emphasis reflects the central importance attached to health promotion initiatives as key interventions in these conditions. As later chapters demonstrate, although NCDs still predominate in high income countries, they are increasing most rapidly in poorer regions of the world. In this chapter therefore, the burden of NCDs is given less detailed coverage than the impact of infectious and parasitic diseases, which receive less attention in most other parts of the book. (Note that SARS figures in Part III, Chapter 14 and HIV/AIDS is the subject of Part II, Chapter 9.)

In the review below, the multiple interactions between infection, unsafe water supply and malnutrition are explored, and prominence is also given to

19

two other global health concerns that generally receive less recognition as subjects for health promotion: mental health problems and traffic-related injuries. Many other sources of illness and disability on the health promotion agenda can only be touched on.

Estimates of morbidity in this chapter are generally presented in Disability Adjusted Life Years (DALYs) an internationally recognised measure that incorporates the years of life lost due to premature death and the years of life lived with disability due to disease or injury, taking into account not only the age at onset and the duration of the condition, but also the severity of disablement. Geographical regions, mortality strata and the categorisation of developed and developing countries are as defined by the World Health Organisation in its most recent annual report (WHO, 2003a).

Major health concerns in different age groups

Data on health status increasingly reflect the striking differences between countries with different levels of income, as many chapters in this book illustrate, but differences between age groups are sometimes submerged. HIV/AIDS ranks fourth globally as a cause of death, but as Table 2.1 shows it heads the ten leading causes of death and the disease burden among adults aged 15–59 years. In 2002, the expectation of life at birth in the African region as a whole would have been greater by 6.1 years, but for the impact of HIV. In the most affected sub-Saharan countries, life expectancy has fallen by 20 years since the epidemic began there in the early 1990s (WHO, 2003a). The resurgence of tuberculosis to third place in the adult mortality ranking is largely a consequence of HIV-related susceptibility to opportunistic infections and the widespread emergence of drug-resistant bacterial strains.

The importance of injuries and violence can be overlooked as a health concern but, as Table 2.1 shows, they account for almost two million deaths a year in this age group and just under 65 million DALYs. Males aged over 15 years are disproportionately subject to injury, as the discussion of traffic-related injuries illustrates later in this chapter. Alcohol misuse also has a male skew and receives rather less publicity than its ranking in the top ten suggests it should merit, both as a direct cause of physical disease, for example, cirrhosis of the liver, and mental health problems, and as a contributor to accidents, self-inflicted injuries and violence. The 1996 Global Burden of Disease project took all these factors into account and estimated that in 1990 alcohol was responsible for 1.5 per cent of all deaths and 3.5 per cent of DALYs. Since that time, the use of alcohol has been increasing rapidly in some non-Islamic low income countries, raising concerns that associated health problems will escalate there as they have done in wealthier nations (WHO, 2001).

It may come as a surprise that unipolar depression is the commonest cause of disabling disease among adult women worldwide, and ranks fourth globally among men, resulting in its second place in the DALYs listed in Table 2.1. The

Table 2.1 The top ten leading causes of death and disability (measured in DALYs) among adults aged 15–59 years, worldwide totals, 2002 (adapted from WHO, 2003, Table 1.3, p.17)

Cause of death		Deaths	Cause of disability		DALYs
1	HIV/AIDS	2,279	1	HIV/AIDS	68,661
2	Ischaemic heart disease	1,332	2	Unipolar depressive disorders	57,843
3	Tuberculosis	1,036	3	Tuberculosis	28,380
4	Road-traffic injuries	814	4	Road-traffic injuries	27,264
5	Cerebrovascular disease	783	5	Ischaemic heart disease	26,155
6	Self-inflicted injuries	672	6	Alcohol-use disorders	19,567
7	Violence	473	7	Adult-onset hearing loss	19,486
8	Cirrhosis of the liver	382	8	Violence	18,962
9	Lower respiratory infections	352	9	Cerebrovascular disease	18,749
10	Chronic obstructive pulmonary disease	343	10	Self-inflicted injuries	18,522

extent of depression and other mental health problems globally is a key health concern for the twenty-first century and is briefly reviewed later in this chapter.

Table 2.1 confirms the pre-eminence of diseases of the heart and circulatory system in all parts of the world. These conditions rank highest in worldwide mortality and disability for all ages combined in low and middle income as well as high income countries (see Part II, Chapter 6). The impact is greatest among adults aged 60 years and above, where the top ten ranking also includes chronic lung diseases and lower respiratory infections, diabetes, dementias and cancers of the respiratory tract, stomach, colon and rectum. The contribution of tobacco smoking to many of these conditions is discussed in Part II, Chapter 9. More than 1.3 billion adults smoke cigarettes and around 5 million deaths annually are attributed to this cause (WHO, 2003a).

In contrast to younger adults, HIV infection rates among people over 60 remain very low, but the indirect impact on older people's lives has been huge in the worst-affected countries, where they have become the principal carers for their orphaned grandchildren, many of whom are themselves HIV positive. Over 90 per cent of childhood mortality occurs under the age of five years and 42 per cent of all child deaths occur in sub-Saharan Africa. In 16 countries, all but two in Africa, mortality rates among under-fives were higher in 2002 than they had been in 1990, largely as a result of HIV infection (WHO, 2003a).

Elsewhere in low income countries, gradual reductions in childhood mortality from some other infectious diseases, for example diarrhoeal diseases and measles, have elevated perinatal conditions including birth asphyxia, other trauma and low birth weight to first place as a cause of death among young children. But communicable diseases still account for seven of the top ten causes (see Table 2.2), as discussed in greater detail shortly.

The increase in proportional mortality from perinatal conditions is a feature of what has been termed the risk transition (WHO, 2002) in which the

Table 2.2 The top ten causes of death among children aged under
five years in developing countries in 2002 (using WHO 2003
country categorisation) (WHO, 2003, Table 1.1, p.12)

Cause of death	Deaths	% of all deaths <5years*
1 Perinatal conditions	2,375	23.1
2 Lower respiratory infections	1,856	18.1
3 Diarrhoeal diseases	1,566	15.2
4 Malaria	1,098	10.7
5 Measles	551	5.4
6 Congenital anomalies	386	3.8
7 HIV/AIDS	370	3.6
8 Pertussis (whooping cough)	301	2.9
9 Tetanus	185	1.8
10 Protein-energy malnutrition	138	1.3
All other causes	1,437	14.0
Total	10,263	

Note: * in developing countries

epidemiological profile of some low and most middle income countries is
shifting towards a pattern that is more typical of North America and Western
Europe. The transition is driven by the gradual reduction in childhood
mortality from some major infectious diseases, coupled with increased food
security, which together improve survival into adulthood and enable the
ageing of the population. At the same time, the consumption of tobacco and
alcohol is rising rapidly in developing countries, an increasing proportion of
dietary calories is coming from saturated fats and sugars, the consumption of
fruit and vegetables is falling, salt intake is rising and the level of physical
activity is going down.

To take one example, lack of physical activity is estimated to cause
1.9 million deaths annually. The attributable risk from physical inactivity as a
contributing cause of several major diseases has been estimated globally at
22 per cent for ischaemic heart disease, 16 per cent for colon and rectal cancers,
14 per cent for diabetes, 11 per cent for ischaemic strokes and 10 per cent for
breast cancer (WHO, 2002, Statistical Annexe, Table 7). Lack of exercise is
strongly associated with becoming overweight (body mass index (BMI) at
least 25 kg/m^2), which in turn contributes a substantial additional risk for all
of the above conditions, some other cancers and osteoarthritis. One billion
adults are now overweight and of these at least 300 million are clinically obese
(BMI at least 30 kg/m^2). The age profile of the obese population is becoming
progressively younger and the epidemic is spreading to lower income
countries (WHO, 2000a).

The prospects for health promotion strategies to intervene in the inevitable
health consequences of this risk transition are explored in many later chapters
in this book. All but the poorest countries are now facing the double jeopardy

of increasing levels of degenerative diseases associated with the risk transition, while still suffering the mortality and morbidity from communicable diseases that dominated their health profiles in the past.

Although the greatest gains for adult health globally may be achieved by directing health promotion at the young to establish lifelong adherence to healthy eating, physical exercise and condom use, among other lifestyle factors, the greatest threat to the lives of the world's children remains the combination of infection and malnutrition. The following brief review illustrates the continuing impact of communicable conditions on global health and raises some considerations for the health promotion agenda.

Infection and parasite-mediated disease

In the 1960s, it was confidently predicted that deaths from infection would be virtually eliminated by the end of the millennium. Yet in 2002, the deaths of 15 million people, 26 per cent of the 57 million who died that year, were attributed to communicable diseases caused by directly or indirectly transmitted bacteria, viruses, protozoa or multicellular parasites. These infectious agents also reduced the years of life lived free from disability in the global population by an estimated 447 million years, 30 per cent of the worldwide DALYs (WHO, 2003a). The burden of life-threatening and disabling infection falls most heavily on the countries of Africa, where they account for 60 per cent of all deaths and DALYs, South East Asia (30 per cent), and the high mortality stratum countries of the WHO's Eastern Mediterranean region, which includes Afghanistan, Iraq, Pakistan, Somalia, Sudan and Yemen (36 per cent).

Table 2.3 shows the ten leading causes of death from infectious or parasitic diseases in 2002, and the disease burden in DALYs associated with these conditions. A comparison between Tables 2.2 and 2.3 immediately reveals the extent to which these diseases disproportionately affect the young. Lower respiratory infections, which include the pneumonias and influenza, are the major infectious causes of death among young children (Williams et al., 2002), and if all ages are combined they kill more people worldwide than any other category of communicable disease, except in those countries worst affected by HIV.

Other sexually transmitted infections (STIs) are also increasing in many parts of the world, particularly syphilis, which is tenth among infectious diseases ranked by cause of death (Table 2.3), and gonorrhoea and chlamydia. In 2002, these STIs accounted for over 11 million DALYs (WHO, 2003a). In addition to the direct effects on the body, the existence of an STI also increases susceptibility to HIV transmission during unprotected sex.

The promotion of safer sex practices has been a global health priority for over a decade. Overcoming opposition to condom use on cultural or religious grounds and the distribution of free condoms are prominent aspects of health

Table 2.3   Deaths and disability (measured in DALYs) attributed to the top six categories of infectious or parasitic diseases, and worldwide totals, 2002 (data derived from WHO, 2003, Statistical Annex, Tables 2 and 3)

Infectious/parasitic disease category (ranked by deaths)	Deaths (x 000)	% of all deaths	DALYs (x 000)	% of all DALYs
1 Lower respiratory infections	3,766	6.7	87,022	5.8
2 HIV/AIDS	2,821	4.9	86,072	5.8
3 Diarrhoeal diseases	1,767	3.1	61,095	4.1
4 Tuberculosis	1,605	2.8	35,361	2.4
5 Malaria	1,222	2.1	44,716	3.0
6 Measles	760	1.3	27,058	1.8
7 Pertussis	301	0.5	13,052	0.9
8 Tetanus	292	0.5	9,398	0.6
9 Meningitis	173	0.3	6,195	0.4
10 Syphilis	157	0.3	4,200	0.3
11 Other infectious/parasitic diseases	2,103	3.7	72,907	4.9
Total	14,967	26.2	447	30.0

promotion programmes to reduce the transmission of HIV and other STIs. But little public attention has been directed to the worldwide shortage of condoms. In sub-Saharan Africa, the total number of condoms available from all sources averages less than five per year for each male aged 15–59 years, around 13 billion condoms less than the estimated annual requirement (Myer et al., 2001; Shelton and Johnston, 2001).

Other structural causes of persistently high rates of infection are more apparent. At the start of the twenty-first century, around 1.1 billion people did not have access to clean water for drinking, washing or cooking, and 2.4 billion (40 per cent of the world's population) lacked adequate sanitation (WHO, 2000b). The countries where these adverse conditions are most prevalent are among those with the highest morbidity and mortality from diarrhoeal diseases such as cholera, salmonellosis, typhoid and shigellosis, which are caused by water-borne bacteria, and other diarrhoeas due to a wide range of viruses and protozoa. Worldwide, there are an estimated four billion episodes of diarrhoea annually, causing over 1.7 million deaths, mostly among children aged under five (WHO, 2003a).

One of the United Nations Millennium Development Goals is to halve the proportion of people without access to safe drinking water by 2015. The *Global Water Supply and Sanitation Assessment 2000* estimated that to achieve this target in Africa, Asia, Latin America and the Caribbean, a safe water supply would have to be provided to an additional 280,000 people every day for the next 15 years (WHO, 2000b). The financial and geological barriers to achieving this goal do not mean that little progress can be made in alleviating the health consequences of contaminated drinking water. The success of health promotion initiatives is evidenced by the increasing use of pre-packaged or home made oral rehydration solutions (ORS), which are thought to be the major factor in the 50 per cent reduction in child deaths from diarrhoeal diseases which has occurred since 1980 (Victoria et al., 2000).

ORS reduces mortality rates without reducing the number of episodes of diarrhoea suffered by the world's children. But another cheap yet unfashionable health promotion strategy could have a very significant impact. A meta review of research studies in countries with high rates of diarrhoeal diseases concluded that washing hands with soap could reduce the risk of infection transmission by 42–47 per cent (Curtis and Cairncross, 2003). The authors estimate that interventions to promote routine hand washing with soap could reduce deaths from diarrhoeal diseases by about one million (range 0.5–1.4 million) in the world's poorest countries. Almost all of these saved lives would be young children.

Drinking water is also contaminated in many parts of the world by the eggs and larvae of parasites that can infect humans. Open water sources provide breeding grounds for parasite vector species including mosquitoes, tsetse flies and snails. Parasites also enter the human population in the food supply and through skin lesions in contact with infected soil. Table 2.4 summarises the estimated number of people suffering from parasite-mediated diseases in the year 2000 (or nearest date).

The importance of health promotion programmes in preventing the transmission of parasites cannot be overstated. For example, in the middle of the twentieth century, guinea worm disease (dracunculiasis) affected 50 million people worldwide, but the parasite is expected to be eradicated globally before the end of this decade and perhaps as soon as 2005. Success has been achieved by systematic data collection to identify all cases, the promotion of filtering drinking water through cloth to remove the parasite vector, and persuading

Table 2.4   Estimated numbers of people affected worldwide by diseases due to common parasites, 2000 or nearest date (adapted from Davey et al., 2001, Table 5.2*)

Parasite/disease: effects	Millions affected
Roundworm (ascaria)/anaemia, weight loss	1,500
Hookworm/severe anaemia, lung disorders	1,300
Whipworm (trichuris)/diarrhoea, weight loss	1,050
Plasmodium/ malaria: fever, vomiting, kidney failure, coma	300–500
Giardia/ diarrhoea, abdominal pain, weight loss	200
Threadworm (strongyloides)/skin and lung disorders	200
Schistosoma/bilharzia: ulceration of bladder and gut; bladder cancer; liver failure	200
Lymphatic filarial worms/elephantiasis: swelling, ulceration of limbs, scrotum	120
Tapeworm/diarrhoea, abdominal pain, weight loss, cysticercosis	100
Amoebae/diarrhoea, abdominal pain, weight loss	50
Onchocerca/river blindness	18
Leishmania/kala-azar: persistent fever, anaemia, skin disorders	12
South American trypanosomes/ Chagas disease: fever, cardiac damage, heart failure	10
African trypanosomes/sleeping sickness: fever, confusion, lassitude	0.5

Source: * Compiled from various WHO sources

infected people not to stand in village water sources while the worms emerge (Cairncross et al., 2002).

Malaria is still the most important parasite-mediated disease, killing over one million young children every year (Table 2.3). But it is being driven back in some parts of the world through health promotion programmes that support the use of bed nets treated with insecticide at fixed intervals. A review of such projects in a number of endemic countries concluded that they had reduced episodes of malaria by almost 50 per cent (Lengeler, 2001). Moreover, child deaths from all causes fell by 17 per cent, a reflection of the increased vulnerability of children with malaria to death from malnutrition and other infections.

Far less attention has been focused on the impact of intestinal worms in children, which are most often transmitted in food and soil. In the poorest developing countries each child is thought to harbour around a thousand intestinal worms on average, causing diarrhoea, anaemia and failure to thrive. This is an important aspect of the cycle of infection resulting in children becoming chronically underweight, which in turn leads to further or more severe infections and accelerated weight loss.

In 2002, the WHO estimated that 27 per cent of the world's children aged under five years were underweight, resulting in 3.7 million deaths annually, all of them in low and middle income countries. The majority of these deaths are due to the increased vulnerability of underweight children to life-threatening infections, with 50–70 per cent of all child deaths from diarrhoeal diseases, malaria, measles and lower respiratory tract infections attributed to the child being underweight (WHO, 2002). Low body weight is also a significant factor in complications of pregnancy and in perinatal and maternal deaths.

Dietary deficiencies of iron, iodine, zinc and vitamin A also increase susceptibility to infection independently of body weight. For example, 18 per cent of deaths from diarrhoeal diseases are attributed to vitamin A deficiency, which is also the leading cause of acquired blindness in children. Iron deficiency is estimated to affect almost one third of the global population and causes 0.8 million deaths annually and 35 million DALYs.

Infections arising from the food supply affect even the richest countries: in the USA, food-borne infections are estimated to cause 76 million illness episodes a year, leading to 325,000 hospitalisations and 5000 deaths (Mead et al., 1999). For a detailed analysis of the impact of food supply on human health and the implications for health promotion, see Part II, Chapter 7.

New threats from infection

This short review has focused on the categories of infectious and parasite-mediated diseases that currently result in the greatest number of deaths and years lived with disability. However, this perspective underplays a feature of interactions between human populations and pathogenic organisms that is increasingly apparent and presents a major challenge to health promotion in the future.

In the last two decades, at least 176 emerging infectious diseases (EIDs) have been identified. EIDs are either new caused by a previously unknown pathogen, for example HIV, or re-emerging as significant threats to health having previously been in decline, like tuberculosis, which now has a reported incidence of over eight million new cases annually, or drug-resistant strains that were formerly susceptible to chemical agents (such as *Mycobacterium tuberculosis*, African trypanosomes, antibiotic-resistant staphylococci). The importance attached to controlling EIDs is reflected in the WHO's decision to establish a Global Outbreak Alert and Response Network in 1998, which sends rapid action teams to reported outbreaks of EIDs worldwide (for a review of activity, see Heyman et al., 2001).

Since HIV was isolated in 1984, many other new viruses have been discovered that cause life-threatening infections, including Ebola haemorrhagic fever, liver disease caused by hepatitis C virus, hantavirus pulmonary syndrome, diarrhoeal disease caused by Norwalk virus and Nipah virus influenza. In 2003, a novel coronavirus was identified as the agent responsible for the first epidemic of Sudden Acute Respiratory Syndrome (SARS), which spread to 30 countries and resulted in 8422 cases and 916 deaths (WHO, 2003a). The response to SARS in Hong Kong, one of the most affected sites, is described in Part III, Chapter 14. Other new infectious agents include the prisons responsible for Creutzfeldt-Jakob Disease (CJD)

The SARS epidemic illustrated the speed with which infection can now travel around the world, bringing to public attention an inevitable consequence of the huge rise in air transport in the last 25 years. SARS is the best-publicised example of a general trend. For example, Japanese encephalitis virus has spread to Australia, possibly via mosquitoes carried in aircraft; malaria frequently 'escapes' from endemic regions by this route. Cases of West Nile fever have occurred in Eastern and Western Europe and the US; the causative virus may have been imported into New York in 1999 with exotic birds purchased for the city's zoo. Merchant shipping is another means by which infection can jump from one continent to another, principally in the transport of food and livestock. The reintroduction of cholera to South America in 1991, after its elimination more than a century earlier, may have occurred when merchant ships flushed the bacteria from their water tanks.

Another contributor to the enhanced threat from infectious disease is global climate change (see Part II, Chapter 10), which is increasing the range of habitats for insect vectors such as mosquitoes, ticks and rodents. Extreme weather events also displace people from their homes into temporary shelters and camps where infection risk is very high, and flooding destroys sewers and contaminates the water supply. A report prepared by the WHO, the World Metereological Organisation and the United Nations Environment Programme estimated that in 2002 over 5.5 million DALYs could be attributed to the effects of climate change (WHO, 2003b).

The rapid evolution of drug-resistant strains of bacteria is a further cause for concern, principally in relation to tuberculosis on a global scale. But resistance is also emerging to the major antibiotics used to treat common bacterial infections in Western hospitals. For example, the first survey of surgical site infections in patients in English hospitals found that 61 per cent were resistant to the antibiotic most commonly used to treat infected wounds (PHLS, 2000). Hospital acquired infections (HAIs) in England alone have been estimated to contribute to around one thousand deaths a year and cost the National Health Service (NHS) close to £1 billion (Plowman et al., 2000).

Another growing health risk is infection resulting from unsafe healthcare practices, including contaminated injections, blood transfusions and organ transplants. About half a million deaths a year are attributed to this cause, primarily involving transmission of blood-borne pathogens such as HIV and the hepatitis B and C viruses (WHO, 2002). The principal route by which the HIV epidemic began in China was via infected blood transfusion equipment.

Finally, a factor that is likely to prove increasingly significant in the future is the rising proportion of the global population with immune deficiencies that make people more susceptible to infection. Would the 2003 SARS epidemic have been contained so quickly, or at all, if the flight taking the virus from Hong Kong to Toronto had instead landed anywhere in sub-Saharan Africa? In high income countries, where HIV prevalence remains relatively low, the ability to resist infection is significantly reduced by radiation and chemotherapy in people diagnosed with cancer, a condition that will affect one in four of the population during their lifetime. Additionally, the recipients of organ transplants and people suffering from certain autoimmune disorders such as rheumatoid arthritis are intentionally immunosuppressed as part of their treatment.

For all these reasons, there can be no complacency about infectious and parasite-mediated diseases as a key global health concern in the twenty-first century, nor any doubt about the potential impact of health promotion strategies.

Traffic-related injuries

In May 2003, the General Assembly of the United Nations recognised traffic-related injuries as a global epidemic. Traffic accidents caused the death of almost 1.2 million people in 2002, 2.1 per cent of all deaths worldwide, and close to 20 million suffered severe injury. As a cause of death and DALYs, road-traffic injuries rank fourth globally among adults aged 15–59 years (Table 2.1); 68 per cent of all traffic-related deaths occur in this age group. In high income countries, the proportion of deaths on the roads has been declining slowly since the early 1990s, particularly among child pedestrians, but the reverse is true elsewhere in the world.

As Table 2.5 shows, over 80 per cent of traffic-related deaths and the burden of disability from injuries occurs in low to middle income countries, where the majority of accidents affect pedestrians, cyclists and passengers on public transport. The distribution of traffic accidents within a population is strongly associated with urban poverty, and males are almost three times more likely

Table 2.5   Deaths and disability (measured in DALYs) resulting from traffic-related injuries in developed and developing regions of the world in 2002, and for males and females of all ages (data derived from WHO, 2003a, Statistical Annex, Tables 2 and 3)

WHO mortality stratum*	Deaths (× 000)	% of all traffic-related deaths	DALYs (× 000)	% of all traffic-related DALYs
Developed	191	16	5,287	13.7
Low-mortality developing	495	41.5	15,425	39.9
High-mortality developing	504	42.3	17,872	46.2
world		% of all deaths		% of all DALYs
both sexes	1,192	2.1	38,660	2.6
Males	869	2.9	27,218	3.5
Females	323	1.2	11,441	1.6

Notes: * For a complete listing, see WHO (2003a) Statistical Annex, p.183; 'developed' includes North America, Eastern and Western Europe, Australia, Japan, New Zealand and Singapore; 'low-mortality developing' includes most countries in South America and the Caribbean, Indonesia, Sri Lanka, Thailand, China, Philippines, Vietnam and many Arab states; 'high-mortality developing' covers the whole of Africa and most countries in Central America and South East Asia, with Afghanistan, Iraq, Korea, Yemen

than females to die or to be injured on the road (WHO, 2003a). Rising trends in the volume of traffic suggest that road-traffic deaths will increase by around 80 per cent in most developing countries by 2020, with even greater increases predicted for China and India. The fatality rates per 10,000 vehicles are already 30–40 times greater in some low income countries, for example Ghana, than in Western Europe (WHO, 2003a).

Road traffic also causes disease and disability indirectly, as a consequence of atmospheric pollution. In 2000, the risk attributed to urban pollution and lead exposure, most of which comes from vehicle exhaust, accounted for over one million deaths and over 20 million DALYs (WHO, 2002, Statistical Annexe, Tables 11 and 12). Studies in some countries in Western Europe have estimated that twice as many people die from the effects of atmospheric pollution emitted by road traffic than die in traffic accidents (WHO, 2003a).

Interventions to reduce deaths and injuries in road accidents understandably focus on structural measures aimed at traffic calming, eliminating road hazards and strengthening vehicles, and on legislation to restrict speed and enforce the wearing of seat belts and helmets. But more progress could be made if safer driving initiatives, particularly among young males, were resourced and promoted as vigorously as safer sex programmes.

Mental health problems

Health promotion as a discipline has always claimed that supporting emotional wellbeing is central to its ethos. This commitment should place mental health problems high on the health promotion agenda, but they have generally received less attention than other categories of noncommunicable disease, except where they are associated with drug or alcohol use.

Yet five categories of mental health problems appear in the top ten causes of disabling disease (measured in DALYs) worldwide in the peak onset age group 15–44 years. The five are unipolar depressive disorders (ranked second in 2000, contributing 8.6 per cent of total DALYs), alcohol use disorders (ranked fifth, 3.0 per cent), self-inflicted injuries (ranked sixth, 2.7 per cent), schizophrenia, (ranked eighth, 2.6 per cent) and bipolar affective disorder (ranked ninth, 2.5 per cent) (WHO, 2001, Figure 2.2).

If the adult age range is extended to 59 years (as in Table 2.1), unipolar depression still ranks second as a cause of DALYs and is revealed as responsible for a greater disease burden among adult women than any other cause. The Global Burden of Disease 2000 survey reported that 5.8 per cent of men worldwide and 9.5 per cent of women in the age range 15–44 years experience an episode of clinical depression in any 12-month period. More than one third of those who recover from their first episode experience a recurrence within two years and 60 per cent do so within 12 years (WHO, 2001).

The extent of domestic and sexual violence against women is one contributing factor in their higher prevalence of depression. It has been estimated (WHO, 1997) that between 16–50 per cent of women, varying with location and circumstances, will experience domestic violence at some point during their lifetime and 20 per cent will suffer a rape or attempted rape. Women exposed to these assaults are also more likely to contemplate suicide (WHO, 2001).

Sexual abuse during childhood is another significant risk factor for mental health problems. Studies in 39 countries found that 11 per cent of females and 2 per cent of males had experienced sexual abuse involving physical contact as children, suggesting that as many as 500 million people worldwide may have suffered this form of abuse (WHO, 2002). An estimated 5–8 per cent of self-inflicted injuries (including suicide), unipolar depression and disorders associated with alcohol and drug use are attributed to sexual abuse during childhood.

The suicide risk among people who suffer from clinical depression is 15–20 per cent and the risk is even higher, around 30 per cent, among people diagnosed with schizophrenia. The incidence of suicide is highest among younger adults aged 15–34 years, where it is in the top three causes of death worldwide and ranks first in some countries, for example in China, and second in the European region. Alcohol use disorders are strongly associated with suicide risk and rates are higher among men than among women. In 2002, self-inflicted injuries, including suicide, were the cause of death for 877,000 people globally, of which 63 per cent were men (WHO, 2003a).

Interacting causes

This short epidemiological review of key global health concerns illustrates the powerful interactions between different causative factors in producing the patterns of disease and disability that have been described. Underweight children are more susceptible to infectious diseases and parasites, which stunt their growth and development. Malnutrition is a concomitant of poverty and poor people are the most likely to be without a safe water supply or adequate sanitation, and thus are more exposed to infection risk. The babies of underweight mothers are themselves of lower birth weight and suffer higher rates of perinatal mortality and disability, and so the cycle goes on into the next generation.

Or to take another example, excessive use of alcohol not only causes cirrhosis of the liver, but is also a risk factor for mental health problems, including suicide and other self-inflicted injuries, road traffic and other accidental injury, ischaemic heart disease, cerebrovascular disease and violence. All of these conditions and others, with few exceptions, are strongly associated with poverty, overcrowding, unemployment, material insecurity and lack of access to the goods and services enjoyed by the more affluent (for a review, see Gray, 2001).

The encouraging message of this book is that health promotion initiatives can intervene effectively at many different points in the web of interacting causes underlying the world's most serious health problems.

References

Cairncross, S., Muller, R. and Zagaria, N. (2002) Dracunculiasis (guinea worm disease) and the eradication initiative. *Clinical Microbiology Reviews*, **15**: 223–46.

Curtis, V. and Cairncross, S. (2003) Effect of washing hands with soap on diarrhoea risk in the community: a systematic review. *The Lancet Infectious Diseases*, **3**: 275–81.

Davey, B., Halliday, T. and Hirst, M. (2001, reprinted with revisions 2004) *Human Biology and Health: An Evolutionary Approach* (3rd edn). Buckingham: Open University Press and McGraw-Hill.

Gray, A. (editor) (2001) *World Health and Disease* (3rd edn). Buckingham: Open University Press.

Heyman, D.L., Ridier, G.R. and the WHO Operational Support Team to the Global Outbreak Alert and Response Network (2001) Hot spots in a wired world: WHO surveillance of emerging and re-emerging infectious diseases. *The Lancet Infectious Diseases*, **1**: 345–53.

Lengeler, C. (2001) Insecticide-treated bednets and curtains for preventing malaria (Cochrane Review). In *Cochrane Library*, **1**. Oxford: Update Software. Linked from *http://www.cochraneconsumer.com/index* last accessed January 2004.

Mead, P.S., Slutsker, L., Dietz, V., McCaig, L.F., Griffin, P.M. and Tauxe, R.V. (1999) Food-related illness and death in the United States. *Emerging Infectious Diseases*, **5**: 607–25.

Myer, L., Matthews, C. and Little, F. (2001) Condom gap in Africa is wider than study suggests. *British Medical Journal*, **323**: 937.

PHLS (2000) *Surveillance of Surgical Site Infection in English Hospitals 1997–1999*. London: Public Health Laboratory Service.

Plowman, R., Graves, N., Griffin, M., Roberts, J.A., Swan, A.V., Cookson, B.D. and Taylor, L. (2000) *The Socio-Economic Burden of Hospital Acquired Infection*. London: Public Health Laboratory Service.

Shelton, J. D. and Johnston, B. (2001) Condom gap in Africa: evidence from donor agencies and key informants. *British Medical Journal*, **323**: 139.

Victoria, C.G., Bryce, J., Fontaine, O. and Monasch, R. (2000) Reducing deaths from diarrhoea through oral rehydration therapy. *Bulletin of the World Health Organisation*, 78: 1246–55.

WHO (1997) *Violence against Women.* Geneva: World Health Organisation (unpublished document WHO/FRH/WHD/97.8).

WHO (2000a) *Obesity: Preventing and Managing the Global Epidemic.* Geneva: World Health Organisation.

WHO (2000b) *Global Water Supply and Sanitation Assessment 2000 Report.* Geneva: World Health Organisation.

WHO (2001) *The World Health Report 2001 – Mental Health: New Understanding, New Hope.* Geneva: World Health Organisation.

WHO (2002) *The World Health Report 2002 – Reducing Risks, Promoting Healthy Life.* Geneva: World Health Organisation.

WHO (2003a) *The World Health Report 2003 – Shaping the Future.* Geneva: World Health Organisation.

WHO (2003b) *Climate Change and Human Health – Risks and Responses.* Geneva: World Health Organisation.

Williams, B.G., Gouws, E., Boschi-Pinto, C., Bryce, J. and Dye, C. (2002) Estimates of worldwide distribution of child deaths from acute respiratory infections. *The Lancet Infectious Diseases*, 2: 25–32.

CHAPTER 3

Inequalities in Health: International Patterns and Trends

DAVID MCDAID AND ADAM OLIVER

This chapter provides an overview of inequalities in health both within individual countries and across the globe, emphasising the need for different approaches to address these inequalities across low, middle and high income countries. Looking at cross-country variations in health status alone is insufficient, in all settings it is important to ascertain the degree of within-country variations in order to fully inform options for policy makers. Factors contributing to variations in health status and international and national policy initiatives are also examined.

What do we mean by the terms health equity and inequalities in health? Equity is a normative concept linked to social justice that can be defined in many, sometimes contradictory, ways (Oliver, 2001). For example definitions of equity include equal access to healthcare for equal need, equal utilisation for equal need, and equity in final health outcomes. Moving towards more equity in final health outcomes requires going beyond healthcare systems, as health promotion strategies need to consider a range of factors including the level and distribution of income, gender, ethnicity, nutrition, housing and lifestyle.

Unlike equity, inequality is an empirical concept that can be measured in many ways, linked for instance to income and wealth, gender, ethnicity or geographical location. Actual measures of health status may be assessed objectively or through self-assessment, which might produce very different values. Importantly, not all inequalities in health status may be inequitable as they may occur as a result of individuals making fully informed choices about the way in which they live, or be due to unavoidable biological factors.

Reducing inequalities in health status or in access to health benefiting services should be distinguished from the concept of improving health. It is possible to reduce inequalities in population health status by reducing the health status of the more affluent, although this may be considered inappropriate or unethical. Inequalities may be of less importance to policy makers than simply ensuring that all of a population reaches some defined minimum level of health.

Nonetheless, policies purporting to promote equity are often likely to focus on reducing avoidable and what society might consider unfair inequalities in health, such as those due to socioeconomic status, gender, ethnicity or country of birth. Measures to alleviate such inequalities may require the use of proactive initiatives and targeting to help specific vulnerable populations, because even in societies where services are universally available and not dependent on ability to pay, some individuals, or groups of individuals, may be much more adept at accessing services than others (Culyer and Wagstaff, 1992). One targeted group might be those in poverty. This term too can have different meanings. There may, for example be a focus on global *absolute* poverty levels, such as the number of people living on incomes of less than US $1 per day, or *relative* levels of poverty recognising the importance of income inequalities even in high income societies.

Equity and inequality concerns should not be considered in isolation. Other factors such as ethics, politics and efficiency require careful consideration. Given that resources are finite, not all inequalities may be alleviated, and investment in strategies reduces funds, in the short term at least, for other public programmes.

Prominence of health inequalities in health policy

Health inequalities have enjoyed varying degrees of prominence within global health policy over recent decades (Gwatkin, 2002a; Braveman and Tarimo, 2002). Emphasis on a primary healthcare strategy intended to reduce inequalities in health arising from the Alma Ata Declaration of Health for All in 1978 (World Health Organisation, 1978) was overtaken by a focus on health sector reform and promotion of long-term sustainability in healthcare systems (World Bank, 1987) before the re-emergence of health inequalities across countries as a key issue in the 1990s following the recognition by the World Bank that poor health is an integral part of poverty (World Bank, 1997) and more recently by the linking of health to economic development by the Commission on Macroeconomics and Health and the World Summit on Sustainable Development in Johannesburg in 2002 (Sarch, 2002). International debt relief has also been linked to a requirement for countries to produce Poverty Strategy Reduction Papers (PSRPs), including strategies to reduce health inequalities. The Millennium Development Goals include specific health related targets while they also concluded that health is an integral part of the economic development process (Sarch, 2002; United Nations Development Programme, 2003b).

In the World Health Report 2003 the new Director General of WHO Dr Lee Jong-Wook called global health gaps unacceptable and referred back to the principles set at Alma Ata, recognising injustices caused by inequalities but setting these alongside the need to *construct sustainable and equitable health systems*, systems that integrate both health promotion and disease prevention strategies with treatments for acute and chronic illness (World Health Organisation, 2003).

Inequalities in health across countries

Over the last 50 years average life expectancy increased worldwide by nearly 20 years to 65.2, while there has been a reduction in the variation in life expectancy for many countries. The greatest increases in life expectancy have been achieved in low and middle income countries, with gains of 17 years reported for countries with high child and adult mortality rates, and 26 years in low mortality countries, compared with nine years in high income countries (World Health Organisation, 2003). In part this reflects a process of catch up in some low and middle income countries in introducing basic improvements such as improved sanitation and access to clean water, mandatory education and the introduction of immunisation programmes.

Despite this welcome improvement in health status, many have not benefited, with the health inequality gap between the poorest low income countries and the rest having widened over the last 20 years, due in no small measure to the spread of HIV/AIDS. Average life expectancy at birth ranges from 81.9 years in Japan to just 34.0 years in Sierra Leone, and of the 50 countries with the lowest rates 44 are to be found in sub-Saharan Africa, with just five in Asia and one in the Caribbean. These variations in life expectancy are seen for both genders: 78.4 years for men in Japan to 32.4 years in Sierra Leone and 32.9 years in Lesotho, and 85.3 years for Japanese women compared to just 35.7 in Sierra Leone and 38.0 years in Zimbabwe.

These inequalities across countries and regions persist when using outcome measures that combine mortality with morbidity, such as the Disability Adjusted Life Year or DALY, thus capturing the consequences of chronic conditions. DALYs combine time lost through premature death with time lived in states of disability. Total disease burden is the difference between observed population health status and that of the ideal population. Another way of expressing this is in terms of healthy life expectancy. This converts total life expectancy into years of full health by taking account of years of life lived with disability and injuries. Life expectancy in the WHO Afro region, which includes all sub-Saharan Africa, is only 43.27 years compared with almost 66 years across the whole EURO region (Table 3.1). Healthy life expectancy in Western Europe is even higher at 71.4 years (World Health Organisation, 2003).

Noncommunicable diseases account for almost 75 per cent of deaths worldwide, but there is significant variation between regions with noncommunicable disease contributing 90 per cent of deaths in high income countries, 75 per cent of some middle and low income regions such as Latin America, Asia and the Western Pacific but only one third of deaths in Africa (see Part II, Chapter 6 for further discussion of the challenge of noncommunicable diseases for global

Table 3.1 Average healthy life expectancy at birth worldwide and in each of the six WHO regions, 2002

WHO region	Probability of dying (per 1000) under 5 years of age	
	Males	*Females*
World	65.61	59.32
AFRO	156.46	143.48
AMRO	31.42	27.11
EMRO	68.14	64.85
WPRO	44.44	38.22
EURO	17.04	13.88
SEARO	71.18	65.81

Key: AFRO (African Region), AMRO (Americas), EMRO (Eastern Mediterranean), WPRO (Western Pacific), EURO (Europe), SEARO (South East Asia)
Source: Source data and a full list of countries in each of the WHO regions is available at www.who.int/evidence/bod

health). Communicable diseases remain of primary importance in sub-Saharan Africa, in particular due to the HIV/AIDS epidemic (World Health Organisation, 2003 and Chapter 9 of this text). Future projections estimate that by 2020 nearly three quarters of the global disease burden would be due to noncommunicable diseases, with only 15 per cent due to communicable disease (Murray and Lopez, 1997). However, the burden of disease experienced by the poorest populations in the world may not follow this trend so closely, and communicable diseases may continue to affect the poor significantly and disproportionately (Gwatkin et al., 1999).

Identifying inequalities within countries

Inequalities exist *within* as well as across countries, although they are complex to measure and explain. They have formed the focus of attention in high income countries, but because of data limitations in low and middle income countries evidence is more limited, and where available predominantly concentrates on issues of child and maternal health.

Measuring such inequalities may be of paramount importance if a goal of policy making is to benefit the less affluent in society. Initiatives not targeted to these groups in low and middle income countries may be subject to an inverse equity law where interventions benefit rich minorities disproportionately compared with the poor (Victora et al., 2000; Gwatkin, 2002b; Victora et al., 2003). In some countries of sub-Saharan Africa the richest quintile in society receive more than twice as much of public expenditure on government health services compared with the bottom quintile (Castro-Leal et al., 2000).

There can also be significant variations in access to healthcare and health promoting services within low and middle income countries where public funding of services may be very limited. Generally healthcare expenditure in these countries remains well below 5 per cent of GDP, and average per capita annual expenditure in the lowest income countries is just US $6. WHO estimates that a minimum of US $35–40 per capita is required for basic services. Even where services are available, and not subject to user fees significant geographical variations in service provision cause problems. Among Cambodians, for instance, 85 per cent of the population live in rural areas, yet 87 per cent of government health workers are located in urban centres (United Nations Development Programme, 2003a).

Inequalities in child health

Child mortality rates remain one of the key indicators used to identify health inequalities between high, middle and low income countries, because much of the variation in overall average life expectancy globally is due to profound differences in mortality rates for children, especially in the first five years of life.

Deaths in children under five globally have decreased from 17.5 million in 1970 to 10.5 million in 2002, but 98 per cent of these occur in low and middle income countries where children are more exposed to many risk factors, including lack of sanitation and clean water, poor housing conditions, malnourishment and a lack of education. Disparities in child health between and within different low and middle income regions are also growing (Victora et al., 2003; World Health Organisation, 2003). Mortality levels are now higher in 16 countries than they were in 1990, 14 of which are in Africa, and overall 35 per cent more African children are at a higher risk of death than they were in 1992. While the average probability of dying before the age of five in the WHO African region is approximately nine times that in Europe (Table 3.2) for the very worst countries the chances of death can vary one hundredfold compared with the best (Table 3.3). Maternal death rates are more than 100 times higher in sub-Saharan Africa than in high income countries. Within countries disparities are again found. The risk of maternal death in Indonesia, for example, is three to four times greater in the poorest income quintile of the population compared with the richest (Graham et al., 2004).

Wang (2002) recently analysed data compiled from standardised World Bank Demographic and Health Survey (DHS) data from more than 60 low income countries, finding a strong negative correlation between the average rate of child mortality and the level of inequality in child mortality rates using concentration indices, so that in countries where mortality rates had decreased, inequalities in mortality by socioeconomic position had increased. Exceptional countries where good improvements in the reduction of mortality rates were accompanied by low inequality within countries could however be found, including China, Ghana, Guatemala and Namibia.

Variations in mortality rates between urban and rural areas within these countries were also identified. Annual under-fives mortality rates in rural areas

Table 3.2   Probability of dying (per 1000) by sex under the age of 5 years in 2002 across the 6 WHO regions

WHO Region	Probability of dying (per 1000) under 5 years of age	
	Males	Females
World	65.61	59.32
AFRO	156.46	143.48
AMRO	31.42	27.11
EMRO	68.14	64.85
WPRO	44.44	38.22
EURO	17.04	13.88
SEARO	71.18	65.81

Key: AFRO (African Region), AMRO (Americas), EMRO (Eastern Mediterranean), WPRO (Western Pacific), EURO (Europe), SEARO (South East Asia)

Source: Adapted from World Health Report 2003, Statistical Annex, Table 1. A full list of countries in each of the WHO regions is available at www.who.int/evidence/bod

Table 3.3   Probability of dying (per 1000) by sex under the age of 5 years in 2002 for top and bottom five countries

Males		Females	
	Probability of dying (per 1000) Under age 5 years		
Finland	4	Finland	3
Iceland	4	Iceland	3
Japan	4	Singapore	3
Singapore	4	Sweden	3
Sweden	4	Monaco	3
Liberia	242	Mali	224
Niger	249	Angola	247
Afghanistan	258	Niger	256
Angola	279	Afghanistan	256
Sierra Leone	332	Sierra Leone	303

Source: Derived from World Health Report 2003, Statistical Annex, Table 1

declined during the 1990s by 2.1 per cent compared with 2.6 per cent in urban communities. The author concluded that this evidence, given that the poorest populations tend to be more heavily concentrated in rural areas, suggested that mortality reduction strategies may not have been successful in targeting the poor (Wang, 2002). Other studies have reported within-country variations by location and wealth. In Zambia in 1996 for example, infant mortality rates across the nine provinces varied from 66 per 1000 to 158 per 1000 (Costello and White, 2001). In Indonesia, under-five mortality is nearly four times higher in the poorest fifth of the population than in the richest fifth while in Bolivia during the 1990s under-five mortality fell by 34 per cent amongst the richest 20 per cent but by 8 per cent amongst the poorest 20 per cent (Wagstaff, 2003b).

An analysis of DHS data from 32 countries looked at the relationship between under fives mortality rates and inequalities between the rich and children living on less than one dollar a day. Generally no correlation was observed between the level of inequality and mortality rates. Niger with the highest rate of under fives mortality had low levels of inequality while Egypt had relatively high levels of inequality and mortality rates. Kazakhstan had both low levels of inequality and very low mortality rates which may be attributed in part to greater public spending on health improving the availability of low cost or free access to health and other services (Wagstaff, 2003a).

Further analysis of the DHS survey data indicates that even when economic status is comparable, poor children in Africa have a much higher risk of mortality compared with those in other low and middle income regions of the world. More affluent children in Africa have a 16 per cent higher chance of mortality than poor children in the Americas (World Health Organisation, 2003). Reducing within-country variations in the risk of mortality although challenging could reduce the overall under fives mortality rates by more than 40 per cent worldwide (Victora et al., 2003). However, progress in tackling within-country variation has been limited; only three out of 24 countries with subnational data on child mortality between the mid-1980s and mid-1990s narrowed the inequality gap in under fives mortality rates over this period (United Nations Development Programme, 2003a).

Inequalities in adult health

Life expectancy has improved overall for those who reach adulthood globally by between two and three years over the last twenty years. There are two notable exceptions to this trend: parts of Africa where life expectancy has reduced by approximately seven years, and the former Soviet Union and parts of Eastern Europe where from the 1990s life expectancy has fallen by almost five years for men, and the risk of death from injuries, including suicide, is now six times higher than that in Western Europe. Of all worldwide deaths related to HIV/AIDS in 2002, 80 per cent occurred in Africa (World Health Organisation, 2003). The decline in life expectancy in Eastern Europe is more complex and is linked to multiple factors which include the collapse of long-standing regimes, economic decline coupled with the introduction of a free market, and reduction of controls on alcohol (Walberg et al., 1998; see also Part III, Chapter 15).

Higher rates of death are still observed between the ages of 15 and 59 years in low and middle income countries compared to high income countries. For men aged over 15 the lowest probability of dying before reaching 59 was found in Kuwait, a rate of 81 per 1000, compared with a rate of 902 per 1000 in Lesotho (Table 3.4). The 50 countries with the highest risk of mortality

Table 3.4   Probability of dying (per 1000) by sex
between ages of 15 and 59 years in 2002 (five best
and worst rates)

Probability of dying (per 1000) between ages of 15 and 59 years			
Males		*Females*	
Kuwait	81	San Marino	31
Sweden	83	Andorra	43
Iceland, San Marino	85	Japan	46
Malta	87	Monaco, Spain	47
Singapore	87	Cyprus, Greece	48
Zambia	700	Zambia	654
Botswana	786	Swaziland	707
Swaziland	818	Lesotho	742
Zimbabwe	821	Botswana	745
Lesotho	902	Zimbabwe	789

Source: Derived from World Health Report 2003, Statistical Annex, Table 1

include six countries formerly part of the Soviet Union: Kyrgyzstan, Turkmenistan, Belarus, Ukraine, Kazakhstan and the Russian Federation that has the worst rate of the six (464 per 1000) (see Part III, Chapter 15 for details of the public health strategies in place to tackle these challenges). The 20 worst performing countries are all in sub-Saharan Africa. While the mortality risks for women are generally lower than for men, in Bangladesh and Tonga they have a higher risk of death. The lowest risk is found in San Marino at just 31 per 1000 compared with 789 per 1000 in Zimbabwe. The risk of dying for women in countries of the former Soviet Union is much better than that of men at 168 per 1000.

Looking for the causes of inequalities in health

Inequalities in health status for both adults and children cannot be attributed to socioeconomic development or poverty alone, as countries such as Sri Lanka, and the Indian State of Kerala have relatively low incomes but similar health outcomes to countries with much higher levels of income (Sen, 1999). In high income countries health inequalities persist and may widen as in the United Kingdom (UK) over the last 30 years (Oliver, 2001). Many different determinants of health inequalities have been identified including income, gender, geographical resource allocation, social class and ethnicity. Some of these are now briefly highlighted.

In some high income countries such as the UK, the Netherlands and Sweden, much research has focused on socioeconomic factors associated with mortality and morbidity. These inequalities are most often measured by (occupational) social class data. The Black Report on social inequalities in health reported growing differences in mortality rates in the UK based on (occupational) social class (Department of Health and Social Security, 1980). More recently the Acheson inquiry, which also looked at factors such as education, gender and ethnicity came to similar conclusions (Department of Health, 1998).

Another factor may be the relative distribution of income within a society. The greater the level of variation in incomes regardless of whether individuals are impoverished, may induce stress and jealousy and reduce the level of social cohesion and social capital in society, which may consequently have adverse effects on health (Wilkinson, 1996; Kawachi and Kennedy, 1997). Studies have also identified the importance of education on health inequalities, and the importance of psychosocial factors (Marmot and Bobak, 2000). Racial variations in health status have been explored in depth particularly in the United States but evidence is also to be found in low income countries. One recent review identified studies from Guatemala, Peru, Sri Lanka, Thailand and parts of Africa that report variations in access to services and outcomes related to ethnicity (Braveman and Tarimo, 2002).

Focus on gender inequalities

The impact of gender on health inequalities has also been widely discussed, and has important implications for the implementation of health promotion strategies, as striking inequalities related to gender can be observed worldwide in a number of low and middle income countries. In 2002 girls were at significant higher risk of mortality before their fifth birthday in China, the Maldives, Nepal, India and Pakistan (Table 3.5). The reasons for these variations are complex, and may be due in part to long-standing cultural and societal values (World Health Organisation, 2003). A recent review identified a number of studies which reported discrimination against female children in Bangladesh and Pakistan, together with evidence of inequalities in access to healthcare

Table 3.5   Selected countries with higher risk of mortality in girls compared with boys under the age of 5 in 2002

	Probability of dying (per 1000) under 5 years of age	
	Males	*Females*
China	31	41
Maldives	38	43
Nepal	81	87
India	87	95
Pakistan	105	115

Source: Derived from World Health Report 2003, Statistical Annex, Table 1

services across a number of countries in Africa, Asia and the Middle East (Braveman and Tarimo, 2002).

The complexity can be illustrated by looking at gender inequalities in India, where northern provinces such as the Punjab and Haryana have for decades had more males than females in the population, and where evidence of systematic discrimination and malnourishment of girls is found (Jatrana, 2003). In the Punjab the rate of female under fives mortality was two to three times higher than that for boys, despite an overall reduction in child mortality rates. Furthermore, this excess mortality rate was most often found in families that already have one surviving daughter. Child mortality rates were higher if mothers are more educated, which may be due to increased ability with education to manipulate family size and structure to that which these women prefer (Das Gupta, 1987). Data from World Bank DHS surveys also indicates that whilst female to male mortality in some Indian states is among the worst in the world, Tamil Nadu is at the other end of the spectrum having one of the lowest female to male mortality rates, bettered by only three countries (Filmer et al., 1998).

Moving away from countries where discrimination against women in society generally is rife, the evidence particularly in high income countries is more complex, contrary to the commonly held perception that women live longer but have higher levels of morbidity than men (Hunt and Annandale, 1999). Evidence from the UK indicates that this is not always the case, and excess female morbidity, with the exception of mental health problems, only coincides with specific diseases and/or at specific points in the life cycle (Macintyre et al., 1996). There is also growing evidence of gender inequalities against men in some settings in high income countries, perhaps notably including highly egalitarian countries such as Finland (Lahelma et al., 1999). This is perhaps of greater significance though for countries of the former Soviet Union. In Kazakhstan male life expectancy has fallen dramatically and the life expectancy gap between men and women is now approximately ten years. Data collected on primary care utilisation indicates that despite increased male morbidity, utilisation rates remain low compared to those for women, and calls have been made to direct more resources to improve male health, particularly by encouraging more frequent contact with primary care services (Cashin et al., 2002).

International moves to tackle health inequalities

A number of international initiatives either directly or indirectly can play a role in tackling inequalities in health. The Millennium Development Goals (MDGs) have a focus on health promoting activities for low income countries including objectives of eradicating extreme poverty and hunger, reducing child mortality, improving maternal health, and combating HIV/AIDs, malaria and other diseases. Other health related benefits to be attained include increasing access to clean drinking water, slum clearance, reducing gender disparities, as well as improving access to primary education and to affordable essential drugs. However can the MDGs be attained and furthermore will they reduce inequalities in health status?

The current situation is discouraging. The World Bank is calling for urgent action from international development partners to make up for lost time if the targets are to be met (World Bank, 2004). There are deteriorating Health Development Indices (HDI), which is an aggregate measure of health, education and living standards, in 21 countries in Africa and Eastern Europe. Only two of the eight MDGs are likely to be met by 2015, halving absolute poverty and improving access to clean drinking water, largely due to progress in India and China. In sub-Saharan Africa at the current rate of progress it will take approximately 150 years to reach targets on child mortality and poverty. The success of other goals such as lowering maternal mortality and HIV/AIDS infection rates will be difficult to measure because of a lack of data (United Nations Development Programme, 2003a).

Access to financial resources to implement strategies across a range of different areas may be problematic, and targets for the reduction in child and maternal mortality require access to health promotion and healthcare services. The WHO Commission on Macroeconomics has called on high income countries to substantially increase annual aid to US $35 billion by 2015 from the current level of US $5 billion (Commission for Macroeconomics and Health, 2001).

The health related targets of the MDGs do not target the least affluent, as most health targets are stated in terms of improvements in societal averages rather than in terms of gains within poor populations. Gwatkin (2002b) looked at the potential consequences of this by comparing two possible implementation scenarios one without targeting where the richest groups benefit first in a low income country (top down) and a second where the poor are targeted (bottom up). Large variations were observed between the top and bottom population quintiles. Inequalities in child under fives mortality rates would be ten times as high using the top-down approach compared with the bottom-up approach. He argues that the drive for more rapid improvements in global averages ignoring targeting may undermine the principle of helping the poor, and it might be better to focus on more challenging efforts targeting the poor, even though it may take longer to reach the MDGs.

Poverty Strategy Reduction Papers (PSRPs), that are required for debt relief, also do not provide a consistent set of health inequality related information; a recent review reported that few included information on tackling financial barriers to access, or the development of strategies to target vulnerable groups. Furthermore noncommunicable diseases were almost always excluded, even though in the poorest of countries they contribute significantly to the burden of disease (Dodd and Hinshelwood, 2002). Again calls for pro-poor targets to be used in PSRPs have been made (Currey, 2002).

The need for specific population targeting can equally be applied to strategies introduced in high income countries, purportedly to tackle inequalities in health. Several targets were introduced in England following the publication of the Acheson report into inequalities in health (Department of Health, 1998). These targets, including goals of reducing deaths from cancer or suicide by 20 per cent, and from cardiovascular disease by 40 per cent were not directed towards the less affluent, but were applied across the whole population, again raising questions as to their suitability for reducing inequalities in health.

The current MDG goals focus very much on issues related to communicable diseases, and are less appropriate for tackling other global health inequalities. The deterioration of health status in eastern Europe and the former Soviet Union, where outcomes are approaching the level observed in some African countries, is not largely due to communicable diseases but to increases in rates of injuries, accidents and violent activities, none of which are covered in the MDG goals on health (Lock et al., 2002).

What next?

While overall health status worldwide, measured simply in terms of life expectancy has continued to improve over the last 50 years, with the greatest gains observed in low and middle income countries, not all countries have benefited. Some sub-Saharan countries in particular now have inferior life expectancy rates than they did a decade ago, in large measure due to the scourge of HIV/AIDS, with 80 per cent of the global disease burden in Africa (see Part II, Chapter 9). Differences of between 40 and 50 years in average life expectancy between countries are highly inequitable and merit action to raise quality adjusted life expectancy levels to at least some acceptable minimum level in all settings.

This focus on cross country differences with its inevitable focus on improving health in areas of the world with high levels of absolute poverty, however, has meant that less international attention has been given to other areas where health promotion can play a vital role in reducing health inequalities. Health status has deteriorated and inequalities risen in parts of eastern Europe and the former Soviet Union, but they may be seen as lower priorities, while in high income countries, although overall health has improved, the level of inequalities across society continue to increase.

Cross country comparisons alone are insufficient to fully identify inequalities, and inform policy making. There is a need to improve data collection systems in low income countries in order to capture more information on geographic, socioeconomic, gender and ethnicity-related variations. Even in high income countries data may not be disaggregated by socioeconomic factors or other possible determinants of health inequalities. Surveys undertaken by the World Bank and others have demonstrated the wide variation in health outcomes in countries with similar economies and expenditure on healthcare. Access to additional data therefore can help identify non-poverty related aspects of health inequalities, elements of best practice, and are essential for determining whether health promoting strategies such as those advocated within the MDGs are reaching their intended target groups.

Improved access to data is also needed to help identify effective approaches to tackling problems associated with economic transition and growth in countries. As nations develop and health status improves, disease patterns change, with a greater burden related to noncommunicable diseases and a need to increase the focus on adult health. Already unipolar depression is the second single contributor to the global burden of disease, and its prevalence across low and middle income countries is growing (see Chapter 2 for further discussion of the global problem presented by mental health issues). One challenge will be to see how knowledge from previous transitions elsewhere, for instance in Europe, can inform development of health promotion strategies. Furthermore, an assessment will need to be made of the extent determinants of health inequalities in high income countries related to noncommunicable diseases can be translated to these transitional settings and of the role cultural factors play.

Promoting health and alleviating health inequalities cannot be done solely by looking at the health sector in isolation, rather a broad approach is needed tailored to specific circumstances. In low and middle income countries the links with development policy need to be strengthened further, and issues such as gender inequalities in terms of health and education need to be addressed. The MDGs are a sound basis for this. In higher income countries the focus needs to be on cross sectoral cooperation to tackle factors influencing health status, whether this be for instance environmental, economic, social or health and safety-related.

A danger to initiatives to tackle inequalities in health status is the time lag between the introduction of policies and their impact. Long-term planning and effective cooperation between all stakeholders including different government sectors, civil society organisations, international donors and local communities is required to overcome political short-termism. One way of strengthening the argument for investing in health promoting and health treating interventions to reduce inequalities and improve health status in all settings is to demonstrate not only that they are effective, but that they can also be highly cost effective, for instance reducing future demand for health services and promoting economic development. Economic evidence is an integral element of a review of the future of public health and health promotion strategies in the UK (Kelly et al., 2004).

Finally it should be emphasised that reducing health inequalities should not be confused with a desire to improve health status. Most measures of health status used in international comparisons are based on population averages. While it is a desirable goal to raise average levels of health status in a population, this may not necessarily reduce health inequalities. Indeed without effective targeting and the reduction of both financial and non-financial barriers to health promotion and healthcare benefits, the chances are that inequalities between the less affluent and the more affluent in societies will increase.

References

Braveman, P. and Tarimo, E. (2002) Social inequalities in health within countries: not only an issue for affluent nations. *Social Science and Medicine*, **54**: 1621–35.

Cashin, C., Borowitz, M. and Zuess, O. (2002) The gender gap in health care resource utilisation in central Asia. *Health Policy and Planning*, **17**: 264–72.

Castro-Leal, F., Dayton, J., Demery, L. and Mehra, K. (2000) Public spending on health care in Africa: Do the poor benefit? *Bulletin of the World Health Organisation*, **78**: 66–74.

Commission for Macroeconomics and Health (2001) *Macroeconomics and health: Investing in health for economic development. Report of the Commission on Macroeconomics and Health chaired by Jeffrey D. Sachs.* Geneva: World Health Organisation.

Costello, A. and White, H. (2001) Reducing global inequalities in child health. *Archives of Disease in Childhood*, **84**: 98–102.

Culyer, A.J. and Wagstaff, A. (1992) *Need, Equity and Equality in Health and Health Care.* York. Centre for Health Economics, University of York.

Currey, M. (2002) Are policies addressing health inequalities? In Oliver, A. (ed.) *International Perspectives on Equity and Health: As seen from the UK.* London: Nuffield Trust.

Das Gupta, M. (1987) Selective discrimination against female children in rural Punjab, India. *Population and Development Review*, **13**: 77–100.

Department of Health (1998) *Inequalities in health: Report of an independent inquiry chaired by Sir Donald Acheson.* London: The Stationery Office.

Department of Health and Social Security (1980) *Inequalities in health: Report of a research working group chaired by Sir Douglas Black.* London: Department of Health and Social Security.

Dodd, R. and Hinshelwood, E. (2002) *Poverty Reduction Strategy Papers – Their Significance for Health.* Geneva: World Health Organisation.

Filmer, D., King, E.M. and Pritchett, L. (1998) *Gender Disparity in South Asia: Comparisons between and within Countries.* Washington DC: Work Bank, Policy Research Working Paper 1867.

Graham, W., Fitzmaurice, A.E., Bell, J.S. and Cairns, J.A. (2004) The familial technique for linking maternal death with poverty. *Lancet*, **363**: 23–27.

Gwatkin, D.R. (2002a) Reducing health inequalities in developing countries. In Detels, R., McEwen, J., Beaglehole, R. and Tanaka, H. (eds). *Oxford Textbook of Public Health* (4th edn), volume 3. Oxford: Oxford University Press.

Gwatkin, D.R. (2002b) *Who would gain most from efforts to reach the Millennium Development Goals for health? An inquiry into the possibility of progress that fails to reach the poor.* Washington, DC: World Bank.

Gwatkin, D.R., Guillot, M. and Heuveline, P. (1999) The burden of disease among the global poor. *Lancet*, **354**: 586–89.

Hunt, K. and Annandale, E. (1999) Relocating gender and morbidity: Examining men's and women's health in contemporary western societies. *Social Science and Medicine*, **48**: 1–5.

Jatrana, S. (2003) *Explaining Gender Disparity in Child Health in Haryana State of India.* Singapore: Asian Metacentre for Population and Sustainable Development Analysis.

Kawachi, I. and Kennedy, B.P. (1997) Socio-economic determinants of health: Health and social cohesion: Why care about income inequality? *British Medical Journal*, **314**: 1037–40.

Kelly, M., McDaid, D., Ludbrooke, A. and Powell, J. (2004) *Economic Appraisal of Public Health Interventions.* London: Health Development Agency.

Lahelma, E., Martikainen, P., Rahkonen, O. and Silventoinen, K. (1999) Gender differences in ill health in Finland: Patterns, magnitude and change. *Social Science and Medicine,* **48**: 7–19.

Lock, K., Andreev, E. M., Shkolnikov, V. M. and McKee, M. (2002) What targets for international development policies are appropriate for improving health in Russia? *Health Policy and Planning,* **17**: 257–63.

Macintyre, S., Hunt, K. and Sweeting, H. (1996) Gender differences in health: Are they really as simple as they seem? *Social Science and Medicine,* **42**: 617–24.

Marmot, M. and Bobak, M. (2000) International comparators and poverty and health in Europe. *British Medical Journal,* **321**: 1124–28.

Murray, C.J.L. and Lopez, A.D. (1997) Alternative projections of mortality and disability by cause 1990–2020: Global burden of disease study. *Lancet,* **349**: 1498–504.

Oliver, A. (2001) *Why Care About Health Inequality?* London: Office of Health Economics.

Sarch, L. (2002) Health at the heart of sustainable development? *Eurohealth,* **8** (5): 23–26.

Sen, A. (1999) Health in development. *Bulletin of the World Health Organisation,* **77**: 619–23.

United Nations Development Programme (2003a) *Health Development Report 2003.* New York: United Nations.

United Nations Development Programme (2003b) http://hdr.undp.org/, New York: United Nations.

Victora, C.G., Vaughan, J.P., Barros, F.C., Silva, A.C. and Tomasi, E. (2000) Explaining trends in inequities: Evidence from Brazilian child health studies. *Lancet,* **356**: 1093–98.

Victora, C.G., Wagstaff, A., Armstrong Schellenberg, J., Gwatkin, D.R., Claeson, M. and Habicht, J.P. (2003) Applying an equity lens to child health and mortality: More of the same is not enough. *Lancet,* **362**: 233–41.

Wagstaff, A. (2003a) Child health on a dollar a day: Some tentative cross-country comparisons. *Social Science and Medicine,* **57**: 1529–38.

Wagstaff, A. (2003b) *Health and Poverty: What's the problem? What to do?* Washington, DC: World Bank.

Walberg, P., McKee, M., Shkolnikov, V.M., Chenet, L. and Leon, D.A. (1998) Economic change, crime and mortality crisis in Russia: Regional analysis. *British Medical Journal,* **317**: 312–18.

Wang, L. (2002) Determinants of child mortality in LDCs: Empirical findings from demographic and health surveys. *Health Policy,* **65**: 277–99.

Wilkinson, R.G. (1996) *Unhealthy Societies: The Afflictions of Inequality.* London: Routledge.

World Bank (1987) *Financing Health Services in Developing Countries: An Agenda for Reform.* Washington DC: World Bank.

World Bank (1997) *Sector Strategy: Health, Nutrition and Population.* Washington DC: World Bank.

World Bank (2004) *Health MDGs at the Crossroads.* Washington DC: World Bank.

World Health Organisation (1978) *Primary health care: Report of the international conference on primary health care, Alma-Ata, USSR, 6–12 September 1978.* Geneva: World Health Organisation.

World Health Organisation (2003) *World Health Report 2003.* Geneva: World Health Organisation.

CHAPTER 4

Global Health Promotion: Challenges and Opportunities

MAURICE MITTELMARK

In order to address the global health challenges described in Chapters 2 and 3 in this section of the book, inter-sectoral collaboration is essential, with new partnerships developed that extend beyond the interest groups and professional alliances that define and shape the orthodoxy of health promotion. This should in theory be feasible. The determinants of good health are essentially the same prerequisites for sustainable development, protection of the environment and a positive business climate. They are also the prerequisites for the advancement of opportunities and rights for women and children, legislative reforms and for the nurturing of inclusive, supportive networks. To accelerate development in enabling people to increase control over and to improve their health, health promoters will have to engage more actively with social progress movements. Health promotion also needs new injections of energy and ideas to stimulate more rapid expansion of its theoretical base. This, too, calls for new alliances with academic disciplines on and beyond the periphery of health promotion.

The need for new alliances for health promotion has been reiterated many times since the 1978 Declaration of Alma Ata emerged from the International Conference on Primary Health Care (World Health Organisation [WHO], 1978). Two decades later, the Fourth International Conference on Health Promotion in Jakarta, Indonesia (WHO, 1997) continued to emphasise the need, with its theme *New Partners for a New Era – Leading Health Promotion into the 21st Century*. The building of multi-sectoral partnerships has therefore become a fundamental task for health promoters (Scriven, 1998).

At all levels from local to international, inter-sector collaboration is a diffi-cult process (Scriven, 1998: 44–45). The main barriers are not centrism and protectionism, but more or less calculated delimitations intended to divide resources and responsibilities into manageable chunks. This gives rise, inevitably, to guild like partitions, each with its associated history, language, customs, associations, books, journals and conferences. Developing a profes-sional identity in this way whilst remaining sufficiently open to multi-professional action is a challenge for health promotion and its natural allies. Seen in this light, it is understandable, though discomforting, that 25 years after Alma Ata, health promotion remains too isolated. Its insularity, however involun-tary, restrains health promotion's full potential to contribute to the global health and social progress agenda. There is potential for improvement in the quality and effectiveness of inter-professional collaboration at both local and regional levels. There is also scope for enhancing collaboration at the macro level with other social progress movements. There are missed opportunities for new academic collaborations to revive and expand the theoretical and research base of health promotion.

The benefits of enhanced collaboration among social progress movements, and a widening of academic collaboration for the advancement of the disciplinary base of health promotion, have received relatively little attention. Compared to the arenas of inter-professional and inter-organisational collaboration, which are extensively addressed in the health promotion literature, they remain unsupported (see especially Dluhy and Kravitz, 1990; Dines and Cribb, 1993; Downie et al., 1996; Baum, 1998; Bracht, 1998; Scriven, 1998 and Green and Kreuter, 1999).

Since not all health promoters may think of themselves as being social activists, the contention that among its various aspects health promotion is also a social movement needs defending. The role of health promotion in global advocacy for social and political change to promote the health of populations is one clear example of this claim. It is manifest, in particular, in the work of the International Union for Health Promotion and Education (IUHPE). As a global professional network of individuals and institutions, the IUHPE has the mission to promote global health and to contribute to the achievement of equity in health between and within countries. The IUHPE has a long record of activism in virtually every part of the world. It conducts advocacy work on several fronts. As one example, the IUHPE advocates for the inclusion of social clauses in trade agreements. Other IUHPE advocacy initiatives underway at the time of writing include work on peace and health, and advocacy for tobacco control (www.iuhpe.org).

Health promotion's insularity

It is a contention of this chapter that health promotion is too insular. For the present purpose, the term health promotion refers to the aggregation of practitioners of various kinds who are self-identified health promoters and people, usually academics, who are developing the theoretical and knowledge base for health promotion. Their common bond is the Ottawa Charter for Health Promotion, a seminal document that represents a distinct way of thinking about health and about how to improve health (WHO, 1986; see also Chapter 1 of this text). Health promotion professionals and academics work in organisations dealing with various specific aspects of health, such as maternal and child health, health in schools and health behaviour change. Gravitating towards health promotion from a handful of disciplines and professional backgrounds with which most continue to identify, their remits are preoccupied with managing practical tasks of their professions and disciplines.

In North America, for example, a large number of health promoters are trained in some aspect of public health or nursing, with others from education, social psychology, and social work. In much of Southeast Asia and Africa, on the other hand, health promotion is managed by professionals, with backgrounds in medical education and formal or informal training in public health, and implemented by communications and health education specialists. In Europe, health educators dominate in France and in the Netherlands, and graduate programmes producing health promotion professionals with master's degrees have been established in many countries. The pattern is much the same in other parts of the world (see Part III of this text for detailed country and regional case studies that expand this analysis). In general, public health and education professions tend to shape health promotion practice and academic health promotion is dominated by the disciplines of public health, health education and health psychology.

Given that the roots of health promotion are in public health and an historical concern with the impact of lifestyle on health status these patterns are predictable and understandable. Highly influential people from other traditions have also made an important contribution to health promotion, including sociologists and policy researchers. It is a testament to their successes that health promotion today is in many places as much a social and political project as a public health project. The WHO, for example, was the cradle of a health promotion that emphasises positive health, inter-sector solutions and capacity building for a more robust society. Nevertheless, leading academic researchers from other disciplines have been few in number. Without their continuing influence there could be a return to a disease prevention emphasis, the targeting of individuals' risk behaviours, and an emphasis on classical public health solutions, all at the expense of the health promotion tradition that the WHO has nurtured.

There are indications of shifting positions that are positive. For a time, Canadians seemed to be replacing the term health promotion with population health, and in other parts of the world, health development started to replace health promotion and education in the names of agencies and organisations. It transpired that in Canada, population health is a welcome reaffirmation of health promotion's emphasis on the determinants of health that are beyond the control of individuals, and the paradigms have largely merged (Millar, 2002; see also Chapter 18, Part III of this text). In places like England and France, where health development replaces health education in the names of key national agencies, it is clear that health promotion remains in focus. The Health Development Agency in England, for example, has at the time of writing produced no less than 27 health promotion effectiveness reviews and many more reports on various aspects of health promotion (www.hda.nhs.uk).

Another positive sign is that the IUHPE enjoys growing membership in every part of the world, holds regional and global health promotion conferences that provide vital professional networking for health promoters, and contributes to improved quality and effectiveness of health promotion through extensive research and publishing activities (www.iuhpe.org). Various elements of the global health promotion infrastructure are working in concert more effectively than ever before, as the Global Programme for Health Promotion Effectiveness illustrates (http://www.who.int/hpr/ncp/hp. effectiveness.shtml).

So, health promotion continues to thrive as a specialist area of global public health activity and, as other parts of this book, particularly Part III, will confirm, it is sufficiently robust to play a part in meeting contemporary and future global health challenges. But health promotion has not been a notable collaborator in the global social progress agenda, nor has it incorporated some academic disciplines that could add considerable vitality to its knowledge and theoretical base.

As will be illustrated next, these are not so much instances of missed opportunities, than of failures to make opportunities.

Corporate social responsibility

Health promoters tend to think of business organisations as suitable settings for implementing health improvement programmes with components both for the workers and for the work environment (O'Donnell and Harris, 1994).

However, workplaces are not just settings presenting intervention opportunities. They are also collective identities with cultures, personalities and ambitions beyond the single-minded achievement of improved efficiency and competitiveness. Although some may suspect their motives, many modern corporations and businesses subscribe to a code calling for socially responsible business practices and relationships with the community (Anderson, 1989; Hopkins, 1999; Crowther, 2003). Corporate social responsibility (CSR) is concerned with treating stakeholders ethically. Since stakeholders exist both within firms and outside, behaving with social responsibility requires businesses to reach beyond their walls to the surrounding community. For global enterprises, the surrounding community is all-inclusive.

It is important not to be too naïve about the CSR movement. Corporate activities can give rise to the suspicion that corporate good works are motivated purely by the pursuit of corporate self-interests. Even those managers that are sincere about good corporate citizenship may not be free to pursue CSR aggressively because of pressure to meet economic and other business targets. Yet, it is important not to be too cynical. Several international CSR networks have a high and sustained activity rate with demonstrable records of accomplishment, and CSR activity in the health domain is evident. For example, the Business for Social Responsibility (BSR) Network, started in 1992, holds CSR conferences and training events that include emphasis on issues of direct relevance to health promotion such as child and forced labour, discrimination, migrant labour and living wages (www.bsr.org). With recent training events in the US, China and Romania, their reach is global. As with other such

CSR networks, the member corporations represent some of the leading names on the stock exchanges of the world. Another example is *CSR Europe*, set up in 1996 by former European Commission president Jacques Delors (www.csreurope.org). With members in 18 European countries, CSR Europe is dedicated to combating social exclusion and promoting social cohesion. CSR Europe works with the Social Fund of the European Union and other partners in managing the European Business Campaign for Corporate Social Responsibility. Since 2001 it has held CSR conferences in 13 countries across the European region. CSR Europe is also one of the networks with explicit interests in health promotion.

The conference and training activities of the BSR Network and CSR Europe, among other similar projects, present opportunities for health promotion to build partnerships with the business world that are entirely different from those involved in workplace health promotion programmes. Such conferences are where motivated business leaders gather specifically to exchange knowledge and ideas on issues that are crucially important to health promotion. Yet there is little indication at present that health promotion networks are linking with CSR networks. This is surely a missed opportunity.

As a final example of the possibilities that CSR offers, in this case with a direct focus on health promotion issues, consider Corporate Marketing Strategies (CMS), a consortium assembled to promote reproductive health, and composed of USAID and non-profit as well as for-profit international consulting, research and social marketing organisations (www.cmsproject.com). CMS forges partnerships with business to mount health projects that have impact in many low income countries and communities. At the time of writing, projects are underway in 12 countries in Africa, Asia, the Caribbean, Latin America and the Near East. In Ghana, for example, CMS works with the private sector on HIV prevention and treatment, increasing access to contraceptives, improving NGO sustainability, and promoting maternal and child health (www.cmsproject.com/country/africa/ghana.cfm).

The suggestion that health promotion should be proactive in developing alliances with CSR organisations will undoubtedly be greeted with scepticism by those who are wary of the mixed motives of businesses engaging in CSR activities (Hopkins, 1999). However, to deny that many business people have a genuine commitment to CSR would be short sighted. The task is to recognise those with a serious sense of responsibility, with whom mutually beneficial collaborative partnerships might be established.

This chapter began by drawing attention to CSR as well as environmental and human rights movements, as health promotion's natural partners for an expanded alliance for social progress. Prominent examples mentioned were movements for sustainable development, protection of the environment, women's and children's opportunities and rights, legal justice reforms and movements for the nurturing of social capital. The need for brevity precludes a description here of the opportunities for alliance-building that these movements represent, and the CSR example must suffice. It is important to note, however, that each of the movements named is a relatively distinct stream in the social progress movement. As a result, each movement, while internally complex and heterogeneous, is nevertheless relatively insular with regard to the other movements. Thus the problem of health promotion's insularity is representative of social movements in general.

However, movement towards better coordination is evident. The Our World is Not for Sale (OWINFS) network is a stimulating example. With its loose grouping of organisations, activists and social movements worldwide, it combats the current model of corporate globalisation embodied in the global trading system (www.ourworldisnotforsale.org). Exemplified by the Columbia University Center for Global Health and Economic Development (www.cghed.columbia.edu), universities worldwide have established social movement research centres that are explicitly interested in the study and stimulation of inter-movement collaboration. The United Nation's Global Forum for Human Development is representative of a growing class of international collaborations that create forums where diverse social movements can gather regularly to exchange knowledge and draw strength and energy from one another (www.undp.org). From centres like these, human development planning and goal-setting activity is starting to function in a distinctly more coordinated, collaborative and inclusive manner (United Nations Development Programme [UNDP], 2003). Health promotion's global organisation, the IUHPE, is committed to a proactive future and acts as a catalyst for such activity.

New academic alliances

Initiatives to tackle global health challenges also require new alliances with academia outside the usual disciplines of health promotion and it is this subject that receives attention in the final part of this chapter. The contention that health promotion must broaden its disciplinary base is perhaps difficult to defend as it is generally recognised as multidisciplinary. Bunton and Macdonald (1992) identify the contributory disciplines of health promotion as being psychology, sociology, education, epidemiology, economics, social policy, marketing and communications. They make little recognition of medicine, nursing, social work or anthropology and other possible academic spheres. Similarly, a popular, brief compilation of common theories and models of health promotion includes reference to theories from social psychology, communications, organisational change, ecology and sociology, with no mention of theories and models from preventive medicine, nursing science, theology or pedagogy (Nutbeam and Harris, 1998).

These patterns of commission and omission reflect the preferences of health promotion practitioners in various parts of the world. Medicine and nursing, for example, have a prominence in North American health promotion texts that is less evident in European texts, and the reverse is true of sociology and critical social theory. Gender studies, feminist scholarship, pedagogy of the oppressed, ethics, community psychology and philosophy exemplify other academic specialisms that receive more or less emphasis in health promotion texts, journals and conferences, depending on traditions in different geographical locations. There are other disciplines and inter-disciplines that have obvious relevance to health promotion that so far have been hardly noticed by the field. Examples include economic development, informatics, international development, cultural epidemiology and political ecology. A particularly good example is the field of community psychology, which demonstrates many opportunities for mutual benefit.

Community psychology

Psychology's main contributions to health promotion are theories of health attitudes, beliefs and behaviour, such as the Health Belief Model, Social Learning Theory, and various theories of reasoned action, planned behaviour and stages of change (Nutbeam and Harris, 1998; Tones and Tilford, 2001). While of obvious importance, such individually oriented health psychology models and associated research by no means represent the only, or even the main possibilities for psychology to enrich health promotion. Perhaps the academic speciality that has the most in common with health promotion is community psychology, yet the field is hardly encountered by most health promoters. This is unfortunate for health promotion. Relating to a number of key constructs in health promotion, such as empowerment, social capital and community development, scholarship of a high calibre has been accumulating in this discipline for decades.

A quarter of a century ago, a founder of the field suggested that 'community psychology is concerned with the right of all people to obtain the material, educational, and psychological resources available in their society. In this regard community psychology is a kind of reform movement ... and its adherents have advocated more equitable distribution of the resources that psychology and the helping professions control' (Rappaport, 1997: 2). Indeed, the founding of community psychology in the 1960's was motivated in no small part by psychologist's desire to reduce social inequality and to right social wrongs (Orford, 1992: 7). Community psychology's ideological synchrony with health promotion is reflected particularly well by its ecological orientation (Catalano, 1979). According to Rappaport (1997: 2–3) it promotes the following ideas:

- The notion that there are neither inadequate persons nor environments, but the fit between the two may be in relative accord or discord;
- The conviction that action for change emphasises the creation of alternatives by developing existing resources and strengths, rather than looking for weaknesses;
- The embracement of a value system based on cultural relativity and diversity.

With its long-standing emphases on person-environment fit in community settings, coping and social support, promotion of social competence, stimulation of citizen participation and empowerment, and organising for community and social change, community psychology today bears a striking resemblance to health promotion (Dalton et al., 2001).

Within the American Psychological Association community psychology is a formally organised branch of psychology, with conferences, journals (*Journal of Community and Applied Psychology, Journal of Community Psychology*), and graduate programmes (www.apa.org/about/division/div27). The European Network of Community Psychologists organises training and conferences on community psychology. The field has active participants in Australia (Bishop, et al., 2001), Latin America (Montero, 1996) and South Africa (Seedat et al., 2001).

Community psychology and health promotion represent an opportunity for mutual enrichment globally. The critical comparison and contrast of how similar constructs and problems are managed in the two fields would undoubtedly be advantageous to both. A synthesis of intellectual interests, opportunities for student and faculty exchange places, and possibilities for collaborative teaching and research are likely to follow.

The argument has focused on community psychology as the exemplar for the case that health promotion theoretical base would be enriched by an expanded academic collaboration. Some of the other promising fields that have not received attention here include environmental psychology (Booth and Crouter, 2001), critical social psychology (Ibáñez and Íñiguez, 1997), economic development (Jack, 1999), political ecology (Stott, 2000), cultural epidemiology (Weiss, 2001), and information technology and pedagogy (Loveless, 2001).

Meeting the challenge of global health

When alliance building for health promotion is being considered the linkages called for here with other social progress movements and with academia may not be the kind that come first to mind. However, they do represent activist and intellectual connections that would benefit health promotion and are beyond the obvious alliance building with which health promotion has been preoccupied. Making it happen will require reaching out. The organisers of health promotion conferences and the publishers of health promotion books and journals will need to extend invitations more widely. Health promoters will have to travel less parochial paths and meet community opportunities where they are. Courses in health promotion will need to break out of over dependence on texts that are the repositories of the received wisdom of health promotion.

All of this requires a proactive frame of mind. If health promotion is to have a realistic hope of making large gains in its effectiveness in the twenty-first century it must keep developing and advancing its discipline and alliance base. The field must not become a technological arena alone, preoccupied with practice and research iterations to refine its repertoire of interventions. To use the term paradigm shift is too grand, but health promotion must continually forge new alliances or risk complacency and a degree of stagnation. Evolving in the ways proposed in this chapter is feasible, and has the potential to assist health promotion to confront effectively the global health challenges it faces.

References

Anderson, J.W. (1989) *Corporate Social Responsibility: Guidelines for Top Management.* New York: Quorum Books.

Baum, F. (1998) *The New Public Health: An Australian Perspective.* Melbourne: Oxford University Press.

Bishop, B.J., Sonn, C.C., Fisher, A.F. and Drew, N.M. (2001) Community-based community psychology: Perspectives from Australia. In Seedat, M., Duncan, N. and Lazarus, S. (eds) *Community Psychology: Theory, Method and Practice. South Africa and Other Perspectives.* Cape Town: Oxford University Press.

Booth, A. and Crouter, A.C. (eds) (2001) *Does it Take a Village: Community Effects of Children, Adolescents and Families.* New Jersey: Lawrence Erlbaum.

Bracht, N. (1998) *Health Promotion at the Community Level.* London: Sage Publications.

Bunton, R. and Macdonald, G. (1992) *Health Promotion: Disciplines and Diversity.* London: Routledge.

Catalano, R. (1979) *Health Behaviour and the Community.* New York: Pergamon Press.

Crowther, D. (ed.) (2003) *Perspectives on Corporate Social Responsibility.* Vermont: Ashgate.

Dalton, J.H., Elias, M.J. and Wandersman, A. (2001) *Community Psychology: Linking Individuals and Communities.* California: Wadsworth.

Dines, A. and Cribb, A. (1993) *Health Promotion Concepts and Practice.* London: Blackwell Science.

Dluhy, M.J. and Kravitz, S.L. (1990) *Building Coalitions in the Human Services.* London: Sage.

Downie, R. S., Tannahill, C. and Tannahill, A. (1996) *Health Promotion Models and Values.* Oxford: Oxford University Press.

Green, L.W. and Kreuter, M.W. (1999) *Health Promotion Planning: An Educational and Ecological Approach.* London: Mayfield Publishing Company.

Hopkins, M. (1999) *The Planetary Bargain: Corporate Social Responsibility Comes of Age.* London: Macmillan Press Ltd.

Ibáñez, T. and Íñiguez, L. (eds) (1997) *Critical Social Psychology.* London: Sage.

Jack, W. (1999) *Principles of Health Economics for Developing Countries.* Washington DC: World Bank.

Loveless, A. (2001) *ICT, Pedagogy and the Curriculum: Subject to Change.* London: Routlege.

Millar, J. (2002) Playing on the same team? Health promotion and population health in Canada. *Health Promotion Journal of Australia,* **13**: 10–12.

Montero, M. (1996) Parallel lives: Community psychology in Latin America and the United States. *American Journal of Community Psychology,* **24**: 589–606.

Nutbeam, D. and Harris, E. (1998) *Theory in a Nutshell*. Sydney: National Center for Health Promotion.

O'Donnell, M.P. and Harris, J.S. (1994) *Health Promotion In The Workplace*. Albany: Delmar Publishers.

Orford, J. (1992) *Community Psychology: Theory and Practice*. New York: John Wiley and Sons.

Rappaport, J. (1997) *Community Psychology: Values, Research and Action*. London: Holt, Rinehart and Winston, Inc.

Scriven, A. (1998) *Alliances in Health Promotion: Theory and Practice*. London: Macmillan Press Ltd.

Seedat, M., Duncan, N. and Lazarus, S. (eds) (2001) *Community Psychology: Theory, Method and Practice. South Africa and Other Perspectives*. Cape Town: Oxford University Press.

Stott, P. (2000) *Political Ecology: Science, Myth and Power*. London: Arnold.

Tones, K. and Tilford, S. (2001) *Health Promotion: Effectiveness, Efficiency and Equity* (3rd edn). London: Chapman Hall.

United Nations Development Programme (UNDP) (2003). *Human Development Report 2003. Millennium Development Goals: A compact among nations to end human poverty*. New York: Oxford University Press.

Weiss, M.G. (2001) Cultural epidemiology: An introduction and overview. *Anthropology and Medicine*, **8**: 5–30.

World Health Organisation (WHO) (1978) *Declaration of Alma-Ata*. Geneva: WHO.

World Health Organisation (WHO) (1986) *Ottawa Charter for Health Promotion*. Geneva: WHO.

World Health Organisation (WHO) (1997) *The Jakarta Declaration on Health*. Geneva: WHO.

CHAPTER 5

The Social Context of Health Promotion in a Globalising World

SEBASTIAN GARMAN

Some two years ago in a letter to the British Medical Journal (Guthrie, 2001) a Glasgow doctor described a labour intensive three-year health promotion initiative to encourage lifestyle changes to pre-empt the increasing risks, in particular, of type 2 diabetes. His efforts proved to be unsustainable. Soon after support was withdrawn from patients they reverted to previous behaviours. His conclusion is that the concept of health promotion is evil and redundant, a convenient device that functions to divert attention from politicians whose policies are the cause of people's problems. It focuses attention on the behaviour of individuals, particularly those in poverty, who are in no position to tackle the circumstances that are damaging them. The letter provoked a spirited response. Citing the WHO (1986) Ottawa Charter Sinclair (2002) pointed out that health promotion is as much about helping people to control their health as efforts to get them to improve it. He pointed to the five main strategies for effective health promotion listed at Ottawa, of which only one is focused directly on clients. The others demand skills in advocacy and effective political mobilisation (see Chapter 1 for an overview of the Ottawa Charter).

This correspondence illustrates a striking dilemma for global public health. On the one hand the rhetoric of health promotion is increasingly preoccupied with upstream (McKinley, 1979) concerns about strengthening the political community, promoting public policy changes and advocacy for legislative reform. On the other the activities of health promoters is often located in downstream settings well out of reach of the decisive causal factors that are shaping people's health and welfare. Perhaps the most important factor that is influencing the promotion of health in the global arena is the deepening public perception of a gap between rhetoric and delivery (for observations on this issue in different regions see Part III of this book).

The upstream/downstream dilemma is only one of several dialectics that have provided a creative tension that drives forward the development of health promotion. They include the historical rift between medicine and the epidemiological and policy thrust of public health, centrally organised public health strategies in contrast to market-led client choice, the biomedical model and the social model, Aesclepius and Hygeia, public health and the new public health, health promotion and population health, allopathic, individualist and secular medicine in contrast to social medicine (Turner, 2000). As a consequence the practice of public health and health promotion is informed by key contradictions that become more apparent as it faces global responsibilities (Kickbusch, 2003). It is only possible to touch on some of these in the confines of this chapter, but other authors pick up these contradictions (see, for example, Chapters 4, 12, 13, 16 and 18).

With ageing population structures and the shift to lifestyle diseases it seems appropriate that people should be mobilised, involved and empowered to take charge of their health. However, public health decision making is often seen to be specialist, esoteric and remote from people's lives (Raeburn and Macfarlane, 2003). For example, a recent study by Lee and Goodman (2002) of the reform of global healthcare financing found a small and tightly integrated network of participants, with a revolving door of career progression. It focused around only two centres, those of Washington DC and London with the involvement of very few institutions. Led by USAID and the World Bank there was surprisingly little involvement of WHO let alone NGOs that might be seen to represent a global citizenship.

Whilst the recent people's health assembly in 2000 reiterated from Dhaka, Bangladesh the people-centred nature of health promotion the actual practice of public health relies on specialists who form epistemic communities (Lee and Goodman, 2002). They develop technical concepts and language so distant from the populations they serve that it has led some to wonder who is the public in public health (Raeburn and Macfarlane, 2003).

The success of global public health initiatives is seen to depend on a consensual model with a negotiated involvement of stake holders, interest groups and citizens (Ziglio et al., 2001; WHO, 2003) and yet global convergence from very inequitable power bases might mean that the interests and values of the powerful are actually being spread by coercion (Hardt and Negri, 2000; Stiglitz, 2003).

By necessity the global health policy has been the initiative of intellectual leadership from wealthy centres of expertise so that the assumptions and solutions are framed in terms more relevant to high income countries (Buse et al., 2002). As the powerful shape and decide whose standards become global the interests and hopes of some peoples and societies become sacrificed. Or in this era of global mass communications they disappear entirely from public view (Schirato and Webb, 2003).

If health promotion is to rise to the challenge of global convergence it will have to attempt to avoid such fault lines through dialogue, compromise and understanding. For example, some argue that the balance of negotiation between individualist market solutions as opposed to collectivist solutions failed in the case of Russia with terrible consequences for its people in terms of death and disease (Walberg et al., 1998; Stiglitz, 2002). Moreover policies encouraging countries to privatise fundamental public services such as water (Hall, 2001) or to increase their wealth by processing products too dangerous for high income workforces, like asbestos (Steele, 2003), can fuel such resentment as to make such policies counterproductive.

Another potential pitfall for health promotion is the dependence on discourses using equity and empowerment orthodoxies based on Enlightenment paradigms of individual freedoms. These, combined with market values, confront peoples with little economic power who cling to identities based on ancient hierarchies (Dumont, 1981). Or perhaps it is worth reflecting on the strategy of secular allopathic individualist medicine in an era of renewed religious revival (Walker, 1999).

Poverty and inequality

The link between health status and poverty has been recorded ever since systematic data was gathered for the emerging nation states of the nineteenth century and the picture remains true today. Globally, the disadvantaged are shorter in stature, experience higher morbidity and higher mortality rates than the advantaged. Moreover, their inequalities in health status seem to be increasing (Macintyre, 1997), an observed trend that has gained increased resonance since the seminal research which suggested that inequality itself was a cause of ill health (Wilkinson, 1996).

In Europe governments of the UK, the Netherlands and Sweden have recently declared an interest in pursuing policies to reduce health inequalities (Macintyre, 2003) and the WHO under the leadership of Gro Harlem Bruntland has encouraged a strategy of investment in health with the aims of both alleviating poverty and helping economic development (WHO, 1999; Ziglio et al., 2001). Nevertheless it is by no means universal for governments to see it as their role to influence health inequalities (Leon et al., 2001) and the attention to the issue by both governments and international agencies has shown considerable variation over recent decades (Townsend and Gordon, 2002).

For global health promotion the factor of inequality is of special significance not only because of the strong links made with health aetiology but also because increased health inequalities between rich and poor countries calls into question the authenticity of the rhetoric of cooperation, participation and empowerment with which it has become associated (for a critical discussion of inequalities, see Chapter 3).

The striking differences in health status of populations in countries of comparable national wealth has redirected attention to the effectiveness of policies in protecting the health of populations (Townsend and Gordon, 2002; Macintyre, 2003). Interesting research suggests that effective social policies can improve health even in low income countries with little economic growth (Sen, 2000). Comparative data from 70 countries shows that just over half have a per capita health expenditure in 1997 of less than US $500. Yet huge variations exist in life expectancy. A similar variation is to be found in middle income and high income countries (Leon et al., 2001).

Ethnicity

Since the processes of globalisation including communications, markets and migrations bring culture groups into new reflexive relationship with each other it is hardly surprising that there is global public health interest in the links between ethnicity, political power and health. Whilst the health damaging consequences of serfdom, enslavement and other forms of bondage are well understood by historians the significance for public health of different forms of political dominance is less often discussed (for one recent discussion see Bashford, 2003). In Europe for example, whilst the Romanies have claims to be one of the largest cultural or ethnic minorities with a terrible history of enslavement and genocide a Medline search on the term gypsy produces more papers on the gypsy variant of the Drosophila fruit fly than on the health of the Roma people (McKee, 1997).

Other dispossessed, damaged or humiliated peoples such as the Dalit of India, the Ju/'hoansi of southern Africa and the Burakumin of Japan have almost entirely disappeared from the public health research record. Nevertheless, following the pioneering work of the journalist Norman Lewis (1988), there have been attempts to record the health experiences of some indigenous peoples (Lewis, 1991; Kunitz, 1994; WHO, 1999; Durie, 2003) including public health initiatives particularly in North America, Australia and New Zealand (see Chapter 17 in Part III of this book for further discussion).

Public health policy and research has been complicated and confused by the uncritical adoption of the socially constructed concept of ethnicity and the even more politically complicated notion of race. Noting the rapid increase of health research in this field, a seminal paper (Sheldon and Parker, 1992) warned of the general lack of consistency in the use of the concepts, the poor understanding in the literature of the cultural and political associations that underpin these categories, the often implied biological or psycho-biological assumptions attending the reporting of findings, and the failure to spell out the implications of the results for improving the health of ethnic minorities. Despite frequent reiteration of these kinds of warnings (Smaje, 1995; Kaplan and Bennett, 2003; Nazroo, 2003) the uncritical use of the concepts is still common in research (Comstock et al., 2004) with damaging consequences for reasoned debate. Nevertheless, the body of research findings on ethnicity and health does suggest a pattern. Differences in health across ethnic groups have been repeatedly documented and socioeconomic inequalities, including the experience of racism, are fundamental causes of ethnic inequalities in health (Nazroo, 2003).

Economic globalisation

It is sometimes suggested that economic growth creates the wealth to improve the health of populations and that this assumption has guided government policies away from a focus on equality (Leon et al., 2001; Townsend and

Gordon, 2002). Certainly one of the justifications for the neoliberal economic climate of the last three decades has been that the willingness of low income countries to open their markets would lead to increased global wealth to the benefit of all (Legrain, 2002). For those that support this view global economic integration improves the income and infrastructure of poor countries and their peoples with no necessary increase in inequalities or health problems. If such disbenefits do occur this is the result of a failure of welfare policies and not of economics (Dollar, 2001). For example, the greater contact between peoples as a result of global market changes can lead to an increase in the speed with which communicable diseases move between population areas if public health systems are not well managed. The usual countries cited as benefiting from globalisation due to such reforming economic policies include China, Vietnam, India and Malaysia.

Others take a much more cautious line (Cornia, 2001; Woodward et al., 2001). The benefits of a neoliberal policy of opening markets only works for low income countries with strong regulatory institutions, good infrastructure and narrow domestic markets. The much-cited success of China and India is interpreted as depending on controls of exchange rates and limits on internal markets (Stiglitz, 2002). However for many, perhaps the majority, of low income countries globalisation has brought uncertain growth and little improvement in health indicators. The conclusion to be drawn from these experiences is that the opening of markets by low income countries should be much more carefully managed (Cornia, 2001). For some it has brought about tragic consequences as with Russia and more recently, Argentina (Stiglitz, 2002).

Whatever the truth might eventually reveal, events have overtaken the debate with the failed negotiations in the World Trade Organisation talks in Cancun, Mexico in September 2003. Backed by a formidable array of NGOs and led by China, India and Brazil, for the first time a coalition of 21 low and middle income countries formed a coalition to confront the US and Europe. The strongly held view of the negotiating representatives of these countries is that Europe and America are guilty of the double standards of preaching market freedoms whilst strongly protecting their own industries and markets with tariff barriers and subsidies (Denny et al., 2003), particularly their agricultural sectors. From this point of view, the greatest stimulus to world health would be for protectionist regimes to open up their markets for agricultural products to low income countries whose poor populations depend on agriculture to survive.

Communications

Of all the recent global transformations in power and social relations none is more significant for the possibilities of public health and health promotion strategies than communications. This is because the information technology paradigm (Castells, 2000) of digitalisation and the microchip has altered the plasticity and speed of the media. Photographs, music, talk and text can now be reconstituted digitally. The technological advance has stimulated massive investment in associated industries that, through merger and privatisation, have become super corporations, shaping the agenda for the global public sphere.

At the same time social model principles, with an emphasis on communication, cooperation and persuasion are increasingly favoured to manage the health challenges of ageing demographic structures of populations and the epidemiological shift from communicable diseases to lifestyle diseases. These strategies are well rehearsed for high income countries where international health agencies are increasingly favouring client control, autonomy, information and education as well as the process of building strategic connections with stake holders such as legislators, food manufacturers, advertisers and media conglomerates (WHO, 2003).

It is interesting to note how fast this pattern has become established in middle and low income regions. In Latin America and the Caribbean, for example, falls in age-adjusted mortality rates and successes in the control of smallpox, poliomyelitis and measles is contrasted with the near epidemic of cardiovascular diseases, an ageing population, a greater dependency ratio, increases in chronic illnesses and heavier treatment costs (Alleyne, 2001). New strategies are being forced upon policy makers who are recommending a greater emphasis on communication, persuasion and behaviour change. An increased importance is being placed on marketing skills and social communication tools, which are becoming as significant for public health as epidemiology and cardiology (Alleyne, 2001: 24). The media technologies are transforming the tools of health promotion available to health workers in low income countries (Alleyne, 2001; Lucas, 2001; Buse et al., 2002). These include the development of sophisticated mechanisms for surveillance, experimentation with telemedicine, almost limitless access to scientific health information and the construction of virtual libraries (for further discussion of the increasing role of the mass media in global health promotion see Chapter 12).

Of course the opportunities for behaviour change and persuasion presented by the new media landscape must work both ways. Yet the health implications of the explosion of communications is poorly understood by health professionals and has not attracted the research funding it deserves (Harrabin et al., 2003; Von Feilitzen, 2002). What research there is suggests for example, that the shift to the consumption of unhealthy imported foods in low income countries is not due to food preferences or lack of nutritional knowledge and is, therefore, not easy to change by educational campaigns (Evans et al., 2001).

The connection is often made between advertising, lifestyle and disease (Jarlbro, 2001) particularly with children (Consumers International, 1999). This is not merely the phenomenon of advertising alone, but the lifestyle package being offered through media conglomerates of style, dress, leisure activities and diet (Von Feilitzen, 2002). In Latin America, for example, the increase in smoking is linked not only to advertising but the whole range of the new communications on offer (Alleyne, 2001). As legislation has closed down the options for tobacco companies in high income countries they have redirected marketing to low income countries where tobacco consumption is rising rapidly. But whether this is in response to developing consumer markets and lack of legislative restriction or, additionally, as has been suggested for Russia, to the fragmenting social networks and rise of stress (Walberg et al., 1998) is difficult to demonstrate. Either way, the health impact for low income countries will be dramatic since death rates from tobacco are predicted to treble over the next twenty years (Brundtland, 2001) to become perhaps the major cause of death (for a detailed discussion of the impact of western tobacco companies on global health see Chapter 8).

Some suggest that the new communications cannot be separated from the larger political changes of which they are a manifestation (Castells, 2000) or that we might be experiencing a new paradigm of capitalism (Hardt and Negri, 2000; Schirato and Webb, 2003; Stiglitz, 2003) with a central role played by knowledge, information, affect and communication. In this account the media and communications industries and health and welfare agencies take on an important role in shaping social relations, subjectivities and dispositions. Nation states began to lose control of the mass media to the fourth estate just at the time when the media became by far the most important means by which the public sphere of life is imagined and defined. Communications, therefore, have become strategic to the process of public health management and the facilitation of health promotion at a time when media ownership and control have become deeply undemocratic.

Research

Next to communications with which it is often linked, good quality and independent research is a key influence in the effectiveness of public health policy and health promotion. It is therefore interesting to note how often the processes associated with globalisation have raised fears about the erosion of the safeguards defending the independence of the research process (Horton, 2003). Within the field of health research, this is not new. As long ago as 1980, in his Reith Lectures, the medical lawyer Ian Kennedy drew on the work of Dubos and McKeown to attract attention to the dependence of medical research on the pharmaceutical industry (Kennedy, 1981). In the UK for example, about half the postgraduate education of doctors is funded by the pharmaceutical industry, which also funds two thirds of clinical trials (MacDonald, 2003).

In low income countries with their smaller research base and less-developed civic culture the power of such lobbying groups is much greater, leaving advocates for health promotion with a serious dilemma. On the one hand partnerships with pharmaceutical industries are welcomed as the means to develop new and improved tools for tackling health problems (Lucas, 2001) yet at the same time such working relationships have their costs (Brugha et al., 2002). These include a changed medical culture with demands of doctors for expensive technologies and a shift in public expectation with exaggerated hopes of improvement from costly hospitals and clinics. Neither the public nor doctors show enthusiasm for cost-effective community-based preventative services. In West Africa a similar conflict arises over capacity development where, except for one or two notable exceptions (Martey and Hudson, 1999 cited by Lucas, 2001), clinical specialists get large resources at the expense of health planners (for further discussion of the negotiation between interest groups in sub-Saharan Africa, see Chapter 12).

With the balance of power shifting against nation states in favour of global market forces (Pollock and Price, 2003), it has been suggested that both universities and national governments have allowed or even encouraged the blurring of boundaries. Groups with commercial interests in particular research findings have grown used to funding research where the research teams are aware that future funding depends on the kind of findings they publicly release (Horton, 2003). Sponsors have been able to negotiate research contracts where they retain ownership of the research with powers to edit the findings or keep the findings private should it prove politically expedient to do so. Commercial lobbying groups have grown used to promoting and financing research groups and government advisory groups that present themselves as independent of financial interest.

One example will illustrate the argument. In June 2001 Dr Norbert Hirschorn, an authority on public health policy who has researched the manner in which tobacco companies have influenced the political process, prepared a confidential report on similar tactics being developed by the food industry in the 1990s which he delivered to the WHO (Williams, 2003). The Guardian newspaper, which obtained a copy summarised Hirschorn's conclusions. These are that representatives of the food industry tried to place scientists with favourable views on WHO and FAO committees, they financially supported NGOs which were invited to formal discussions with UN agencies, and they financed research, policy groups and individuals who promoted a point of view favourable to their position (Boseley, 2003a).

When asked later about Hirschorn's report WHO officials downplayed it as being of largely historical interest (Williams, 2003) because it referred to a period in the 1990s before the organisation had brought in stronger ethical guidelines. It was suggested that dialogue with all interested parties on the issue of diet and disease was welcome and that unlike the tobacco industry, those of food and beverages were part of the solution to world health problems. Indeed, it was in the interests of food industries to partner health workers in improving health. Attention was drawn to the WHO policy of keeping an open dialogue with all interested parties. 'By keeping the work on strategy open' the spokesman is quoted as saying 'there is not need for anyone to seek to influence the process' (Yach, cited Williams, 2003).

Yet less than three months later, when WHO was playing a crucial and successful role in coordinating a worldwide and difficult campaign to manage the SARS epidemic, the Sugar industry through its pressure group the *Sugar Association* wrote to the Director General of WHO threatening to persuade the US Congress to withdraw its US $404 million funding of the agency. It was acting in response to the WHO making public for the purposes of consultation the draft of its report *Diet, Nutrition and the Prevention of Chronic Illness*. At the same time the *Sugar Association* with six other food production groups wrote to the US Health Secretary asking him to get the WHO report withdrawn (Boseley, 2003b).

The perception has grown of a compromised health research process (Horton, 2003) so that scientific and medical journals have had to change their rules about the acceptance of articles where the interests of sponsors is not transparent. Moreover the ownership of scientific journals is a contentious issue due to the costs on knowledge that they impose. Finally an impression has been allowed to take root that universities and other leaders of research have bartered their independence. There is a new interest in policy on the relationship between science, integrity and the mass media (Harrabin et al., 2003; Royal Society, 2003).

A recent King's Fund report finds that the media have an influential effect on policy makers and public alike in ways that are mutually reinforcing and often damaging to public health (Harrabin et al., 2003). The authors find that there is a serious imbalance in the reporting of health issues. For example, news media in particular tend to focus on stories about health services and health scares. In contrast stories about public health such as measures to improve health, prevent illness or tackle inequalities are rare. They recommend changes in practice by journalists and health professionals alike including a more sophisticated training and awareness by health workers and policy makers of the ways the media works, and how news is constructed. They suggest that policy makers should pay more attention to how the public perceive and interprets risks. They make a case for stronger advocacy in public health at all levels and a more sophisticated presentation of health issues by health experts and policy makers including a greater readiness to track patterns of risk reporting over time.

Alliances and networks

The rapid transformations of the global economic climate have led to a noticeable change in business behaviour towards alliance formation not only with other corporations (Gomes-Casseres, 1996; Hamel and Prahalad, 1996) but also between business and government (Dunning and Boyd, 2003). Moreover an enormous expansion in the numbers and influence of NGOs is changing the politics of development (Clarke, 1998) and the possibilities of health alliances (Akukwe, 1998). The response to these global changes within the fields of public health and health promotion seems to be still in the process of emergence. In the last decade there was interest in healthy alliances (Scriven, 1998) particularly for single issues such as AIDS (Aggleton, 1997). In the field of welfare, too, the benefits of alliances and networking are increasingly recognised (Trevillion, 1999). Yet given the sophistication and dynamism of the alliances of private industry and NGOs it is perhaps surprising there is not more research on the impact of alliances on global health policy (for the insularity and isolation of global health promotion and the need for alliances, see Chapter 4).

The need to build alliances is widely recognised in global public health (Akukwe, 1998). As noted above, some policy makers have stressed the increased possibilities of networks and alliances to tackle health issues provided by the new technologies, particularly in low income countries where limited infrastructures and small research base is given as reasons for failure. For example, the African region has pioneered a number of working relationships with programmes such as the Council for Health Research and Development (COHRED), the European Commission Programme for Health Research with Developing Countries, and the Global Forum for Health Research (GFHR) able to draw on the research and expertise of richer institutions (Lucas, 2001). The benefits include the sharing of expertise, access to research, the linkage with sophisticated managerial infrastructures, and the sharing of marketing and production skills. Other examples include the designing of modular programmes for African ministries by WHO and UNICEF and the prescribed list of cost-effective public health interventions provided by the World Bank (further examples of these are discussed in Chapters 4, 11, 12, 13 and 18).

A recent initiative that is built around alliances is the *WHO Global Strategy on Diet, Physical Activity and Health* that aims to improve public health through healthy eating and physical activity (WHO, 2003). Of the four guiding principles of the process by which the strategy will be prepared for presentation to the World Health Assembly in May 2004, two involve the building of links with stakeholders including the food, sport and advertising industries. Another recent instance was that of the European Union in 2001, at the time of the Swedish presidency, to debate in Europe the extension of Swedish national policy of limiting the targeting of television advertising at children. That it came to little at the time might be due to a political realisation that there was a more effective organised alliance of economic interests against it (Garman, 2001).

Any alliance involves negotiated power relationships. If global inequalities are not reversed then as public health and health promotion attempts a global role the issue of power is likely to become ever more apparent. For health promoters who see themselves as advocates of the poor and dispossessed it is not at all clear that a consensual model of stakeholder involvement will suffice. In the African region (Lucas, 2001) the costs of alliances can endanger self-determination and the conflicting aims of interested parties can lead to policies that might be against the interest of citizens. The remarkable threat by the Sugar Association of America to the Director General of the WHO and the expansion of tobacco manufacturers from high income countries into low income countries must lead to questioning the implications of stakeholder involvement in the *Global Strategy on Diet, Physical Activity and Health*.

Disrupted social fabrics and war

Global public health strategies must be underpinned by a social fabric supported by law and the state, yet the comforting modernist paradigm of the twentieth century that war is a condition of international disorder to be remedied by the development of international law is being challenged by a bleaker vision in an era of globalisation (Bobbitt, 2003). It is suggested that instead of the nation state forming the basis of legitimacy and international law, it is itself the creation of war. Electronic communications and the possibilities the technology offered for the fluidity of capital means that the nation state is giving way to market states (Bobbitt, 2003) or empire (Hardt and Negri, 2000). For large areas of the world including the Balkans, the Middle East, much of Africa, and Southeast Asia state building is always problematic whilst war has never gone away.

During the last half-century almost all wars have been in low income countries and many have been of long duration (Amnesty International and Oxfam International, 2003). By the year 2000, for example, war had lasted 12 years in Somalia, 22 years in Afghanistan and 35 years in Angola. With fragile or non-existent states paramilitary factions are the effective power brokers, often backed by elaborate market economies, such as the diamond trafficking of Angola or the opium trade of post Taliban Afghanistan (Southall and O'Hare, 2002). During the last decade low income countries have become swamped with arms. There are thought to be over 600 million small arms circulating in the world, the majority of which are privately owned. They are the most deadly current weapons of mass destruction killing half a million people a year. The US is the most important manufacture and exporter of arms with the UK following as a distant second. Since the US led war on terror many countries have relaxed their controls on arms sales so that the situation is deteriorating further (Southall and O'Hare, 2002). The major cost is to non-combatants. Between 1986 and 1996 countless women and over two million children were killed and over six million children were disabled. The indirect effects of war include food deprivation, disruption of public health, spread of disease, psychological and emotional damage, disability, separation of families, loss of education, sexual abuse of children, child abduction, torture and slavery, and child soldiers, and displaced populations (Southall and O'Hare, 2002).

It is impossible to stop war as political communities emerge and transform themselves but it might be possible to reduce the health damage to their populations. By drawing upon the fact that the wealthiest countries are the source of the weapons and profit from the trafficking that supports the war economies, it makes sense to focus activity in countries where social fabrics are robust, with defined legal structures and the means to hold people to account for their actions. For example, the attempt to develop an ethical foreign policy in the UK has resulted in annual reports of licences granted for the export of arms being published. In 1998 a European Union code of conduct on arms exports was agreed as well as a moratorium on the trading of small arms into West Africa. (Southall and O'Hare, 2002). Amnesty International and Oxfam International (2003) have launched a new global campaign by NGOs incorporating an international arms trade treaty to control exports to regions where wars are causing such violations of humanitarian law. The treaty is to be put before a United Nations conference on small arms in 2006.

Rapid global changes in politics and communications are transforming the opportunities for health promotion and public health. As nation states lose control of policy new alliances are continually emerging. It is possible that the vertical representation of the WHO is giving way to a more horizontally managed plethora of interest groups (Walt, 2003). New players in global public health, such as private corporations and NGOs are increasingly influential. Some such as the World Bank and the Bill and Melinda Gates Foundation have budgets that rival and in certain cases surpass that of the WHO. Properly managed the benefits can be striking, as with collaborative activities to eradicate disease such as the Global Alliance for Vaccines and Immunisation, Roll Back Malaria, the International AIDS Vaccine Initiative and Stop TB (Richards, 2001). There are, however, concerns about accountability, inequity and the excessive influence of particular interests that could damage health (Bettcher et al., 2000). In 1986 a pioneer of upstream approaches in health promotion, the head of the semi-autonomous Health Education Council in London, Dr David Player, not only lost his job but also had the unenviable experience of witnessing the organisation closed down around him (Player, 1988). On reflection Player concluded that he had failed to hold the interested parties together. It is a daunting challenge for those working in health promotion in the global arena to do better.

References

Aggleton, P. (ed.) (1997) *AIDS: Activism and Alliances*. London: Taylor and Francis.

Akukwe, C. (1998) The growing influence of non governmental organisations (NGOs) in international health: challenges and opportunities. *Journal of the Royal Society of Health*, **118**, 2: 107–15.

Alleyne, G.A.O. (2001) Latin America and the Caribbean. In Everett Koop, C., Pearson, C.E. and Schwarz, M.R. (eds) *Critical Issues in Global Health*. San Francisco: Jossey-Bass.

Amnesty International and Oxfam International (2003) *Shattered Lives*. Eynsham: Information Press.

Bashford, A. (2003) *Imperial Hygiene*. Basingstoke: Palgrave.

Bettcher, D.W., Yach, D. and Guindon, G.E. (2000) Global trade and health: key linkages and future challenges. *Bulletin of the World Health Organisation*, **78**(4): 521–34.

Bobbitt, P. (2003) *The Shield of Achilles*. London and New York: Allen Lane, Penguin Press.

Boseley, S. (2003a) WHO 'infiltrated by food industry'. *The Guardian*, 9 January: 1.

Boseley, S. (2003b) Sugar industry threatens to scupper WHO. *The Guardian*, 21 April: 1.

Brugha, R., Starling, M. and Walt, G. (2002) GAVI, the first steps: lessons for the Global Fund. *Lancet*, **359**(9304): 435–8

Brundtland, G.H. (2001) The Future of the World's Health. In Everett Koop, C., Pearson, C.E. and Schwarz, M.R. *Critical Issues in Global Health*. San Francisco: Jossey-Bass.

Buse, K., Drager, N., Fustukian, S. and Lee, K. (2002) Globalisation and health policy: trends and opportunities. In Lee, K., Buse, K. and Fustalkian, S. (eds) *Health Policy in a Globalising World*. Cambridge: Cambridge University Press.

Castells, M. (2000) *The Rise of the Network Society* (2nd edn). Oxford: Blackwell.

Comstock, R.D., Castillo, E.M. and Lindsay, S.P. (2004) Four year review of the use of race and ethnicity in epidemiologic and public health research. *American Journal of Epidemiology*, **159**(6): 611–19.

Consumers International (1999) *A Spoonful of Sugar*. Brussels: Consumers International.

Clarke, G. (1998) Non-governmental organisations and politics in the developing world. *Political Studies*, **46**: 36–52.

Cornia, G.A. (2001) Globalisation and health: results and options. *Bulletin of the World Health Organisation*, **79**(9): 834–41.

Denny, C., Elliott, L. and Vidal, J. (2003) Alliance of the poor unites against west. *The Guardian*, 14 September: 16.

Dollar, D. (2001) Is globalisation good for your health? *Bulletin of the World Health Organisation*, **79**(9): 827–33.

Dumont, L. (1981) *Homo Hierarchicus: The Caste System and its Implications*. Chicago: Chicago University Press.

Dunning, J.H. and Boyd, G. (eds) (2003) *Alliance Capitalism and Corporate Management*. Northampton MA: Edward Elgar.

Durie, M.H. (2003) The health of indigenous peoples (Editorial). *British Medical Journal*, **326**(7388): 510–11.

Evans, M., Sinclair, R.C., Fusimalohi, C. and Liava'a, V. (2001) Globalisation, diet, and health: an example from Tonga. *Bulletin of the World Health Organisation*, **79**(9): 856–62.

Garman, S.P. (2001) *Pressure Group Politics and Advertising Targeted at Children*. Paper presented at the Inaugural International Media Conference, Institute of Education, London, UK, 24 July.

Gomes-Casseres, B. (1996) *The Alliance Revolution: The New Shape of Business Rivalry*. Cambridge MA: Harvard University Press.

Guthrie, C. (2001) Prevention of type 2 diabetes: health promotion helps no one. *British Medical Journal*, **323**(7319): 997.

Hall, D. (2001) *Water Privatisation and Quality of Service: PSIRU Evidence to the Walkerton Inquiry, Toronto, July 2001*. London: Public Services International Research Unit, University of Greenwich.

Hamel, G. and Prahalad, C.K. (1996) *Competing for the Future*. Boston: Harvard Business School.

Hardt, M. and Negri, A. (2000) *Empire*. Cambridge MA: Harvard University Press.

Harrabin, R., Coote, A. and Allen, J. (2003) *Health in the News: risk, reporting and media influence*. London: King's Fund.

Horton, R. (2003) *Doctors, Diseases and Decisions in Modern Medicine*. Cambridge: Granta.

Jarlbro, G. (2001) *Children and Advertising: the players, the arguments and the research during the period 1994–2000*. Stockholm: Swedish Consumer Agency.

Kaplan, J.B. and Bennett, T. (2003) Use of race and ethnicity in biomedical publication. *Journal of the American Medical Association*, 289(20): 2709–16.

Kennedy, I. (1981) *The Unmasking of Medicine*. London: Allen and Unwin.

Kickbusch, I. (2003) The contribution of the World Health Organisation to a New Public Health and Health Promotion. *American Journal of Public Health*, **93**(3): 83–388.

Kunitz, S. (1994) *Disease and social diversity the European impact on the health of non-Europeans*. New York: Oxford University Press.

Lee, K. and Goodman, H. (2002) Global policy networks: the propagation of health care financing reform since the 1980s. In Lee, K., Buse, K. and Fustalkian, S. (eds) *Health Policy in a Globalising World*. Cambridge: Cambridge University Press.

Legrain, P. (2002) *Open World: The Truth About Globalisation*. London: Abacus.

Leon, D.A., Walt, G. and Gilson, L. (2001) International perspectives on health inequalities and policy. *British Medical Journal*, **322**: 591–94.

Lewis, N. (1988) *The Missionaries*. London: Secker and Warburg.

Lewis, N. (1991) *A Goddess in the Stones*. London: Jonathan Cape.

Lucas, A.O. (2001) *Africa*. In Everett Koop, C. et al. (eds) *Critical Issues in Global Health*. San Francisco: Jossey-Bass.

MacDonald, L. (2003) The ties that bind. *The Guardian*, 12 August.

Macintyre, S. (1997) The Black Report and beyond; what are the issues? *Social Science and Medicine*, **44**: 723–46.

Macintyre, S. (2003) Evidence based policy-making: impact on health inequalities still needs to be assessed. *British Medical Journal*, **326**(7379): 5–6.

Martey, J.O. and Hudson, C.N. (1999) Training specialists in the developing world: ten years on, a success story for West Africa. *British Journal of Obstetrics and Gynaecology*, **106**: 91–94.

McKee, M. (1997) The health of gypsies. (Editorial) *British Medical Journal*, 315(7117): 1172–73

McKinley, J.B. (1979) A case for refocusing upstream: the political economy of health. In Jaco, E.G. (ed) *Patients, Physicians and Illness* (3rd edn). New York: Free Press.

Nazroo, J.Y. (2003) The structuring of ethnic inequalities in health: economic position, racial discrimination, and racism. *American Journal of Public Health*, 93(2): 277–84.

Player, D. (1988) Dr David Player in interview with Max Blythe. February. *The Royal College of Physicians and Oxford Brookes University Medical Science Video Archive MSVA 032*.

Pollock, A.M. and Price, D. (2003) The public health implications of world trade negotiations on the general agreement on trade in services and public services. *Lancet*, **362**: 1072–75.

Raeburn, J. and Macfarlane, S. (2003) Putting the public into public health. In Beaglehole, R. (ed.) *Global Public Health; A New Era*. Oxford: Oxford University Press.

Richards T. (2001) New global health fund: Must be well managed if it is to narrow the gap between rich and poor countries. *British Medical Journal*, **322**(7298): 1321–22.

Royal Society (2003) Royal Society to investigate how research results are communicated. Media Release. London: Royal Society, 11 August.

Schirato, T. and Webb, J. (2003) *Understanding Globalisation*. London: Sage.

Scriven, A. (1998) *Alliances in Health Promotion: Theory and Practice*. Basingstoke: Macmillan.

Sen, A. (2000) Economic progress and health. In Leon, A. and Walt, G. (eds) *Poverty, Inequality and Health: An International Perspective*. Oxford: Oxford University Press.

Sheldon, T.A. and Parker, H. (1992) Race and ethnicity in health research. *Journal of Public Health Medicine*, 14(2): 104–10.

Sinclair, A. (2002) Don't strangle health promotion, redefine it. *British Medical Journal*, 324(7334): 427.

Smaje, C. (1995) *Health, Race and Ethnicity: Making Sense of the Evidence*. London: King's Fund Institute

Southall, D.P. and O'Hare, B.A.M. (2002) Empty arms: the effect of the arms trade on mother and children. *British Medical Journal*, 325(7378): 1457–61.

Steele, J. (2003) The cancer business. *The Guardian*, 23 September.

Stiglitz, J.S. (2002) *Globalisation and its Discontents*. London: Allen Lane, The Penguin Press.

Stiglitz, J.S. (2003) *The Roaring Nineties*. London and New York: Allen Lane, The Penguin Press.

Townsend, P. and Gordon, D. (2002) *World Poverty: New Policies to Defeat an Old Enemy*. Bristol: Policy Press.

Trevillion, S. (1999) *Networking and Community Partnership*. Ashgate: Arena.

Turner, B.S. (2000) Changing concepts of health and Illness. In Albrecht, G.L., Fitzpatrick, R. and Scrimshaw, S.C. (eds) *The Handbook of Social Studies in Health and Medicine*. London: Sage.

Von Feilitzen, C. (2002) *Outlooks on Children and Media: Child Right, Media Trends, Media Research, Media Literacy, Child Participation Declarations*. Philadelphia: Coronet Books Inc.

Walberg, P., McKee, M., Shkilnikov, V., Chenet, L. and Leon, D.A. (1998) Economic change, crime, and mortality crisis in Russia: regional analysis. *British Medical Journal*, 317(7154): 312–18.

Walker, A. (1999) *The Third Schism*. London: Hodder and Stoughton.

Walt, G. (2003) *The Global Health Fund and public health*. Paper presented to the Globalisation and Health Policy conference at the Society for Social Medicine, London. 14 November.

Wilkinson, R.G. (1996) *Unhealthy Societies*. London: Routledge.

Williams, F. (2003) WHO denies food lobby influence. *The Financial Times*, 10 January.

Woodward, D., Drager, N., Beaglehole, R. and Lipson, D. (2001) Globalisation and health: a framework for analysis and action. *Bulletin of the World Health Organisation*, 79(9): 875–81.

World Health Organisation (1986) *Ottawa Charter*. Geneva: WHO.

WHO Committee on Indigenous Health (1999) *The Geneva Declaration on the Health and Survival of Indigenous Peoples*. Geneva: WHO. WHO/HSD/00.1.

World Health Organisation (1999) *World Health Report 1999. Making a Difference*. Geneva: WHO.

World Health Organisation (2003) *Process for a Global Strategy on Diet, Physical Activity and Health*. February. WHO/NMH/EXR.02.2.

Ziglio, E., Hagard, S. and Levin, L. S. (2001) Investment for health: developing a multi-faceted appraisal approach. In Rootman, I., Goodstdt, M. and Hyndman, B. (eds) *Evaluating Health Promotion: Principles and Perspectives*. Copenhagen: World Health Organisation.

PART II

GLOBAL HEALTH CHALLENGES: AN OVERVIEW

Angela Scriven

We are confronted with formidable public health challenges at the beginning of the twenty-first century. Changing demographic trends and increased longevity, social changes that include increased sedentary lifestyles, shifting patterns of food consumption and increased uses of tobacco and alcohol are resulting in a mounting burden of chronic diseases. New infectious diseases, environmental degradation, transnational factors involved in the integration of the global economy, financial markets and trade are also having significant negative impacts on the health and wellbeing of populations. This section of the book highlights five of the most significant global public health challenges, namely *noncommunicable diseases, food and diet, tobacco, HIV/AIDS, environment.* Together, these five are responsible for the majority of the mortality rates, DALYs and the health inequalities discussed in Part I, and as such are the most pressing problems that those working to promote health have to overcome. A chapter is devoted to each, offering a critical examination of causal factors and an assessment of the health promoting approaches that might be employed in addressing the issues that emerge.

The section begins with an examination of noncommunicable diseases (NCDs). The considerable global challenge that these present is made evident through the figures demonstrating that NCDs are the leading cause of death globally and a major contributor to health inequalities. Many of the risk factors identified are lifestyle-orientated (see the point made by Mcdaid and Oliver about lifestyle choices associated with inequity and inequality in Chapter 3, Part I). However, there is a strong link made to risk transition resulting from globalisation processes, particularly the marketing of anti-health products in new markets. Whilst there is a strong suggestion that there is insufficient global heath promotion targeting NCDs, there is also an assessment of where health promotion interventions have succeeded in reducing disease rates, so there is much to be gleaned from this analysis.

Chapter 7 on food and diet contextualises one of the determinants of NCDs, and explores the concept of risk transition through the notion of nutritional transition. Robust arguments are made in demonstrating the negative impact of globalisation on diet. There are radical suggestions for action that

73

include increasing the role of food governance and for health promoters to actively confront the food industry and its practices by adopting an advocacy role in influencing national and international policies to curb the excesses of massive food corporations.

The discourse around determinant of NCDs continues with Chapter 8 on tobacco consumption. There are some disturbing trends identified, with projected increases in smoking-related mortality and DALYs. Whilst a comprehensive approach to promoting health around tobacco use is suggested, it is the political, fiscal and legislative action and the Framework Convention for Tobacco Control (FCTC) that directly targets the powerful global tobacco industry and in so doing reflects the types of approaches suggested in earlier chapters.

The chapter on HIV/AIDS (Chapter 9) clearly illustrates the serious nature of the pandemic. Recent figures of 40 million people living with HIV/AIDS indicate that there is much to be done by primary preventative health promotion, with an increase in global health inequalities predicted unless effective action is taken. Insights are offered in to what health promotion can learn from preventative action targeting HIV/AIDS, and what those with a responsibility for delivering the preventative actions can learn from health promotion. Recommendations include a call for increased efforts involving multi-professional approaches.

Environmental degradation is distinct from the other public health challenges in this section in that the threats to health are in one sense, outside the control of individuals, although at a population level it is human activity and lifestyle that is disrupting environmental stability. An examination of the broad nature of environmental health concerns demonstrates that a significant determinant is the same as in many other chapters in this section, namely rampant consumption-based economic development. As with many health challenges, there is a long lead in time to future detrimental health impact, which might result in complacency and lack of action. There are strong recommendations, therefore, for new partnerships for health and for the international community to take preventative action before serious and non-reversible adverse consequences take hold.

Concluding remarks

The chapters in this section establish a number of key arguments in relation to the significant global public health challenges that need to be addressed. The increase in noncommunicable diseases and their link to globalisation and lifestyle choices are major issues creating complex problems in terms of health promotion action. The targeting of the underlying causes is a considerable challenge because of their multifaceted nature. As Davey demonstrates in the first chapter of the previous section (Chapter 2), there is a complex mesh of interrelating determinants of NCDs, making it inappropriate to single out lifestyle choices as the causal factor for these twenty-first century health challenges. The socioeconomic environment in which the lifestyle choices are made is clearly a dominant issue and this has to be addressed in radical ways that includes establishing new forms of health governance and social reforms and investments. In this sense, the conclusions drawn here mirror those of Part I. Tackling the challenges highlighted in Part II has to involve international endeavours and a resilient system of global governance for health, as so eloquently argued by Kickbusch in the Foreword to this book.

The overall conclusion from this part of the book, therefore, is that these are complex global health challenges and whilst different, they require similar solutions. There are strong recommendations for new and radical responses to deal with the multifaceted array of determinants identified. In essence, as in Part I of this book, all the authors are advising that international and national cooperation is essential with the creation of new partnerships for health on an equal footing between the different sectors at all levels of governance. The challenge will be to break through traditional boundaries within and between governments and non-government organisations so that new international political and economic action for health can take place.

CHAPTER 6

Globalisation and Noncommunicable Diseases

DEREK YACH, ROBERT BEAGLEHOLE AND CORINNA HAWKES

Noncommunicable diseases (NCDs) are the leading cause of death in the world. Out of an estimated 56 million deaths globally in 2000, NCDs accounted for 60 per cent. The leading NCDs are cardiovascular disease (CVD), especially ischaemic heart disease (IHD) and stroke (16 million deaths); cancer (seven million deaths); chronic respiratory disease (3.5 million deaths); and diabetes (almost one million deaths). Mental health problems are also important contributors to the burden of disease in many countries (WHO, 2001).

Table 6.1 illustrates that of WHO's six regions, only in the African region are communicable diseases more frequent as causes of death than NCDs. NCDs are major causes of premature adult mortality (between the ages of 15 and 59 years) with the highest levels being in central and eastern European countries (WHO, 2001). NCDs are an important contributor to health inequalities within and between countries. The burden is higher on poorer populations. In the year 2000, 2.8 million CVD deaths occurred in China and 2.6 million in India. In the future, NCDs will continue to dominate the global pattern of death and disability. In the year 2020, IHD and stroke are expected to be the first and third leading causes of death, and third and fourth cause of disability adjusted life years lost (DALYs) (revised estimates based on data in WHO, 2002). HIV/AIDS is predicted to be second leading cause of death (see Chapter 9 in this section for a detailed examination of the global challenge of HIV/AIDS) and could overtake CVD if treatment access does not rapidly improve; it is already the leading cause of lost DALYs (WHO, 2003a).

Global risk factors for noncommunicable diseases

The current burden of NCDs reflects the cumulative exposure to past risks to health. The future burden will be largely determined by current population exposures to the major risk factors listed in Table 6.2. These risk factors are

Table 6.1 Ten leading causes of deaths – globally, in developing and developed countries, estimates for 2000 (as percentage of total deaths)

	World		Developed Countries[a]		Developing Countries	
1	Ischaemic heart disease	12.4	Ischaemic heart disease	22.6	Ischaemic heart disease	9.1
2	Cerebrovascular disease	9.2	Cerebrovascular disease	13.7	Cerebrovascular disease	8.0
3	Lower respiratory infections	6.9	Trachea, bronchus, lung cancers	4.5	Lower respiratory infections	7.7
4	HIV/AIDS	5.3	Lower respiratory infections	3.7	HIV/AIDS	6.9
5	Chronic obstructive pulmonary disease	4.5	Chronic obstructive pulmonary disease	3.1	Perinatal conditions	5.6
6	Perinatal conditions	4.4	Colon and rectum cancers	2.6	Chronic obstructive pulmonary disease	5.0
7	Diarrhoeal diseases	3.8	Stomach cancer	1.9	Diarrhoeal diseases	4.9
8	Tuberculosis	3.0	Self-inflicted injuries	1.9	Tuberculosis	3.7
9	Road traffic accidents	2.3	Diabetes	1.7	Malaria	2.6
10	Trachea, bronchus, lung cancers	2.2	Breast cancer	1.6	Road traffic accidents	2.5

Note: [a] Developed countries includes European countries, former Soviet countries, Canada, USA, Japan, Australia, New Zealand.

Source: WHO (2002)

Table 6.2 Contribution (%) of ten selected risk factors to burden of disease by level of development and mortality

Developed countries* (population:1.4 billion)		Developing countries*			
		High mortality (population: 2.3 billion)		Low mortality (population: 2.4 billion)	
Tobacco	12.2	Underweight	14.9	Alcohol	6.2
Blood pressure	10.9	Unsafe sex	10.2	Blood pressure	5.0
Alcohol	9.2	Unsafe water, sanitation and hygiene	5.5	Tobacco	4.0
Cholesterol	7.6	Indoor smoke from solid fuels	3.7	Underweight	3.1
Overweight	7.4	Zinc deficiency	3.2	Overweight	2.7
Low fruit and vegetable intake	3.9	Iron deficiency	3.1	Cholesterol	2.1
Physical inactivity	3.3	Vitamin A deficiency	3.0	Indoor smoke from solid fuels	1.9
Illicit drugs	1.8	Blood pressure	2.5	Low fruit and vegetable intake	1.9
Unsafe sex	0.8	Tobacco	2.0	Iron deficiency	1.8
Iron deficiency	0.7	Cholesterol	1.9	Unsafe water, sanitation and hygiene	1.7

Source: WHO, 2002. See WHO, 2002 for full list, Developed countries include the USA, Japan and Australia; low-mortality developing countries include China, Brazil and Thailand; and high-mortality developing countries include India, Mali and Nigeria.

well known and explain the occurrence of almost all new events within populations (Stamler et al., 1999; Magnus and Beaglehole, 2001). Most of these risk factors are common to the main categories of NCDs and all are modifiable, albeit with some difficulty. Although there are some quantitative differences between countries, the relationship between the major risk factors and NCDs can be applied globally.

The contribution of the major NCD risk factors to the burden of disease is summarised in Table 6.2. In high income countries these risk factors constitute seven of the ten leading risk factors contributing to the burden of disease, compared to six of ten among low-mortality developing countries, and three of ten in high-mortality developing countries. In most low and middle income countries, the secular trend for NCD risk factor levels has been negative over the last decade portending a massive increase in the occurrence of NCDs over the next two decades in these countries.

Risk factors and health inequalities

The distribution of major NCD risk factors explains to a large extent the disproportionate burden of NCDs on poorer populations (Kunst et al., 1998; Evans et al., 2001; Leon and Watt, 2001). In high and some middle income countries where risk factors have been established for decades, inequalities in CVD, cancer and diabetes by social class and ethnicity are well established (Kogevinas et al., 1997; Mackenbach et al., 2000; Aboderin et al., 2001; Batty and Leon, 2002). There are also inequalities by gender (Brands and Yach, 2002). In most lower middle income countries, where risk levels have been high for years, there is a steep gradient favouring the more affluent and educated groups with respect to risk prevalence, but a mixed picture with respect to diseases and causes of deaths. In lower income countries, NCDs initially increase among those with the highest levels of disposable incomes. But evidence shows that as economies develop, risks such as tobacco use, physical inactivity and obesity become higher among the poorest groups (see Chapter 3 in Part I of this book for a fuller discussion of international patterns and trends in inequalities in health).

Tobacco and diet/physical activity complex of risk factors

Key contributors to the burden of disease in all categories of countries are tobacco and the diet/physical activity related complex of risks: overweight or a high body mass index, lack of physical activity, low fruit and vegetable consumption, alcohol consumption, high blood pressure and cholesterol levels. The global spread of these risk factors can explain in part the growing significance of NCDs around the world, and their disproportionate burden on disadvantaged groups.

Tobacco

There were about 1.235 billion smokers in 1999, one-third of the world's population aged over 14 years (Corrao et al., 2000). Tobacco consumption now kills five million people per year, and rates are rising. The toll will double in 20 years unless known and effective interventions are quickly and widely adopted (WHO, 2003b). In China alone, annual smoking deaths are expected to rise from one million to three million in 2050 (Murray and Lopez, 1996). Smoking rates are rising amongst children, adolescents and women, and initiation is increasingly at a younger age.

The distribution of disease caused by tobacco is shifting from high income to lower middle and low income countries, thus increasing the burden on poorer nations. These countries are expected to see significant increases in tobacco-related deaths over the next twenty years, in contrast to a steadying percentage in established market economies (Wipfli et al., 2001). Chapter 8 in this section offers a fuller discussion of the global challenge for heath promotion of tobacco consumption.

Food

Globally, dietary and nutrition transitions are well underway in all but the poorest populations (Popkin, 2002). Diets are becoming characterised by a higher proportion of fatty and sugary foods, and lower consumption of whole-grains and vegetables. Subsequently, energy intake from nutrients associated with NCDs, such as fats and sugars, are increasing while consumption of protective factors such as dietary fibre and micronutrients is declining. These trends are emerging in countries as diverse as Brazil, Malaysia, China and South Africa. Although under nutrition remains a massive problem and demands continued and increased investment, it is possible that this too is associated with NCDs. Some evidence, albeit controversial, suggests that children with low birth weight are at highest risk for heart disease, hypertension and diabetes in adulthood (Aboderin et al., 2001). The rapidity of the transitions and the reductions in the energy expended on physical activity, especially in urban areas, are reflected in the rapid rise of urban obesity. In China, for example, the prevalence of obesity in urban children aged two to six years increased from 1.5 per cent in 1989 to 12.6 per cent in 1997 (Luo and Hu, 2002). This has significant economic costs. One estimate put the health and productivity costs of diet-related NCDs in China as high as US \$15.1 billion in the year 1995 (Popkin et al., 2001). For a more detailed analysis of issues around food and health please refer to Chapter 7.

Globalisation processes and noncommunicable diseases

Globalisation is discussed in a number of chapters in this text. See, for example Part I, Chapters 1 and 5. It can be defined as a process whereby increasing economic, political, and social interdependence and global integration take place as capital, traded goods, persons, concepts, images, ideas and values diffuse across state borders (Yach and Bettcher, 1998). The economic, political and social forces that drive the globalisation process are important in the global spread of the risk factors related to tobacco and food. Key processes are the production, distribution, including cross-border trade, and marketing of tobacco and food products. These processes encourage the entrenchment of the risk factors for NCDs in all regions.

Production

The globalisation of the world economy has facilitated the ability of the tobacco industry to locate production in countries where costs are cheaper. These shifts reduce production costs and maximise access to countries with weaker tobacco control measures. Dietary and nutrition transitions are also influenced by the increasingly globalised nature of food production processes (Goodman and Watts, 1997). Commodities such as oilseeds and corn are produced in one country to sell as vegetable oils, livestock feed and sweeteners in another, facilitating the abilities of transnational corporations (TNCs) to create cost and production efficiencies (see, for example, Micek, 1999; Prokopanko, 1999 and Caraher et al., in Chapter 7 of this part of the book). Production of livestock has increased dramatically in China, South Korea, South Africa and many other countries, with simultaneous declines in human consumption of cereals and grains (Gale et al., 2002; FAOSTAT, 2003).

Distribution

Expanded distribution of tobacco through global trade has been a key driver in promoting demand. Facilitating greater tobacco trade is the recent wave of international trade liberalisation. Membership of the World Trade Organisation (WTO) has grown, while the Uruguay Round of trade negotiations included the liberalisation of unmanufactured tobacco for the first time and the new Multilateral Agreements of the WTO significantly reduced tariff and non-tariff barriers to tobacco trade (Chaloupka and Corbett 1998; Wipfli et al., 2001). Research suggests a link between increased cross-border trade and smoking. Lower trade barriers have the potential to reduce the price of imported cigarettes and, in the absence of government regulation, may increase the expenditure on cigarette advertising. A study in the late 1990s found a substantial rise in the market share of American cigarettes in countries in which the US aggressively pursued market-opening measures (Chaloupka and Laixuthai, 1996). Smoking in the affected countries was 10 percent higher than it would have been if markets had remained closed to US cigarettes. Related research suggests that while reduced trade barriers have no significant impact on smoking in high income countries, it has a small but significant impact on consumption in middle income countries, and a significant impact on low income countries (Bettcher et al., 2001).

In addition to trade liberalisation, the transnational tobacco industry has also taken advantage of more open conditions for foreign direct investment (FDI) in low and middle income countries (Taylor and Bettcher, 2000). The same applies to the food sector. Broader global distribution has increased the availability of foods associated with risk factors for NCDs. This in part arises from greater trade between international borders. The amount of food traded has tripled in the last 40 years, arising in part from more liberal trade policies, with implications for health (Halweil, 2002). Trade policy reform in India, for example, has resulted in increased imports of palm oil, an oil linked with higher rates of CVD (Dohlman et al., 2003; WHO, 2003c). FDI has probably had even more significant impacts, along with the development of national transportation networks and new patterns of retailing. Food distribution is increasingly controlled by TNCs that have gained efficiency through vertical and global integration (Bonanno et al., 1994). US food processing firms, for example, generated an estimated US $150 billion in 2000 through FDI. This compares with US $30 billion generated by food exports. It is often economically advantageous to invest capital in overseas production than ship the product from a domestic source (Bolling and Somwaru, 2001). TNCs also have the capital to invest in distribution networks and refrigeration. Global soft drinks companies, for example, invest in transportation networks to ensure their products are as widely available as possible (Hawkes, 2002). Meanwhile, the globalisation of supermarket retailing is changing consumption patterns, as well as transforming the food supply chain (Reardon and Berdegué, 2002).

Marketing

Promotional marketing is at the interface between production, distribution and consumers. As such, it plays a key role in encouraging greater consumption of tobacco and certain food products. Marketing campaigns by multinational tobacco and food companies leverage a global brand to target all consumption occasions, but are tailored to local communities. Commonly used techniques include advertising, sales promotions, sponsorship and philanthropy. Food companies use these methods to take share away from other foods and drinks, including traditional products, thus boosting category and brand consumption. Young children and teenagers are targeted directly via strategies such as sponsorship of television shows, sporting activities and music events (Hawkes, 2002). Among the most heavily marketed products are foods and beverages usually classified under the eat-least category in dietary guidelines. Boosted by huge expenditure, marketing thus creates an environment where healthy choices are the more difficult choices, especially for children. As such, marketing of energy dense, micronutrient poor foods and sweetened drinks is considered a probable cause of weight gain and obesity (WHO, 2003c).

Tobacco companies are also renowned for their marketing activities. Although the exact figures for global advertising are not known, in the US alone, tobacco companies spend over US $10 billion a year on promotion (Campaign for Tobacco-Free Kids, 2003). Marketing is known to contribute to the global spread of tobacco use. Numerous studies have shown how advertising and point-of-sales promotions increase average tobacco sales, to both adults and children (World Bank, 1999). Although many countries have now imposed restrictions on the promotion of tobacco, new advertising techniques pose a challenge at a global scale. Online marketing by major tobacco manufacturers has increased substantially over the past three years. RJR Reynolds, for example, began advertising a new brand Eclipse, solely through the Internet (Beaglehole and Yach, 2003). Moreover, transnational tobacco companies aggressively target marketing campaigns at young people and children using marketing strategies that have long been banned in many developed countries. Free samples are a case in point. In some countries, up to 25 per cent of teenagers have been offered free cigarettes by tobacco company representatives (Warren et al., 2000).

Noncommunicable diseases and health promotion: the challenges

1 *Limited global health promotion for prevention and control of noncommunicable diseases* There is only limited advocacy at the global level for the prevention and control of noncommunicable diseases, and what there is tends to be fragmented and risk factor or disease specific. Many of the potential advocacy groups have their origins in specialist health professional organisations and have not yet coalesced to become strong promoters of broad prevention and control policies (Beaglehole, 2001). This lack of strong voices for disease prevention and health promotion programmes is in contrast to the growing dominance of commercial and consumer groups who have placed treatment at the centre of health policy debates and funding priorities. Because of their origins the most effective advocates for prevention have concentrated on single risk factors or specific diseases, often with great success, for example national tobacco control advocacy groups. Stronger and broader alliances of major health professional bodies, consumer groups, enlightened industries and academics are now needed to effectively prioritise the prevention of major risk factors for chronic diseases. Slowly this is happening with the World Heart Federation, the World Medical Association and its associated health professional's alliance that includes nurses, pharmacists and dentists, and the International Cancer Control Union (UICC) increasingly working together on chronic disease promotion issues. Full activation of their national associations would bring a powerful global voice to a neglected area of public health.

2 *Failure to invest in global prevention and control of noncommunicable diseases* The capacity at the national level for NCD prevention and control is weak in terms of personnel, infrastructure and resources (Alwan et al., 2001). There is a need for a significant investment in the capacity of countries to plan and manage health projects for infectious diseases and even more for chronic diseases (Berwick, 2002; Morrow, 2002). Unfortunately, donors and governments have been reluctant to invest in national institutions and infrastructure for health promotion for NCD prevention. A global commitment is needed if sustainable progress in policy development and implementation for chronic diseases, as well as other aspects of public health, is to be assured. WHO's Tropical Disease Research programme funded by a consortium of donors has developed over the last two decades an impressive network of communicable disease researchers and provides many useful lessons for chronic disease control efforts (Nchinda, 2002). The US National Institutes for Health through their Fogarty International Center, and Canada's IDRC have begun to invest

modestly in tobacco control research in developing countries and this needs to be expanded to other aspects of chronic diseases.

Noncommunicable diseases and health promotion: the successes

Despite the shortfalls of global advocacy and investment, effective health promotional activities do exist at a local, national and global level. This has led to sustained declines in NCD mortality in most OECD countries over the last two decades. A combination of educational, legislative, fiscal and intersectoral policies over many years have driven the process. These national successes usually were started when NCD risks were ubiquitous and NCD death rates were already high. In contrast, for many poorer countries the policy challenges are different: how to avoid an increase in risks and NCD outcomes. In this regard, two national examples that have the potential to be scaled up for global application are Finland and Thailand.

Health promotional efforts in Finland began in 1972 in the province of North Karelia, where rates of heart disease were double that of the rest of the country and at a time when Finland was not the wealthy country it is now. Taking a population-wide approach, the North Karelia project encouraged change across sectors, including diversification of agriculture away from meat and dairy; encouragement of individual lifestyle shifts to better diets, more exercise and less smoking; training of medical professionals to increase monitoring of blood pressure. The programme was expanded to the rest of Finland in 1977. Although drugs that lower cholesterol may also have played a role, in the past 30 years deaths from heart disease and deaths from lung cancer in North Karelia have fallen by around 70 per cent each. Male life expectancy has increased, as has per capita vegetable consumption. The integrated approach of this form of health promotion has global application. Under the auspices of the WHO, pilot projects based on North Karelia have been developed in regions of China, Chile, Iran and Oman.

Another example comes from Thailand, which has identified health promotion as a priority area to reduce the incidence of NCDs (WHO Thailand, 2000). As part of their efforts, the Thai government set up the Thai Health Promotion Foundation (ThaiHealth) in April 2001. By funding health promotion campaigns, research projects, networking, media development and education, ThaiHealth has become a major player in health promotion in Thailand. The foundation is sustained by a dedicated 2 per cent surcharge tax on alcohol and tobacco products. Although inevitably prone to shifts in the tax regime, the funding provides a relatively sustainable source of revenue and has allowed ThaiHealth to gain prominence in the international arena.

There are also examples of leadership, the global level of efforts to promote health to reduce NCDs. The WHO noncommunicable disease division has initiatives such as Move for Health and Quit and Win. They are also in the process of developing a global fruit and vegetable promotion initiative (WHO, 2003d). Another recent and major initiative taken to promote health by reducing tobacco use was the Framework Convention on Tobacco Control (FCTC), also mentioned in Chapter 8 of this part of the book. The FCTC, adopted by the WHO in May 2003, requires countries to promote and strengthen public awareness of tobacco control issues, using all available communication tools, as appropriate (WHO, 2003e).

Global progress on tobacco is now being matched by emerging global efforts to promote healthy diets and increased physical activity. The Global Strategy on Diet, Physical Activity and Health, developed by the WHO in consultation with stakeholders from the UN and inter-governmental agencies, civil society and the private sector, calls for the development of national strategies on diet and physical activity (WHO, 2004). The aim is to encourage healthy choices through the implementation of policies on dietary guidelines, the information environment around food, and prevention initiatives built into health services.

As infectious diseases eventually decline in low and middle income countries, it would be a great public health tragedy if these successes were eroded by a rising toll of NCDs. At exactly the same time as infectious diseases are being addressed, urgent attention should be given to NCD prevention and control. Given that exposure to risks over the life course are cumulative, a life-course perspective to prevention and health promotion is needed to yield benefits over the next 50 years (Aboderin et al., 2001). Putting effective treatment and prevention programs for NCDs into health systems as they are scaled up to address AIDS, malaria and TB would be cost-effective and reduce the burden of current disease in many populations. Acting globally to address the transnational dimensions of NCD risks and policy development through rapid implementation of the FCTC and the new global strategy on diet and physical activity could significantly alter the risk environment in which people live for the better; and working with colleagues in infectious diseases to ensure greater overall investment in health by countries and development agencies would make it possible to achieve health for all.

References

Aboderin, I., Kalache, A., Ben-Shlomo, Y., Lynch, J.W., Yajnik, C.D., Kuh D. and Yach, D. (2001) *Life course perspectives on coronary heart disease, stroke and diabetes: key issues and implications for policy and research.* Geneva: World Health Organisation.

Alwan, A., MacLean, D. and Mandil, A. (2001) *Assessment of National Capacity for Noncommunicable Disease Prevention and Control.* Geneva: World Health Organisation.

Batty, G.D. and Leon, D.A. (2002) Socio-economic position and coronary heart disease risk factors in children and young people. *European Journal of Public Health*, **12**: 263–72.

Beaglehole, R. (2001) Global cardiovascular disease prevention: time to get serious. *Lancet*, **358**: 661–63.

Beaglehole, R. and Yach, D. (2003) Globalisation and the prevention and control of non-communicable disease: the neglected chronic disease of adults. *Lancet*, **362**: 903–08.

Berwick, D.M. (2002) A learning world for the Global Fund. *British Medical Journal*, **325**: 55–56.

Bettcher, D., Subramaniam, C., Guidon, E., Perucic, A-M., Soll, L., Grabman, G. and Joosens, J., WTO Secretariat and Taylor, A. (2001) *Confronting the Tobacco Epidemic in an Era of Trade Liberalisation*. Geneva: World Health Organisation.

Bolling, C. and Somwaru, A. (2001) U.S. food companies access foreign markets through direct investment. *Food Review*, **24**: 23–28.

Bonanno, A., Busch, L., Friedland, W.H., Gouveia, L. and Mingione, E. (eds) (1994) *From Columbus to ConAgra: The Globalisation of Agriculture and Food*. Lawrence, KS: University Press of Kansas.

Brands, A. and Yach, D. (2002) *Women and the Rapid Rise of Noncommunicable Diseases*. NMH Reader No. 1. Geneva: World Health Organisation.

Campaign for Tobacco-Free Kids (2003) *Tobacco marketing that reaches kids: point-of-purchase advertising and promotions*. Campaign Factsheet. Washington DC: Campaign for Tobacco-free Kids.

Corrao, M.A., Guindon, E., Cokkinides, W. and Sharma, N. (2000) Building the evidence base for global tobacco control. *Bulletin of the World Health Organisation*, **78**: 884–90.

Chaloupka, F.J. and Laixuthai, A. (1996) *U.S. Trade Policy and Cigarette Smoking in Asia*. Cambridge, MA: NBER.

Chaloupka, F. and Corbett, M. (1998) Trade policy and tobacco: towards an optimal policy mix. In Abedian, I., van der Merwe, R., Wilkins, N. and Jha, P. (eds) *The Economics of Tobacco Control: Towards an Optimal Policy Mix*. Cape Town: Applied Fiscal Research Centre.

Dohlman, E., Persaud, S. and Landes, R. (2003). *India's Edible Oil Sector: Imports Fill Rising Demand*. Electronic Outlook Report from the Economic Research Service. Washington DC: United States Department of Agriculture.

Evans, T., Whitehead, M. and Diderichsen, F. (eds) (2001) *Challenging Inequities in Health: From Ethics to Action*. New York: Oxford University Press.

FAOSTAT (2003). Database on Agricultural Production – Livestock Primary. Accessed 31, October 2003 http://apps.fao.org/cgi-bin/nph-db.pl?subset= agriculture.

Gale, F., Tuan, F., Lohmar, B., Hsu, H.H. and Gilmour, B. (2002) *China's Food and Agriculture: Issues for the 21st Century*. ERS Agricultural Information Bulletin No. AIB775. Washington DC: United States Department of Agriculture.

Goodman, D. and Watts, M.J. (1997) *Globalising Food*. London: Routledge.

Halweil, B. (2002) *Home Grown: The Case for Local Food in a Global Market*. World Watch Paper #163. Washington DC: Worldwatch Institute.

Hawkes, C. (2002) Marketing Activities of Global Soft Drink and Fast Food Companies in Emerging Markets: a Review. In *Globalisation, Diets and Noncommunicable Diseases*. Geneva: World Health Organisation.

Kogevinas, M., Pearce, N., Susser, M. and Boffetta, P. (eds) (1997) *Social Inequalities and Cancer*. IARC Scientific publications No 138. Lyon: IARC Press.

Kunst, A.E., Groenhof, F. and Mackenback, J.P. (1998) Mortality by occupational class among men 30–64 years in 11 European countries. *Social Science and Medicine*, **46**: 459–76.

Leon, D.A. and Watt, G. (2001) *Poverty, Inequality and Health: An International Perspective.* Oxford: Oxford University Press.

Luo, F. and Hu, F.B. (2002) Time trends of obesity in pre-school children in China from 1989 to 1997. *International Journal Obesity Related Metabolic Disorders,* **26**: 553–56.

Mackenbach, J.P., Cavelaars, A.E.J.M., Kunst, A.E. and Groenhof, F. (2000) Socioeconomic inequalities in cardiovascular disease mortality. An international study. *European Heart Journal,* **21**: 1141–51.

Magnus, P. and Beaglehole, R. (2001) The real contribution of the major risk factors to the coronary epidemics: time to end the 'only 50%' claim. *Annals of Internal Medicine,* **161**: 2657–60.

Micek, E. (1999) Global agriculture: working toward a sustainable food system. *The Cargill Bulletin,* 7(4): 1–8.

Morrow, R.H. (2002) Macroeconomics and health. *British Medical Journal,* **352**: 53–54.

Murray, C.L. and Lopez, A.D. (eds) (1996) *The Global Burden of Disease: a Comprehensive Assessment of Mortality and Disability From Diseases, Injuries and Risk Factors in 1990 and Projected to 2020.* Cambridge, MA: Harvard School of Public Health on Behalf of the World Health Organisation and the World Bank.

Nchinda, T. (2002) Research capacity strengthening in the South. *Social Science and Medicine,* **54**: 1699–711.

Popkin, B.M. (2002) An overview on the nutrition transition and its health implications: the Bellagio meeting. *Public Health Nutrition,* **5**: 93–103.

Popkin, B.M., Horton, S., Kim, S., Mahal, A. and Shuigao, J. (2001) Trends in diet, nutritional status, and diet-related noncommunicable diseases in China and India: the economic costs of the nutrition transition. *Nutrition Review,* **59** (12): 379–90.

Prokopanko, J. (1999) *Laying the Foundation for a Prosperous Agriculture in the New Millennium: A Cargill Perspective for the Northern Great Plains.* Speech given at a Conference of Northern Great Plains Inc. Knowledge Management – Practice & Promise in an eBusiness World. Winnipeg, Manitoba, Canada – 16–17 October 2000.

Reardon, T. and Berdegué, J.A. (2002) The rapid rise of supermarkets in Latin America: challenges and opportunities for development. *Development Policy Review,* **20**: 371–88.

Stamler, J., Stamler, R. and Neaton, J.D. (1999) Low risk-factor profile and long-term cardiovascular and non-cardiovascular mortality and life expectancy. Findings for 5 large cohorts of young adult and middle-aged men and women. *Journal of the American Medical Association,* **282**: 2012–18.

Taylor, L. and Bettcher, D.W. (2000) WHO Framework for Tobacco Control: a global 'good' for public health. *Bulletin of the World Health Organisation,* **78**: 920–29.

Warren, C.W., Riley, L., Asma, S., Eriksen, M.P., Green, L., Blanton, C., Loo, C., Batchelor, S. and Yach, D. (2000) Tobacco use by youth: a surveillance report from the Global Youth Tobacco Survey Project. *Bulletin of the World Health Organisation,* **78**: 868–76.

Wipfli, H., Bettcher, D.W., Subramaniam, C. and Taylor, A.L. (2001) Confronting the global tobacco epidemic: emerging mechanisms of global governance. In McKee, M., Garner, P. and Stott, R. (eds) *International Health Cooperation.* Oxford: Oxford University Press.

World Bank (1999) *Curbing the Epidemic: Governments and the Economics of Tobacco Control.* Washington DC: World Bank.

World Health Organisation Thailand (2000) *WHO Country Cooperation Strategy for Thailand*. Nonthaburi, Thailand: World Health Organisation. http://w3.whothai. org/EN/Section3/Section14.htm.

World Health Organisation (2001) *World Health Report, 2001*. Geneva: World Health Organisation.

World Health Organisation (2002) *World Health Report, 2002*. Geneva: World Health Organisation.

World Health Organisation (2003a) World Health Organisation says failure to deliver AIDS medicines is a global health emergency. *Press Release* (22 September 2003) Geneva: World Health Organisation.

World Health Organisation (2003b) *World Health Report 2003*. Geneva: World Health Organisation.

World Health Organisation (2003c) *Diet, Nutrition and the Prevention of Chronic Diseases*. WHO Technical Report Series 916. Geneva: World Health Organisation.

World Health Organisation (2003d) *Fruit and Vegetable Promotion Initiative: A Meeting Report* (25–27 August, 2003). Geneva: World Health Organisation.

World Health Organisation (2003e) *WHO Framework Convention on Tobacco Control*. Geneva: World Health Organisation. http://www.fctc.org/

World Health Organisation (2004) *Global Strategy on Diet, Physical Activity and Health*. Geneva: World Health Organisation.

Yach, D. and Bettcher, D. (1998) The globalisation of public health, 1: threats and opportunities. *American Journal of Public Health*, **88**: 735–38.

CHAPTER 7

Food, Health and Globalisation: Is Health Promotion Still Relevant?

MARTIN CARAHER, JOHN COVENEY AND TIM LANG

This chapter explores the value of health promotion for food and health policy. Questions immediately arise: Is there one approach? Does health promotion influence food policy, or does food policy frame health promotion? Addressing such questions requires practitioners and researchers to negotiate the interface between ideology or framing assumptions, on the one hand, and policy delivery on the other. Perceived and actual positions on the value of engagement with the food system are almost proxy indicators for an approach to health promotion: are health promoters for or against the food sector as potential allies, confounders or enemies?

Over the twentieth century, many indicators on food and health improved dramatically, a testament to interventions and improved incomes. Globally, for example, life expectancy rose; people have grown taller; malnutrition rates have dropped; fat intake as a percentage of total energy has fallen. But against these gains, other indicators have dramatically worsened or been stubbornly resistant to positive change, for instance, obesity, physical activity levels, consumption of fresh fruit and vegetables, food security and inequalities both within and between countries. Taken together, the positive and negative indicators on food and health suggest that far from being resolved, the problems of food policy seem merely to have shifted and become more complex (Millstone and Lang, 2003; Lang and Heasman, 2004).

Where is health promotion practice to stand while these complex issues are to be researched and clarified? For the last 20 years practice has tended to engage with the food industry as partners. The search for solutions has tended to be downstream, focused on what consumers can do (Labonte, 1998, 2003). This approach deserves tougher scrutiny. In many high income countries where resources have been expended on health promotion, the diet-related indicators are mixed.

Rapid changes in the food supply chain are outpacing what health promotion can do to ameliorate dietary failings. Health promotion needs to build practice on a better understanding of who controls, distributes and markets

90

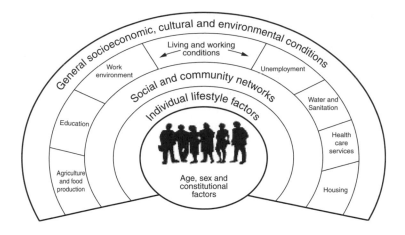

Figure 7.1   Spheres of influence on health, adapted from Dahlgren and Whitehead (1992)

what the food consumers eat, as changes in the food supply chain strongly influence the context within which consumer choice occurs. Globally, the range of goods on sale and the cultural determinants of choice influence whether consumers freely *choose* or merely *select* between preordained packages.

The model proposed by Dahlgren and Whitehead (1992) (see Figure 7.1) illustrates the policy divide. Health promotion has tended to focus on the inner rings of influence, with a concentration on individuals, families and communities, while largely ignoring the outer determinants of choice. This strategy has allowed the food supply chain to position itself as just another sector of the wider economy, increasingly concerned, not about health, but about regional and global competitiveness and survival in fiercely fought over sectors.

The nutrition transition

Part of the challenge for a reinvigorated health promotion is what might be termed its geo-spatial boundaries. Health profiles are not restricted to national geographical limits. In this volume the terms low, middle and high income is used to depict the status of countries. The classification is useful but limited when exploring nutrition transition, a term used to describe a process of rapid change of diet. Established and researched by Popkin and colleagues, it refers to a consistent pattern of dietary change in societies, from eating local or national foods and traditional diets to one characterised by higher fat, salt and sugar intake, more consumption of pre-processed foods, a limit in intake of fruit and vegetables and decline in fibre. Liquid intake also shifts from water sources to carbonated, sweetened soft drinks, high in energy (Popkin, 1998; Caballero and Popkin, 2002).

Nutrition transition is associated with national food markets opening up to global marketing and the arrival of highly processed foods in countries where they were previously unknown or too expensive for mass consumption. The transition is driven by rising income and consumer aspirations and is linked to urbanisation and the departure from rural life and more traditional food cultural mores. The implications of the nutrition transition are considerable. It is associated with a rise of degenerative diseases such as cardiovascular diseases, type 2 late onset diabetes and obesity occurring among the population at large. Diabetes, more usually associated with middle age and older people, begins to appear among younger members of society and to increase in prevalence. As a result, within the same society, there can be simultaneous exhibition of diseases of under, mal and over consumption. The diet related health profile becomes more complex and more pernicious, with diseases associated with low income and high income existing side by side (Wilkinson, 1996).

As emphasised in Chapter 1, global classifications such as low, medium and high income countries can disguise the inequalities inherent *within* countries. Diet and styles of food consumption are heavily associated with both relative and absolute levels of income. World Bank estimates suggest widening inequality gaps in some regions of the world (World Bank, 2003). Most projections for the early twenty-first century suggest that low income and poor health indicators will particularly burden sub-Saharan Africa, while the East Asian economies and the Middle East and North Africa should show greater improvements (see Part I, Chapter 3 for a detailed analysis of health inequalities). The Millennium Development Goals are unlikely to be met, on current projections. For improvements to occur income rises and rates of growth will have to be considerable, with the projected rate of GDP growth in some regions having to be remarkable if they are to reduce hunger dramatically, as promised at the World Food Summit 1996 (see Table 7.1). The Newly Independent States in the former USSR, for instance, would have to achieve growth rates of 7 per cent up to 2025 and of 3.9 per cent up to 2050 to banish hunger, when they only achieved a growth rate of 0.1 per cent between 1975 and 1999 (see Chapter 15 for a fuller discussion on the former Soviet Union). The focus on GDP, moreover, suggests that for policy, the main concern is absolute hunger, when there is already evidence that this alone is not the sole source of diet-related ill health. Food can also be a source of social exclusion, a social wedge within societies.

Popkin's (1998) analysis of the dietary shifts associated with nutrition transition shows that fat consumption increases in low income countries with resultant upsurge in prevalence of obesity and chronic diseases more associated with affluence and therefore more prevalent in high income countries in the past. Partly responsible for this shift is the greater availability of cheap fats as a result of global trade. One indication of the nutrition transition is mass change in food preparation, with a decline of traditional cooking and the rise of

Table 7.1 Annual average growth rates in GDP per capita needed to end hunger and actual 1975–99 rates

Country/region	1975–99 GDP per capita in constant 1995 US$	2025 (%)	2050 (%)
Sub-Saharan Africa	0.5	6.3	3.5
East Asia	1.8	7.0	3.9
China	7.5	7.0	3.9
South Asia	3.2	6.8	3.7
Latin America	1.5	7.0	3.9
Middle East/North Africa	1.1	6.6	3.7
Newly Independent States	0.1	7.0	3.9

Source: Runge, Senauer, Pardey and Rosegrant (2003). Reprinted with permission from the International Food Policy Research Institute www.ifpri.org and Johns Hopkins University Press www.press.jhu.edu

processed and pre-prepared foods. First exhibited in affluent countries as they industrialised, it is now manifest in those countries rapidly industrialising in the Asia Pacific, Latin America, Middle East and Africa. One implication of this change to convenience foods is that the control over ingredients is located with food designers, factory recipe manager and cost controllers sited elsewhere, sometimes at a considerable distance. Product labelling may not compensate for consumer awareness of a product's nutritional impact. Health claims and dubious marketing confounds real information and value. Once incomes rise, populations seem inevitably to enter into the nutrition transition. The health costs associated with the transition can be considerable. The costs of poor nutrition, obesity and low physical activity for Europe, calculated in Disability Adjusted Life Years (DALYs), a measure of health burden, is 9.7 per cent, which compares to 9 per cent due to smoking (World Health Organisation, 2000b). In low income countries where healthcare budgets and facilities can be limited these costs are unacceptable. There is an opportunity here for a reinvigorated and globally aware health promotion strategy. A recent analysis has suggested that strategies to promote healthy eating and dietary change were among the most cost-effective of methods of preventing cardiovascular disease (Brunner et al., 2001).

In a world with lowered barriers to cross-border trade, noncommunicable diet-related disorders (NCDRDs) also spread quickly across national borders. In this respect, although not contagious in formal medical terms, the lifestyle acts as though it is. The causes of ill health are not infectious agents but the new vectors of culture and behaviour change. These are different mechanisms than communicable diseases. Whereas the latter usually spread by infection, the former tend to spread in ways that reflect changes in food supply, culture and lifestyle related to food (Lang and Caraher, 2001). For example, obesity and coronary heart disease (CHD) have until relatively recently been seen as less of a problem in low income countries than in high income ones. CHD and some food-related cancers, such as cancer of the bowel (World Cancer Research Fund [WCRF], 1997) are on the increase in low income countries, where the more affluent social groups are changing lifestyles, eating different foods and taking less exercise. The irony is that the new pattern of disease in low income countries is first manifest among the more affluent, whereas in high income countries, it is the poor that have the worse diet-related health profiles (Dowler et al., 2002). The new pattern is represented in Table 7.2.

An illustration is given for the coexistence of over- and under-consumption, represented by obesity and under-nourishment figures, by world region, in Figure 7.2.

Table 7.2   Types and effects of malnutrition

Type of malnutrition	Nutritional effect	No. people affected globally (billion)
Hunger	Deficiency of calories and protein	At least 1.2
Micronutrient deficiency	Deficiency of vitamins and minerals	2.0–3.5
Over-consumption	Excess of calories, often accompanied by deficiency of vitamins and minerals	At least 1.2–1.7 billion

Source: Gardner and Halweil 2000, based on WHO, IFPRI, ACC/SCN data. Reprinted with permission from the International Food Policy Research Institute, www.ifpri.org and Johns Hopkins University Press www.press.jhu.edu

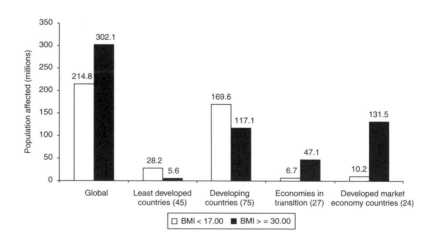

Figure 7.2   Global population affected by underweight and obesity in adults for year 2000, by level of development

Source: WHO (2000a)

There is a reminder in Table 7.2 and Figure 7.2 of the continued existence of serious under consumption in the world. According to the United Nations Children's Fund, one in five persons in the low income countries suffer from chronic hunger, 800 million people in Africa, Asia and Latin America. Over two billion people subsist on diets deficient in the vitamins and minerals essential for normal growth and development, and for preventing premature death and such disabilities as blindness and mental retardation (UNICEF, 1996). While such facts are sobering, inadequacies of income also affect dietary intake in affluent countries (Dowler and Rushton, 1993). While the Food and Agriculture Organisation (FAO) (FAO, 1999) estimates for the period 1995–97 that 790 million people in the low income countries did not have enough to eat, the same report points out that in high income countries there were eight million people undernourished and suffering serious food deprivation. In Eastern Europe this figure is estimated to be four million and in the newly independent states of the former Soviet Union 22 million, 7 per cent of the population. These figures refer to under nourishment as opposed to the availability of culturally and socially appropriate foods. The emergence of global consuming and under consuming classes is extending the globalisation of inequalities.

The hidden costs of the globalisation of food

In addition to the direct impact on health of changes in food supply there are a number of other costs that are referred to as hidden, these include impacts on the environment, local economies and the social fabric of societies (Barling et al., 2001; Bové and Dufour, 2001).

In Europe, the increases in fruit consumption extolled by health promotion campaigns can be largely accounted for by the increase in purchases of fruit juice, which does not provide equivalent nutrition to its fresh counterpart. This fruit juice consumption is often of juices from long distant fruit, such as oranges from Brazil. Transportation carries a measurable environmental burden (Garnett, 2003). The Wupperthal Institute in Germany calculated that 80 per cent of Brazilian orange production is consumed in Europe. Annual German consumption accounted for 370,000 acres of Brazilian productive land, three times the land down to fruit production in Germany. If this level of German orange juice consumption were to be replicated worldwide, 32 million acres would be needed just for orange production (Kranendonk and Bringezau, 1994). The increasing range of fruit available throughout the year also contributes to this rise in consumption. Together such developments result in an increase in food miles with food travelling greater distances, an increase in pollution and a reduction in local indigenous crops as they are replaced by foods for export. These are indirect costs of the regionalising and globalising food market with implications for health through increased fumes and pollution, road accidents, amenity loss and inter-generational damage to the environment through energy use and reliance on non-renewable sources.

The twentieth-century food revolution was latterly driven and characterised by remarkable changes in distribution. This not only gave retailers key power over the entire food system by use of contracts and specifications, but also directly affected what the farmer grows and how they grow it. Due to economies of scale and cheap energy, consumers get the advantage of cheaper foods, but for low income consumers the costs of getting to more distant stores, as local shops close is an additional cost burden. The supply chain determines the consumer experience. Shops sell vegetables that can and were grown locally that are now brought thousands of miles. Consumers gain a seasonality of choice but monoculture spreads on the land.

Another feature of current global food supply is its high degree of concentration. Small companies are squeezed; giant corporations emerge in processing, retailing and foodservice. More farmers in Europe, for example, now market wholesale produce through fewer buying channels dominated by a concentration of supermarket chains (Institute of Grocery Distribution [IGD], 2001; Grievink, 2003). The emergence of global food retailers, as well as retail buying consortia, is likely to shape the food system in the early twenty-first century, with the turnover of top global chains already considerable (see Table 7.3).

To put this in context Wal-Mart serves more than 138 million customers on a weekly basis drawn from 85 per cent of American households. It is the biggest employer in 21 US States and the single biggest employer in the US, with more people in uniform than the US army (Norman, 1999). The company employs 1.3 million associates with an average wage of US $15.000 for a full-time employee. Compare this average wage to five members of the Wal-Mart family, who are among the 10 richest people in the world. Wal-Mart is the world's biggest corporation with sales of US $244.5 billion in the fiscal year ending 31 January 2003. This corporate power ensures that companies of this size can control different aspects of the food system from growing to the choices available to the consumer in the aisles of a supermarket.

Food citizenship rights and responsibilities

One effect of this emergence of new food market powers is that *de facto* there is a dual system of regulation and control; one is the State's, the other private corporations. The vertical control of food supplies means that the major retailers control what is grown and how, which may have an impact on local food security. A debate about the implications of this for governance and food governance, is now urgently required (Lang, 2003a). In many low to middle income countries the development of neoliberal economies has focused on the growth of cash crops for export (Griffiths, 2003). In Latin America, the power of the supermarkets and fast food chains are changing the horticultural and agri-food systems of countries in the region, their supply chains, the face of local retailing and consumer behaviour (Chavez, 2002; Gutman, 2002; Reardon and Berdegué, 2002; Rodríguez et al., 2002).

Table 7.3   World top 30 food retailers, 2002

Rank	Company	Country	Turnover ($m)	No. countries	Foreign sales (%)	Ownership
1	Wal-Mart	US	180,787	10	17	Public
2	Carrefour	France	59,690	26	48	Public
3	Kroger	US	49,000	1	0	Public
4	Metro	Germany	42,733	22	42	Public/family
5	Ahold	NL	41,251	23	83	Public
6	Albertson's	US	36,762	1	0	Public
7	Rewe	Germany	34,685	10	19	Co-operative
8	Ito, Yokado (incl. Seven Eleven)	Japan	32,713	19	33	Public
9	Safeway Inc.	US	31,977	3	11	Public
10	Tesco	UK	31,812	9	13	Public
11	Costco	US	31,621	7	19	Public
12	ITM (incl. Spar)	France	30,685	9	36	Co-operative
13	Aldi	Germany	28,796	11	37	Private
14	Edeka (incl. AVA)	Germany	28,775	7	2	Co-operative
15	Sainsbury	UK	25,683	2	16	Public/family
16	Tengelmann (incl. A&P)	Germany	25,148	12	49	Private/family
17	Auchan	France	21,642	14	39	Private/family
18	Leclerc	France	21,468	5	3	Co-operative
19	Daiei	Japan	18,373	1	0	Public
20	Casino	France	17,238	11	24	Public
21	Delhaize	Belgium	16,784	11	84	Public
22	Lidl & Schwartz	Germany	16,092	13	25	Private
23	AEON (formerly Jusco)	Japan	15,060	8	11	Public
24	Publix	US	14,575	1	0	Private
25	Coles Myer	Australia	14,061	2	1	Public
26	Winn Dixie	US	13,698	1	0	Public
27	Loblaws	Canada	13,548	1	0	Public
28	Safeway plc	UK	12,357	2	3	Public
29	Lawson	Japan	11,831	2	1	Public
30	Marks & Spencer	UK	11,692	22	18	Public
	TOTAL		**930,537**			

Source: IGD (2002)

The World Bank and others have encouraged low income countries to jettison long-held commitments to national self-reliance and to specialise and buy on world markets to meet food needs, with cash and markets forming the new policy definition of food security (Lang, 2003b). This allows wealthy consumer societies to source elements of their diet globally. But for less affluent consumers or countries, cheap food for the consumer in high income countries does not necessarily equate with fair prices for the producer. The new policy regime is risky (Watkins, 2002) as the world market for stable goods such as maize or rice is subject to fluctuations. Local subsistence agriculture has acted as the bulwark against famine or want. A shortage of food followed by a famine indicates the emerging problems, such as in Lesotho in 2000–02. This was compounded by the weather but aggravated by the fact that the World Bank had pursued a policy of encouraging the growing of potatoes as a cash crop for export to South Africa. The collapse of the export market resulted in money not being available to buy goods and the shift from growing of maize as a subsistence crop meant there was little to fall back on. This is a feature of famines across the globe, where the issue is not always the lack of food but the lack of entitlement to that food (Watkins, 2002).

Sen (1981) the Nobel Laureate and economist argued that local production is not the key issue. Famines occur despite plenty, and in the face of demand. The key variable, he argued, is entitlement, a notion he used to explain culturally embedded rights and expectations. A famine is a deficiency that occurs when a society allows some to go without, as opposed to there not being enough food to eat. This is an important distinction as in the old global order the nation states had some commitment to their citizens by ensuring entitlement, however this was manifested, in food welfare schemes (Riches, 1997). The new order owes no such allegiance and the reaction by the public health community often suggests that famines are new phenomena as opposed to age-old occurrences influenced by environmental conditions and by political expectations, the structure of markets and the state of global trade (Davis, 2001).

Regulation of global food supply chains

Trade is a key influence of the food supply chain and its impact on inequalities. World history suggests richer countries use others as their grain store; this applied as much to ancient Rome as it did to the British Empire. The logic is the pursuit of cheaper land and labour, not just better climates. The modern world, however, is entering new policy arenas with the agreement by national governments of a commitment to globalise food trade, or more specifically to reduce protection and import tariffs. Since the 1994 General Agreement on Tariffs and Trade (GATT), nation states have signed up to the neoliberal experiment that market rigours will yield improved food security. The case for high subsidies supporting uneconomic production is now widely agreed to be unwarranted. In the early 2000s, President George W. Bush reversed Americas' commitments when he hugely increased farm support for US farmers. This became a subject of heated exchange and contributed to the collapse of the World Trade talks at Cancun, Mexico in 2003 (Rice et al., 2003).

Key issues of citizen consumer rights to food and State responsibilities to ensure its availability are at stake. It is not sufficient that an individual country has an adequate food supply, it must look at the way it sources its food and if it is self-sufficient in food production, the way it exports its surplus. Australia with a population of 18 million grows enough to feed 60 million people (Bawden, 1999). For many items it is self-sufficient and could be seen to be a model of agricultural prudence. The consequences of this surplus are three hidden impacts. The first is the impact of intensified food production systems in the vast amounts of once arable land now laid barren by loss of top soil and salinity problems, and waterways and rivers polluted by toxic algal bloom produced by fertiliser run off (Coveney, 2000). The second is the impact on the internal communities in Australia where the intensification of agriculture has meant that remote rural and aboriginal communities are dependent on food being brought to them at a price. The third impact is on the economies receiving the exported. Australian food exported to South East Asia displaces rather than supplement local food production. The globalising effects of Australian food production and export have far-reaching effects on the local economies of Asian countries (Caraher and Coveney, 2004).

The number of people directly working on the land worldwide is declining as a proportion of the total labour force, this is accompanied by a concentration of power into the hands of a relatively few companies off the land. Nestle (2002) contends that 80 per cent of the US food dollar, the sum paid by end consumers, goes to categories other than the farm value of the food itself. As food systems get more complex and value is added to the food so that variations emerge in who makes money from food, the farmers' percentage declines as the processors and retailers rise. This is a situation repeated globally. The pressure is on processors to use cheap, readily available ingredients and to add value where possible. This more complex picture of the new food economy contrasts with the more ideological claims that food liberalisation will automatically bring benefits to the grower of cash crops. In reality nearly 80 per cent of food expenditure goes on the alleged added value to the food itself such as processing, packaging, transport, advertising and taxes. In addition, the growers and producers of healthy foodstuffs are less likely to receive their fair share of the retail cost of the food. The producers of foods such as beef receive 50–60 per cent of the retail cost of the food as opposed to vegetable producers who receive as little as 5 per cent.

Transnational corporations (TNCs) account for 70 per cent of total world trade in all goods, not just food. Of those TNCs, the top 350 account for around 40 per cent. In food, such power had emerged by the 1970s, according to early research by the now abolished United Nations Centre on Transnational Corporations (Sen, 1981). Since then, already high levels of concentration increased throughout the food system, not just among processors. Much of this is hidden from consumers who may recognise product brand giants such as Nestle or Kellogg but will rarely be aware of Cargill, which is a family-owned commodity trader that by the early 1990s had 60 per cent of world cereal trade (Lang and Hines, 1993). Low income countries encouraged to specialise, and to export to generate cash have been put into a trade double bind. The biggest five corporations control 77 per cent of the cereals trade; the biggest three have 80 per cent of the banana market; the biggest three have 83 per cent of cocoa; the biggest three have 85 per cent of the tea trade (Vorley, 2003).

Implications for health promotion

There are two ways of interpreting the global epidemiological diet and health data. One is that marginal improvements have been won by a health promotion effort that was poorly funded, and that thus health promotion deserves more not less resources. The other is that so drastic are the needed changes in diet-linked health indicators that health promotion cannot possibly succeed in tackling the complex determinants of food-related morbidity and mortality.

The financial wealth of individual countries or blocks of countries is not totally within the control of national governments (Labonte, 2003). The emerging dual system of governance, State and Corporate, means that health promotion is increasingly influenced by corporate behaviour, product development, marketing, branding, corporate social responsibility initiatives established outside national parameters. National governments might find commitments to health education programmes convenient because the onus is on consumers to improve their diets, without them having to place upstream pressure on food companies marketing unhealthy processed products and threatening the relationship between political parties and the companies who may be large contributors to their funds (Nestle, 2002).

What is required however is a radical approach that targets food itself, its production and trade links (Bettcher et al., 2000; Hertz, 2001; Ollila, 2003). As Coveney (1990) has noted, there is a need to understand the pre-swallowing health issues of food, its production, transport and distribution, as well as the post-swallowing aspects, nutrition and diet-related diseases. It is the latter that has traditionally received the attention of health promotion practice, whereas the diverse nature of the global food system provides potentially confounding problems of complexity that health promotion must engage with, including issues of governance. When changes in lifestyles are directly influenced by huge investment in food advertising, health promotion with limited funds will struggle to have any impact. Despite these resource inequalities, an optimistic scenario can be drawn. The sudden awareness and debate about obesity is an indication of changing agendas. After years of food industry arguments about obesity being a lifestyle choice or a matter for personal responsibility, the enormity of the health challenge has been recognised globally, resulting in new health promotion initiatives, such as the debate about television food advertising directed at children. Other worrying trends in food supply and their impact on human and ecological health are also policy opportunities. Target areas include insecure water supply, climate change, rising meat consumption's demand for animal feedstuffs (Lang and Heasman, 2004).

A critical question for health promotion is whether it should be advocating for health against the excesses of the food supply chain and associated marketing and information. In a world where the largest fast foodservice company expends over US $1.5 billion on global marketing, it is difficult for health promotion to compete with the resources and the creativity applied to the food industry's advertising and marketing. In the UK, for instance, one soft drink manufacturer spent £23 million on advertising in 2002, about ten times the entire national nutrition budget on food and health (Lang, 2003a). Between January and July 2003, a leading crisp and snack manufacturer spent on advertising around five times the annual food budgets of the leading consumer advocacy groups in the UK, heavily targeting the after-school eating market.

Campaigns about food and health have shown that consumers see food as a public good, expecting it to be safe and nutritious. Food is both a public good in that it contributes to the health of a population and also a private good in that it is subject to the law of supply and demand. The notion of rights is likely to continue to be important in food and health thinking. But unless ordinary consumers own this right, it remains legalistic and abstract (Lang and Heasman, 2004). The entitlement to food occupies both the realms of citizenship, where communities have a right to an adequate amount of safe wholesome food; and at the same time food is a consumer good where the entitlement may be mediated by trade and financial rights (Sen, 1981).

Governments and corporations regulate the food supply chain within regionalising and globalising supply and value chains. This poses difficulties for health promotion. Largely funded by and a creation of government, health promotion has entered into partnerships with companies to try to bridge this regulatory divide. Yet, it is governments and states that have the ultimate capacity to change how the supply chain works. Contracts and specifications are the new regulators of standards, but the State dictates the framework in which they operate. Of course, companies can have budgets, resources and influence greater than national governments, but health promotion as an arm of the State has an integrity and vision that has considerable potential.

The notions of public goods and citizenship within public health are likely to become important for health action (Smith et al., 2003). An indication of this is the heated debate about the liberalisation of service industry regimes in healthcare at the World Trade Organisation 2000–03, the General Agreement on Trade in Services (GATS). The GATS proposals were largely framed to benefit service corporations but the opposition was centred on a re-assertion of the public or civic nature of rights and services (Lee et al., 2002). Health promotion, in this respect, takes an ethical position.

But is health promotion in a strong enough situation to argue such cases? Is its weakness a symbol of a wider weakness of public health movements? In the late twentieth century, public health did tend to be marginalised by macro-economic restructuring. Partly, this was due to faulty models, but also to lack of political influence. The current emphasis and language in health promotion is on capacity building, but there is a danger that this approach places responsibility on local communities and at risk to protect themselves. A central flaw in this approach is its reliance on consumer power. This can be effective, but consumers are notoriously fissiparous and fragmented. It might be more fruitful to consider health promotion as advocating the health of citizens, rather than consumers (Gabriel and Lang, 1995).

Health citizenship requires a commitment to enhance citizens' representation. Already there are some important tussles to democratise global food governance. One such is the Codex Alimentarius Commission, the UN's food standards forum. Given a more central role by the 1994 GATT, Codex lacked full accountability. Consumer groups have campaigned hard to improve its transparency and to rein back the influence of corporate powers (Lang and Hines, 1993; Lee et al., 2002).

There have been powerful calls for health promotion to recover some of its fundamental principles (Baum, 2002). This means reconsidering the Ottawa Charter as a mandate for progressive health improvements (World Health Organisation, 1986). The platform provided by the original Ottawa Charter has been built on progressively with international conferences, such as those in Adelaide (1988), Sundsvall (1991) and Jakarta (1997). Throughout this time, several key principles aimed at lifting the health status of people, improving their quality of life, and providing cost-effective solutions to tackling health problems, have been clarified (see Chapter 1 of this book for further details on Ottawa). Some authors in this text argue for public–private partnerships for health promotion (see, for example, Part I, Chapter 4) but these do not always lead to positive public health outcomes when the partnerships are with food corporations. A recent review of marketing partnerships between food companies and health associations and charities in the UK found that overall benefits to consumers were often dubious, that previously good reputations of health organisations were often sullied, and that public health benefits were frequently limited (Food Commission, 2002). Nestle's description of industry–professional relationships in the US highlights numerous difficulties with partnerships with the food industry (Nestle, 2002). Strong links with food industry dented the reputation and credibility of the American Dietetic Association, a professional association with over 70,000 members. In Australia, industry partnerships have created a division within the Dieticians' Association of Australia, with some senior members resigning (Correy, 2001). So while the financial advantages of industry sponsorship of health promotion and health professional activity may seem attractive to those trying to achieve food-related health goals, there are associated difficulties. Health promotion, and health promoters, should never lose sight of the primary responsibility of advancing public health through socially just and publicly accountable means.

Food and health policy suggests that health promotion's policy terrain can be fraught and delicate but that there are grounds for optimism. A way forward is to acknowledge the wider context of health promotion and to get back to basics, for example by reviewing practice in relation to the original five principles in the Ottawa Charter, as suggested earlier. These stressed the importance of settings and the role of health promotion as a key investment and essential element of social and economic development. If, as has been suggested, the food supply chain has rapidly concentrated, transnationalised and increased in power, the ground on which health promoters work has been reconfigured. Careful thought is needed. Health promoters need to be advocates for health in and on that process; this is ripe with tensions but rich in possibilities (Barber, 1995).

References

Barber, B. (1995) *Jihad vs. McWorld: How The Planet is Both Falling Apart and Coming Together And What This Means for Democracy.* New York: Times Books.

Barling. D., Lang, T. and Caraher, M. (2001) Food, social policy and the environment: towards a new model. *Social Policy and Administration*, **35** (5): 538–58.

Baum, F. (2002) *The New Public Health: An Australian Perspective* (2nd edn). Oxford: Oxford University Press.

Bawden, R. (1999) Eating into the environment. Paper presented at the conference, Eating into the Future, Adelaide, Australia. http://pandora.nla.gov.au/tep/10511

Bettcher, D., Yach, D. and Guindon, G.E. (2000) Global trade and health: key linkages and future challenges. *Bulletin of the World Health Organisation*, **78** (40): 521–34.

Bové, J. and Dufour, F. (2001) *The World Is Not For Sale: Farmers Against Junk Food.* London: Verso.

Brunner, E., Cohen, D. and Toon, L. (2001) Cost effectiveness of cardiovascular disease prevention strategies: a perspective on EU food-based dietary guidelines. *Public Health Nutrition*, **4** (2B): 711–15.

Caballero, B. and Popkin, B. (2002) *The Nutrition Transition: Diet and Disease in the Developing World.* London: Academic Press.

Caraher, M. and Coveney, J. (2004) Public health nutrition and food policy. *Public Health Nutrition*, **7** (5): 591–8.

Chavez, M. (2002) The Transformation of Mexican retailing with NAFTA. *Policy Development Review*, **20** (4): 503–14.

Correy, S. (2001) Australian Broadcasting Commission, Radio National, Background Briefing, Drugs or Dinner? http://www.abc.net.au/rn/talks/bbing/stories/s381313.htm

Coveney, J. (1990) Towards 2000 – planning the dietetic odyssey. *Dietitians Association of Australia National Conference Proceedings*, No9.: 33–36, Melbourne: Dietitians Association of Australia.

Coveney, J. (2000) Food security and sustainability: Are we selling ourselves short? *Asia Pacific Journal of Clinical Nutrition*, **9**: S97–S100.

Dahlgren, G. and Whitehead, M. (1992) *Polices and Strategies to Promote Equity in Health.* Copenhagen: WHO.

Davis, M. (2001) *Late Victorian Holocausts: El Niño Famines and the Making of the Third World.* London: Verso.

Dowler, E., Turner, S. and Dobson, B. (2002) *Poverty Bites.* Child Poverty Action Group: London.

Dowler, E. and Rushton, C. (1993) *Diet and Poverty in the UK.* London: Centre for Human Nutrition, University College London.

Food and Agriculture Organisation (1999) *Enabling development. Policy Issues Agenda item no 4.* Rome: Food and Agriculture Organisation.

Food Commission (2002) *Cause or compromise? A survey into marketing partnerships between food companies and health charities or medial associations.* London: Food Commission.

Gabriel, Y. and Lang, T. (1995) *The Unmanageable Consumer.* London: Sage.

Gardner, G. and Halweil, B. (2000) *Underfed and Overfed: The Global Epidemic of Malnutrition.* Worldwatch paper 150. Washington DC: Worldwatch Institute.

Garnett, T. (2003) *Wise Moves*. London: Transport2000/Department for Transport.

Grievink, J.W. (2003) The changing face of the global food supply chain. Paper presented at OECD Conference on Changing Dimensions of the Food Economy, The Hague, 6–7 February. Paris: Organisation for Economic Co-operation and Development.

Griffiths, P. (2003) *The Economist's Tale: A Consultant Encounters Hunger and the World Bank*. London: Zed Books.

Gutman, G.E. (2002) Impact of the rapid rise of supermarkets on dairy products. *Policy Development Review*, **20** (4): 409–28.

Hertz, N. (2001) *The Silent Takeover: Global Capitalism and the Death of Democracy*. London: Heinemann.

Institute of Grocery Distribution (2001) *European Grocery Retailing*. Letchmore Heath, Herts: Institute of Grocery Distribution.

Institute of Grocery Distribution (2002) *Global Grocery Retailing*. Letchmore Heath, Herts: Institute of Grocery Distribution.

Kranendonk, S. and Bringezau, B. (1994) *Major Material Flows Associated with Orange Juice Consumption in Germany*. Wupperthal, Germany: Wupperthal Institute.

Labonte, R. (1998) Healthy public policy and the World Trade Organisation: a proposal for an international health presence in future world trade/investment talks. *Health Promotion International*, **13** (3): 245–56.

Labonte, R. (2003) *Dying For Trade: Why Globalisation Can Be Bad for Our Health*. Toronto: The CSJ Foundation for Research and Education.

Lang, T. (2003a) Food Wars: the modern drama of consumer sovereignty. Economic and Social Research Council Cultures of Consumption lecture. London: Royal Society, 17 November. www.esrcConsume.bbk.ac.uk

Lang, T. (2003b) Food industrialisation and food power, *Development Policy Review*, **21** (5): 30–39.

Lang, T. and Caraher, M. (2001) International public health. In Pencheon, D., Guest C., Melzer, D. and Muir Gray, J. (eds) *Oxford Handbook of Public Health Practice*. Oxford: Oxford University Press.

Lang, T. and Heasman, M. (2004) *Food Wars*. London: Earthscan.

Lang, T. and Hines, T. (1993) *The New protectionism: Protecting the Future Against Free Trade*. London: Earthscan.

Lee, K., Buse, K. and Fustukian, S. (2002) *Health Policy in a Globalising World*. Cambridge: Cambridge University Press.

Millstone, E. and Lang, T. (2003) *The Atlas of Food*. London: Earthscan.

Nestle, M. (2002) *Food Politics: How The Food Industry Influences Nutrition And Health*. California: California State University Press.

Norman, A. (1999) *Slam-dunking Wal-Mart!* New Jersey: Raphel Marketing.

Ollila, E. (2003) Global health-related public private partnerships and the United Nations. Helsinki: Globalism and Social Policy Programme. Also available on the Globalism and Social Policy Programme Website www.gasp.org.

Popkin, B. (1998) The nutrition transition and its health implications in lower-income countries. *Public Health Nutrition*, **1** (1): 5–21.

Reardon, T. and Berdegué, J.A. (2002) The rapid rise of supermarkets in Latin America: challenges and opportunities for development. *Policy Development Review*, **20** (4): 371–88.

Rice, T., Green, D., Wiggerthale, M. and Reichert, T. (2003) *Post-Cancun Reflections on Agriculture. Policy Recommendations*. London: Action Aid/CAFOD/ Germanwatch/WWF.

Riches, G. (ed.) (1997) *First World Hunger: Food Security and Welfare Politics*. Basingstoke: Macmillan Press.

Rodríguez, E., Berges, M., Casellas, K., Di Paola, R., Lupín, B., Garrido, L. and Gentile, N. (2002) Consumer behaviour and supermarkets in Argentina. *Policy Development Review*, **20** (4): 429–40.

Runge, C.F., Senauer, B., Pardey, P.G. and Rosegrant, M.W. (2003) *Ending Hunger in Our Lifetime: Food security and Globalisation*. Baltimore: John Hopkins University Press.

Sen, A. (1981) *Poverty and Famines: An Essay on Entitlement and Deprivation*. Oxford: Oxford University Press.

Smith, R., Beaglehole, R. and Woodward, D. (eds) (2003) *Global Public Goods for Health*. Oxford: Oxford University Press.

UNICEF. (1996) *Food, Health and Care: the UNICEF Vision and Strategy for a World Free from Hunger and Malnutrition*. New York: United Nations Children's Fund.

United Nations Centre on Transnational Corporations (1981) *Transnational Corporations in Food and Beverage Processing*. New York: United Nations.

Vorley, B. (2003) *Food, Inc., Corporate Concentration from Farm to Consumer*. London: UK Food Group.

Watkins, K. (2002) *Rigged Rules and Double Standards: Trade, Globalisation, and the Fight Against Poverty*. Oxford: Oxfam International.

Wilkinson, R. (1996) *Unhealthy Societies: The Afflictions of Inequality*. London: Routledge.

World Bank (2003) http://www.developmentgoals.org/Poverty.htm

World Cancer Research Fund (WCRF) in association with American Institute for Cancer Research (1997) *Food, Nutrition and the Prevention of Cancer: a Global Perspective*. Washington DC: World Cancer Research Fund/American Institute for Cancer Research.

World Health Organisation (1986) Ottawa Charter for Health Promotion. *Health Promotion*, **1** (4): i–v.

World Health Organisation (2000a) *Nutrition for Health and Development, A Global Agenda For Combating Malnutrition*. Geneva: WHO.

World Health Organisation (2000b) *Food and Nutrition Action Plan for Europe*, August 2000. Copenhagen: WHO European Regional Office.

CHAPTER 8

Tobacco: The Global Challenge for Health Promotion

SAMIRA ASMA, PRAKASH GUPTA AND CHARLES W. WARREN

Tobacco use is one of the major causes of premature disease and death and is an emerging detriment to world economic progress. There are billions of smokers worldwide and by 2030 it is estimated that another billion young adults will have started to smoke (Peto and Lopez, 2000). If current smoking patterns persist, the annual number of tobacco related deaths worldwide will rise from a current 4.9 million to more than ten million deaths a year by 2030 (Peto and Lopez, 2000). More than seven million of these deaths are projected to occur in the low and middle income countries that cannot afford the costly health consequences of tobacco use (Peto and Lopez, 2000; see also Chapter 9 of this text). Effective health promotion strategies exist to prevent tobacco use, and low, middle and high income countries could put these strategies in place (Jha and Chaloupka, 2000). The challenge is to translate these strategies into practical actions to build effective and sustainable health promotion programmes.

Patterns of tobacco use

Data from the Global Youth Tobacco Survey (GYTS) suggests that one out of ten children in the world has smoked their first cigarette by the age of ten. The estimated prevalence of tobacco use among school children aged 13–15 ranges throughout the world from 10 per cent to as high as 60 per cent (GYTS Collaborating Group, 2002).

The global prevalence of tobacco use among adults is estimated to be 29 per cent and rising (Peto and Lopez, 2000). It is still much higher among men, at 47 per cent as compared to 12 per cent among women in high income countries and 48 per cent of men and 7 per cent of women in low and middle income countries (Jha and Chaloupka, 2000). The difference in smoking prevalence among the WHO regions is great, especially among women. The highest prevalence of smoking is 60 per cent in males in the Western Pacific Region; about 30 to 40 per cent of males smoke in other regions. The highest prevalence of smoking in females is in the Americas and Europe where over 20 per cent of women are regular smokers. In the Asian and Eastern

Mediterranean regions the prevalence of smoking in females is lower, at about 4 per cent (World Health Organisation, 1997).

Though fewer women than men are smokers, an increasing number of young women are taking up cigarettes. It is estimated that the number of women smokers will triple over the next generation (World Health Organisation, 1997). Already, recent evidence points to an alarming increase in smoking rates among women (US Department of Health and Human Services, 2001; World Health Organisation, 2001). The latest report from the GYTS shows that on average, 15 per cent of boys and over 6 per cent of girls aged 13–15 worldwide smoke cigarettes (GYTS Collaborating Group, 2003).

This recent GYTS report (GYTS Collaborating Group, 2003) shows smoking among both boys and girls was highest in Europe, with over a third of the boys and 29 per cent of the girls reporting they are current smokers. The lowest rate for boys was in the African region, at 10.4 per cent. For girls, Southeast Asia had the lowest rate, at just over 3 per cent. The GYTS report also spotlighted a very disturbing trend. The survey found that the traditional gap in cigarette smoking rates between girls and boys is narrowing in most regions of the world. In over half the sites included in the survey, the data showed no gender difference in cigarette smoking. The report also showed that girls and boys are using non-cigarette tobacco products, including spit tobacco, bidis and water pipes, at similar rates, and that these rates are often as high as or higher than cigarette smoking rates (GYTS Collaborating Group, 2003). Given the GYTS results, it is very possible the estimates of future deaths and disease from tobacco use are an undercount. If the gender gap in smoking continues to narrow as shown in the GYTS data, then more adult women than originally estimated may well drive up tobacco morbidity and mortality statistics in the years ahead (GYTS Collaborating Group, 2003).

The growing percentage of girls smoking may be due in part to the tobacco industry's efforts to target women in the low and middle income countries. These efforts include focused marketing tactics aimed at women and girls by linking smoking to independence and glamour, promoting false images of health, fitness and beauty, and producing products specifically for women, by advertising directly to the female populations through fashion magazines and by sponsoring sport and fashion events for women (US Department of Health and Human Services, 2001). The main targets of the industry and associated marketing campaigns are women and young people (Brands and Yach, 2002). Tobacco companies have also consistently denied the adverse effects of tobacco, especially via passive smoking (Ong and Glantz, 2001; Yach and Bialous, 2001).

Health consequences of tobacco use

The health impact of tobacco use is widely known and established. Tobacco use is a known or probable cause of more than 25 specific diseases. Prolonged smoking causes many diseases in addition to lung cancer including other cancers and chronic respiratory and cardiovascular disease, in particular ischaemic heart disease. In populations where cigarette smoking has been common for several decades, about 90 per cent of lung cancer, 15–20 per cent of other cancers, 75 per cent of chronic bronchitis and emphysema, and 25 per cent of deaths from cardiovascular disease at ages 35–60 years are attributable to tobacco (Peto et al., 1994).

Exposure to secondary smoking is associated with lung cancer and ischaemic heart disease, and several other important health ailments in children such as sudden infant death syndrome, low birth weight, and children's respiratory disease (California Environmental Protection Agency, 1997; US Department of Health and Human Services, 2001).

Benefits of reducing tobacco use

Reduced smoking prevalence has been demonstrated to have a positive benefit on chronic disease morbidity and mortality. Studies have estimated that reduced smoking prevalence decreased the number of hospitalisations for acute myocardial infarctions (AMI) by nearly 1000 and the incidence of stroke by over 500 in the United States (Lightwood and Glantz, 1997). Reports from the US indicate that decreased smoking prevalence produces lower rates of lung cancer and mortality from heart disease (Fichtenberg and Glantz, 2000). The reasons for the decline in Cardio Vascular Diseases (CVD) mortality are complex and include improved management of high risk populations, particularly in the US, and in some countries, such as Finland, prevention programmes for reducing population risk levels in combination with other environmental changes (Beaglehole and Dobson, 2003).

The application of existing knowledge could have a major impact and cost-effective contribution to the prevention and control of the tobacco epidemic. Appropriate strategies do exist. However, their implementation is still at a very early stage in many low and middle income countries.

Health promotion strategies to prevent and reduce tobacco use

Strategies to prevent and reduce tobacco use are most effective when they are comprehensive in nature addressing four major goal areas: (i) preventing initiation of tobacco use among young people, (ii) promoting quitting among young people and adults, (iii) eliminating nonsmokers' exposure to second-hand smoke, and (iv) identifying and eliminating the disparities related to tobacco use and its effects among different population groups. The following is a brief review of selected intervention strategies targeting reduction of tobacco use, prevention of initiation and reducing environmental tobacco smoke. A combination of interventions, including bans on tobacco advertising, strong warnings on tobacco packages, controls on the use of tobacco in public indoor locations, high taxes on tobacco products, health education and tobacco use cessation programmes have the greatest chance for success. The success of tobacco control will be facilitated by monitoring the course of the tobacco epidemic through improved surveillance systems, challenging and changing the social norms regarding tobacco use and tobacco's role in society. Finally, international agencies play a major role in defining principles and goals, setting priorities for global tobacco control. The WHO Framework Convention on Tobacco Control (FCTC) is a major initiative engaging multi-sectors to respond to the global tobacco epidemic.

Although there are numerous strategies implemented throughout the world to address the tobacco epidemic, those that have been evaluated on the basis of effectiveness and feasibility have the greatest potential for being scaled up to encompass larger populations. Below is a brief summary of strategies with the greatest effectiveness. Surveillance systems to monitor the tobacco epidemic and tobacco control strategies remain the corner stone of a comprehensive strategy.

Taxation: Higher tobacco prices reduce the prevalence and consumption of tobacco products among adults, young adults and youth (The World Bank, 1999). Studies have reported that higher tobacco prices are associated with lower tobacco use. Cumulatively, price elasticity for tobacco product use was −0.41, meaning that a 10 per cent increase in the price of cigarettes would result in 4.1 per cent decline in tobacco use prevalence (The World Bank, 1999). Half of the decline is a result of people quitting and the other half is due to lower consumption among continuing smokers. Equally important is the effect of higher cigarette prices on revenues accruing to government to be used for tobacco use prevention programmes.

Comprehensive bans on advertising of tobacco products through legislation: One of the principal reasons for banning tobacco advertising is that it prevents marketing to young people, thereby reducing tobacco use initiation. Comprehensive legislation to ban tobacco advertising should include advertising in print, broadcasting and other mass media in public areas as well as at point of sale. The sponsorship of sports and other cultural events should also be forbidden, in addition to prohibiting the distribution of free promotional items (US Department of Health and Human Services, 1994, 2001).

Smoking bans and restrictions: Exposure to second hand smoke (SHS) can take place in homes, workplaces and public places. Policies that control smoking in public places, including workplaces, can be effective in reducing tobacco-related morbidity and mortality by reducing exposure to SHS, encouraging smokers to quit or to reduce tobacco consumption, and changing public perceptions of smoking as normative behaviour. Studies reporting on the impact of controlling smoke in public have shown that implementing a ban or restriction on public smoking resulted in a median relative reduction of 72 per cent of SHS components. Furthermore, reduced consumption of cigarettes was reported at a median absolute change of -1.2 cigarettes per day in response to bans or restrictions (Hopkins et al., 2001). With its mutual benefit of preventing second hand smoke and encouraging reduction of tobacco use, expanding smoke free public and workplaces is a defining programme for tobacco control.

Cessation assistance: Another component of a comprehensive tobacco control programme is cessation assistance by a trained healthcare provider. Studies have reported increased rates of quitting tobacco use when a provider is reminded to advise the patient to quit and the provider educates the patient on cessation. Quit Lines have also shown considerable effectiveness in facilitating cessation. Though an expensive intervention, Nicotine Replacement Therapy (NRT) has been shown to be an effective aid for quitting, but more effective are policies that help reduce out of pocket costs for patients for these cessation aids (Hopkins and Fielding, 2001).

Education for the public: In addition to healthcare provider education, mass media campaigns warning the public about the consequences of tobacco use have proved effective. Studies have reported a decline in initiation of tobacco use as well as a decrease in the number of tobacco products consumed due to mass media campaigns and when compared with groups not exposed (Hopkins and Fielding, 2001).

While each of these tobacco control strategies have been studied and reported as effective, their greatest effect is produced when they are implemented concurrently. By aiming for a decline in initiation of tobacco use, reduction of exposure to SHS, and increase in cessation, a comprehensive programme for tobacco control can produce the synergistic effect of reducing overall prevalence of tobacco use.

Global tobacco surveillance systems

The effectiveness of interventions to reduce the burden of the tobacco epidemic depends on the quality and timeliness of data. The World Health Organisation and the Centers for Disease Control and Prevention (CDC) are collaborators for the development and maintenance of a Global Tobacco Surveillance System (GTSS). The GTSS will function to improve the ability of countries to monitor the tobacco epidemic and to develop, implement and evaluate their own tobacco control programmes. The GTSS has the three components: The Global Youth Tobacco Survey, the Global School Personnel Survey, and the Global Health Professional Survey.

Table 8.1 Status of the Global Youth Tobacco Survey (GYTS) by WHO Regions, as of January 2004

WHO regions	Number of countries			
	Completed	In field	Preparing for field	Training planned
AFRO	27	2	3	14
AMRO	36	1	1	0
EMRO	17	4	1	0
EURO	19	7	3	0
SEARO	6	2	0	2
WPRO	15	2	1	10
Total	120	18	9	26

Note: In addition, repeat GYTS have been completed in 14 countries, 10 are in the field, and 11 are preparing for the field.

The Global Youth Tobacco Survey: GYTS captures tobacco related information on prevalence, access, exposure to second hand smoke, media and advertising exposure, cessation and school curriculum for youth. The GYTS was developed to provide systematic global surveillance of youth tobacco use. The GYTS provides data, which can be used by countries to evaluate their country specific tobacco control programme, monitor trends in global youth tobacco use and compare tobacco use among countries and regions (see Table 8.1 for further details on the global spread of GYTS).

The GYTS has, for the first time, documented a serious problem in youth tobacco use that is global in nature. The problem is of equal concern in developed and developing countries. Of the 120 countries and regions that have completed GYTS, not a single site had a prevalence rate of current *any tobacco use, current smoking*, or *other tobacco use* equal to zero. In addition, almost one in four students who ever smoked cigarettes smoked their first cigarette before the age of ten. Thus, future health consequences of tobacco use and dependency on tobacco appear to be a significant problem facing countries throughout the world. These findings suggest that immediate attention needs to be given to the development of both global and country specific tobacco control programmes.

The Global School Personnel Survey: GSPS collects information on tobacco use, knowledge and attitudes from adult school personnel. The objectives are to obtain baseline information on tobacco use by school personnel; evaluate the existence, implementation and enforcement of tobacco control policies in schools; understand personnel's knowledge about and attitudes toward tobacco control policies; and assess training and material requirements for implementing tobacco prevention and control interventions in the schools. Over 20 countries have completed the GSPS and two articles have been published (Sinha et al., 2002, 2003).

The Global Health Professional Survey: GHPS collects information on tobacco use, knowledge and attitudes regarding tobacco, and school curricula concerning instruction on harmful effects of tobacco from third year students attending medical, dental, nursing and pharmacy schools. The GHPSS is being pilot tested in each of the six WHO Regions during 2004.

These three surveillance systems have been developed using consistent survey designs and data processing methodologies. This consistency will allow changes over time to be monitored and programme effects to be measured in a standardised way across the countries, regions and the world. The GTSS is a successful example of monitoring tobacco use among youth and selected adult populations that will provide significant data to inform comprehensive global health promotion approaches employed against tobacco use.

Framework Convention on Tobacco Control (FCTC)

The Framework Convention on Tobacco Control (FCTC) is the first international treaty directed towards the control of tobacco use adopted after three years of negotiations (Taylor and Bettcher, 2000). Tobacco use is perhaps the only health problem that is being promoted by a powerful and rich global industry necessitating this approach. On 24 May 1999 the 191 member World Health Assembly, the governing body of the World Health Organisation unanimously adopted a resolution calling for work to begin on the FCTC.

The purpose of the FCTC is to block the advance of the tobacco problem and limit the spread of tobacco into new markets, empowering governments to resist the tobacco industry and put human life ahead of tobacco industry profits. The treaty aims to accomplish this by requiring countries within five years of ratification, unless constitutional barriers exist, to enact comprehensive legislation to restrict advertising, require a higher standard of health warnings on product packaging, reduce second hand smoke by prohibiting smoking in public places, raise tobacco taxes to increase prices, reduce cigarette smuggling and diversify agriculture away from tobacco (Taylor and Bettcher, 2000). The framing, enactment and enforcement of comprehensive laws in each country will engage a cross section of areas of governance: health, finance, trade, labour agriculture and social affairs.

The FCTC negotiations process has led to a coherent United Nations system-wide approach to tobacco control. The non governmental organisations played an important role by providing facts, science and expert support. Despite many hurdles health ministers from around the world made history on 21 May 2003 by adopting the FCTC. The process of signing and ratification is on going and at the time of writing 109 countries have signed and five countries have ratified the treaty (Lee, 2004). The treaty will become enforceable when 40 countries ratify it.

Resources

The challenge of responding to the global tobacco epidemic cannot be met without new, additional and sustained resources. There is a need for sustained national and global funding for tobacco control. Governments need to formulate active funding plans which should be supported by a sound process of priority setting for health promotion, prevention and treatment; effective systems for estimating the costs of these interventions and effective, transparent mechanisms for funding allocations and accountability, and monitoring and evaluating services and programmes.

The political commitment that emerged during the FCTC negotiations is helping to motivate the involvement of people from various walks of life and sectors of society. The pace for reversing the escalating tobacco epidemic is improving with existing knowledge for implementing strategies to prevent tobacco use coupled with a dynamic surveillance system and a strong international and national political commitment. The challenge is now to keep that momentum going and to capitalise on the many opportunities it provides. Sustained progress will occur when tobacco prevention and control strategies are scaled up with coherent and intensified investments at national and international levels. The approaches recommended in this chapter reflect a wealth of knowledge and experience gained through many years of efforts by people working at global, regional, national and community levels. The first steps in taking the strategy forward are for national health ministries, with the active participation of their health-sector partners, to examine planning for tobacco control. The way forward for the global tobacco control strategy is not easy. Nevertheless, globally there are many examples of real progress resulting from innovation and partnership, and lessons should be drawn from these initiatives.

References

Beaglehole, R. and Dobson, A. (2003) The contributions to change: risk factors and the potential for prevention. In Marmot, M. and Elliott, P. (eds) *Coronary Heart Disease Epidemiology* (2nd ed). Oxford: Oxford University Press.

Brands, A. and Yach, D. (2002) *Women and the Rapid Rise of Noncommunicable Diseases*. NMH reader no 1. Geneva: World Health Organisation.

California Environmental Protection Agency (1997) *Health Effects of Exposure to Environmental Tobacco Smoke – Final Report and Appendices*. Sacramento, CA: California Environmental Protection Agency, Office of Environmental Health Hazard Assessment.

Fichtenberg, C.M. and Glantz, S.A. (2000) Association of the California Tobacco Control Program with declines in cigarette consumption and mortality from heart disease. *New England Journal of Medicine*, **343**: 1772–77.

GYTS Collaborating Group (2002) Tobacco use among youth: a cross country comparison. *Tobacco Control*, **11**: 252–70.

GYTS Collaborating Group (2003) Differences in worldwide tobacco use by gender: findings from The Global Youth Tobacco Survey. *Journal of School Health,* August, **73**: 207–15.

Hopkins, D.P. and Fielding, J.E. (eds) (2001) The guide to community preventive services: tobacco use prevention and control. Reviews, recommendations, and expert commentary. *American Journal of Preventive Medicine,* **20** no. 2S.

Hopkins, D.P., Briss, P.A., Ricard, C.J., Husten, C.G., Carande-Kulis, V.G., Fielding, J.E., Aloa, M.O., McKenna, J.W., Sharp, D.J., Harris, J.R., Woollery, T.A. and Harris, W. (2001) Reviews of evidence regarding interventions to reduce tobacco use and exposure to environmental tobacco smoke. *American Journal of Preventive Medicine,* **20**(2S): 16–56.

Jha, P. and Chaloupka, F.J. (2000) *Tobacco Control in Developing Countries.* New York: Oxford University Press.

Lee, J.W. (2004) *Framework Convention on Tobacco Control* [Online] Available at *http://www.who.int/tobacco/fctc/en/*

Lightwood, J.M. and Glantz, S.A. (1997) Short term economic and health benefits of smoking cessation. *Circulation* **96**: 1089–96.

Ong, E.K. and Glantz, S.A. (2001) Constructing 'Sound Science' and 'Good Epidemiology': Tobacco lawyers and public relation firms. *American Journal of Public Health,* **91**: 1749–57.

Peto, R. and Lopez, A.D. (2000) The future worldwide health effects of current smoking patterns. In: Koop, E. C. and Schwarz, R. M. (eds) *Global Health in the 21st Century.* New York: Jossey-Bass.

Peto, R., Lopez, A.D., Boreham, J., Thun, M. and Heath, C.Jr. (1994) *Mortality from Smoking in Developed Countries 1950–2000: Indirect Estimates from National Vital Statistics.* Oxford: Oxford University Press.

Sinha, D.N., Gupta, P.C. and Pednekar, M. (2003). Tobacco use among school personnel in eight North-eastern states of India. *Indian Journal of Cancer.* **40**(1): 3–14.

Sinha, D.N., Gupta, P.C., Pednekar, M.S., Jones, J.T. and Warren C.W. (2002) Tobacco use among school personnel in Bihar, India. *Tobacco Control,* **11**: 82–83.

Taylor, A. and Bettcher, D. (2000) A WHO framework convention on tobacco control: a global public health good for health. *Bulletin of the World Health Organisation,* **78**: 920–29.

The World Bank (1999) *Curbing the Epidemic: Governments and the Economics of Tobacco Control.* Geneva: World Bank.

US Department of Health and Human Services (1994) *Preventing Tobacco Use. Report of the Surgeon General.* Rockville: US Department of Health and Human Services.

US Department of Health and Human Services (2001) *Women and Smoking: A Report of the Surgeon General.* Rockville: US Department of Health and Human Services, Public Health Service, Office of the Surgeon General.

World Health Organisation (1997) *Tobacco or Health: A Global Atlas Report.* Geneva: World Health Organisation.

World Health Organisation (2001) *Women and the Tobacco Epidemic: Challenges for the 21st Century.* Geneva: The World Health Organisation.

Yach, D. and Bialous, S.A. (2001) Junking science to promote tobacco. *American Journal Public Health,* **91**: 175–48.

CHAPTER 9

HIV/AIDS: Lessons for and from Health Promotion

PETER AGGLETON

In the space of 20 years, HIV/AIDS has grown from being something of a curiosity, supposedly affecting only minority communities such as injecting drug users, sex workers and gay men, to becoming the most serious pandemic the world has ever known. At the same time, it has moved from being something of an outside field within health promotion to being an issue from which others can learn. This chapter reviews these dual transitions, with a view to identifying where the future might lie.

At the end of the year 2003, UNAIDS and WHO (2003) estimated that approximately 40 million people were living with HIV/AIDS. Globally, HIV infected an estimated five million people in that same year, and three million people died as a result of AIDS. There continues to be no vaccine to protect against infection, and while anti-retroviral treatment offers hope to those who receive it, only a relatively small proportion of people globally are able to access the treatment drugs they need.

Against this backcloth, primary prevention remains of fundamental importance. Yet prevention efforts are frequently hampered by responses of stigma and denial. Nations, communities, households and individuals persist in denying that they are at risk. This makes facing up to the epidemic extremely difficult. There has also been something of a tendency for health promotion specialists to avoid engagement with the epidemic. Relatively few attend the biennial international or regional conferences on HIV/AIDS, and their voices remain muted in national fora where the epidemic is addressed.

Why is this, and how can we move beyond the present situation? Part of the problem stems from the fact that AIDS is sexually transmitted, and like all sexually transmitted infections (STIs), HIV carries with it connotations of wrong doing and shame. All over the world, individuals have been blamed for acquiring the virus and for infecting others. These negative responses have led to discrimination and the abuse of human rights: as individuals, their families and communities have been denied access to schooling, health services, freedom of movement, insurance and employment (Maluwa et al., 2003).

Importantly, the stigma and discrimination associated with the epidemic reinforces existing social inequalities. Thus, HIV/AIDS has reinforced racism through the view, common in Europe, that AIDS is a disease of Africa, as well as through the view, common in parts of Africa and Asia, that AIDS is a disease of Westerners. Likewise, HIV/AIDS has reinforced gender divisions. In some parts of the world, women are routinely blamed for transmitting HIV, whereas in other regions the finger is pointed at men. Divisions of sexuality have also been reinforced, with gay and other homosexually active men being held responsible for HIV/AIDS even in countries where the bulk of transmission occurs through unprotected heterosexual sex (Parker and Aggleton, 2003).

Clearly, therefore, the global epidemic of HIV/AIDS is as much a social as a biomedical phenomenon. This was pointed out nearly two decades ago when the late Jonathan Mann drew attention to the three epidemics associated with AIDS. The first is that of HIV infection, which enters a community largely unseen and un-noticed. The second is that of AIDS, which emerges typically some ten years later. The third is the epidemic of negative social responses to HIV/AIDS including stigmatisation, discrimination and denial (Mann, 1987).

So what can health promotion offer? And what can health promotion learn from success against the epidemic, nationally and internationally? Following an overview of the pattern and structure of the global epidemic, this chapter will offer a description of the different types or models of health promotion that have been brought to bear on the epidemic. It will describe the achievements of different frameworks for planning and delivering health promotion, as well as some of their limitations.

The global picture

Sub-Saharan Africa

To characterise HIV/AIDS as a global disaster or pandemic that has impacted evenly upon different nations and regions is misleading, in that it conceals the existence of numerous local epidemics, each with its own dynamics and growth characteristics. Without doubt, the hardest hit region of the world to date is sub-Saharan Africa, where some 25–28 million adults and children were living with HIV/AIDS at the end of 2003, and where there is an estimated mean prevalence among adults aged 15–49 of between 7.8–8.5 per cent. While a few countries have made progress when it comes to reducing the number of new infections, the overall picture is bleak, with prevalence rates of 16 per cent, 20 per cent and even 40 per cent being reported among pregnant women in Malawi (Blantyre), Zambia (Lusaka) and Botswana (Gaborone) respectively (UNAIDS and WHO, 2003).

Uganda, Senegal, Zambia and Rwanda are countries where there is evidence of some headway being made against the epidemic. HIV prevalence fell to 8 per cent in Kampala, Uganda in 2002, in contrast to a prevalence among pregnant women in two urban antenatal clinics in the city of 30 per cent a decade ago. In Senegal, sustained prevention programmes have stabilised HIV prevalence among pregnant women at around 1 per cent since 1990, with these levels holding fast through 2002, but HIV prevalence among sex workers has increased slowly over the past decade. And in Kigali, Rwanda the proportion of pregnant women found to be HIV positive in antenatal clinic sites has fallen to 13 per cent from a high of almost 35 per cent in 1993 (UNAIDS and WHO, 2003).

Asia and the Pacific

HIV infected over one million people in Asia and the Pacific in 2003, and an estimated 7.4 million people are now living with HIV/AIDS in this part of the world. Asia contains some of the most populous nations on earth. Among them are India and China. Although national adult HIV prevalence in India is currently below 1 per cent, the total estimated number of people living with HIV/AIDS in India was estimated at between 3.82 and 4.58 million by the end of 2002.

Injecting drug use and sex work is common in some Asian countries. As a result, countries with currently low infection levels could see epidemics surge suddenly. In parts of China, for example, high rates of HIV prevalence have been found among injecting drug users, 35 to 80 per cent in Xinjiang and 20 per cent in Guangdong, while a severe HIV epidemic affected communities where unsafe blood collection practices occurred in the 1990s (UNAIDS and WHO, 2003).

With effort, some countries in Asia and the Pacific have been able to bring their national epidemics under control. They include Thailand, Australia and Cambodia. In Cambodia, adult HIV prevalence has remained stable at about 3 per cent since 1997, thanks to broad-based efforts to control the epidemic. In Thailand, the vigorous promotion of condoms in sex work has done much to control the domestic epidemic, whereas in Australia pragmatic, broad-based programming and the involvement of heavily affected communities (gay men, injecting drug users and sex workers) has made significant progress against HIV/AIDS.

Having said this, there are rapidly developing epidemics of HIV/AIDS in countries such as Indonesia and Papua New Guinea, and there is evidence too from both Thailand and Australia that prevention approaches that worked well in the past may need to be re-invigorated, if lasting effects are to be obtained.

The Americas

More than two million people are living with HIV/AIDS in Latin America and the Caribbean, including the estimated 200,000 that contracted HIV in the past year. At least 100,000 people died of AIDS in the same period, the highest regional death toll after sub-Saharan Africa and Asia. HIV/AIDS has a national prevalence of at least 1 per cent in 12 countries, all of them in the Caribbean. HIV prevalence among pregnant women has reached or exceeded 2 per cent in six of them: the Bahamas, Belize, the Dominican Republic, Guyana, Haiti, and Trinidad and Tobago (UNAIDS and WHO, 2003).

All the main modes of transmission exist in most. In the Caribbean, heterosexual transmission predominates, but elsewhere in Latin America, sex between men is a major cause, accounting for some 50 per cent of AIDS cases in Mexico and 40 per cent of cases in Brazil and the Southern Cone. In the US, the epidemic remains largely uncontrolled. The US Centers for Disease Control estimates that between 850,000 and 950,000 US citizens are currently living with HIV, and a quarter of these remain unaware of their infection. An estimated 40,000 new HIV infections continue to occur in the US each year, of which African Americans account for more than half, 55 per cent (Centers for Disease Control, 2003).

Having said this, there are signs of prevention success in countries such as Brazil, where strong political support, sustained investment in prevention and care, NGO and civil society involvement, support for human rights, and the promotion of treatment drug access, are key factors underpinning this success (Centro Brasileiro de Estudos de Saude, 2003; UNAIDS and WHO, 2003).

Europe and Central Asia

Europe presents a mixed pattern when it comes to understanding the nature and impact of the epidemic. In Western Europe, deaths as a result of AIDS are steadily declining under the impact of anti-retroviral therapy, yet at the same time there is evidence that prevention activities in several high income countries are not keeping pace with treatment advance. The resurgence of other sexually transmitted infections, however, points to a revival of high-risk sexual behaviour. In England and Wales, for example, diagnoses of gonorrhea at sexually transmitted infection clinics rose by 102 per cent between 1995 and 2000, with the steepest increases occurring among young people aged 16–19. Reported gonorrhea cases have also increased in the Netherlands, Sweden and Switzerland (UNAIDS and WHO, 2003).

In Eastern Europe and Central Asia, over 230,000 people became infected with HIV in 2003. Approximately one million people aged 15 to 49 are living with HIV/AIDS in the Russian Federation. In this part of the world, HIV transmission is facilitated by widespread injecting drug use and unsafe sex, especially among young people. Recent estimates suggest that there are as many as three million injecting drug users in the Russian Federation alone, more than 600,000 in Ukraine and up to 200,000 in Kazakhstan. Most are male and many are very young. The use of unclean injecting equipment, together with unprotected sex, is the main means of transmission (UNAIDS and WHO, 2003).

Health promotion and HIV/AIDS

Internationally, there exist a variety of frameworks or models within which health promotion and HIV/AIDS can be carried out. Four of these, distinguished relatively early on in the epidemic, have their counterparts in more general approaches to the promotion of health and wellbeing. These have been described as (i) behaviour change (ii) empowerment (iii) community-oriented and (iv) socially transformatory models respectively (Homans and Aggleton, 1987; Aggleton, 1989, 1993). While the first two focus largely upon the individual, seeking to bring about changes in behaviour or feelings of self-empowerment respectively, the latter two emphasise the role of community and broader social structures in the determination of health.

The first two models will be familiar to perhaps everyone involved in health promotion and health education about HIV/AIDS. The *behaviour change model*, in particular, sees the origins of the epidemic as lying within the risky behaviours of individuals: behaviours that have to be changed in order to manage the epidemic and bring it under control. It is the model that, in the US, has given rise to the study of interventions for prevention: actions to increase the knowledge, skills and self-efficacy of groups with respect to condom use, for example, or the use of clean syringes and needles. It is also the model that largely sees individuals as possessing deficits to be corrected through public health intervention.

Empowerment models, on the other hand, can be of varying types. Many focus upon the individual, and her or his capacity to see clearly and take control in sometimes, difficult circumstances. Approaches to safer sex education that have emphasised communication and negotiation, expressing one's feelings and exploring the possibilities for change, fall within such an approach, as do certain forms of counselling where the emphasis is on the development of self-understanding and self-growth. Gay men, for example, have been encouraged through group work to examine the extent to which self-understanding and sometimes self-damaging behaviours may be motivated by early experiences of rejection and abuse. Similar approaches have been utilised with injecting drug users as part of psychotherapeutic and other traditions.

Community-oriented models move away from the idea that health is largely a matter of individuals and their behaviour. Instead, the emphasis is placed on groups, group norms and community structures. Community-oriented approaches seek to utilise the resources that exist within communities, and the degree of connectedness between community members, to achieve desired goals. Within the field of HIV/AIDS-related health promotion, such approaches have been used to effect within the gay communities of cities such as Sydney, London and New York. They have also influenced outreach and community development work undertaken with sex workers and injecting drug users.

Socially transformatory models of HIV/AIDS-related health promotion argue that far reaching social change is needed if HIV/AIDS is to be controlled and affected communities supported in ways that promote social justice. Divisive ideologies of race, class, age, gender and sexuality, through which the epidemic is constructed and reproduced, must be challenged if stigmatisation and discrimination are to be reduced, and human rights upheld. Such approaches have informed the actions of groups all over the world working to challenge the racism, sexism and homophobia the epidemic has triggered. They have also informed the agendas of grass roots organisations campaigning for treatment drug access.

Models in action

Before examining how different models of health promotion have informed actions against the epidemic, a word of caution is necessary. Within the field of HIV/AIDS, as in other areas of health promotion, actions, programmes and interventions are rarely planned with one particular theoretical framework in mind. More usually, they arise as national and local responses to pressing needs and are frequently mixed mode, both in their structure and in their method of delivery. While, after the event, it may be possible to construe actions as having been influenced by a particular theoretical paradigm or approach, this does not mean that, at the time, such had been directly intended. This important *proviso* should be borne in mind when reflecting on the examples and evidence that follows.

Behaviour change approaches

Perhaps the majority of activities and programmes described in the international literature to date have sought to bring about behaviour change on the part of individuals. In a recent review of prevention programmes for young people, for example, Hughes et al. (2001) describe a wide range of initiatives designed to increase awareness of HIV/AIDS and their capacity to act on the basis of what they know. They identify two individual determinants as important in promoting safer sex: (i) intentions and motivations, and (ii) skills and abilities. Both are essential to risk reduction. However, they also point to the importance of there being an enabling environment for sexual risk reduction and good access to health and social service infrastructure.

Likewise, and in relation to work to promote condom use among sex workers, Vuylsteke and Jana (2001) stress the importance of targeted information and behaviour change messages for both sex workers and their clients. Citing their own earlier work in Abidjan among the clients of women sex workers, they show that despite the men having good general knowledge of HIV/AIDS, 36 per cent *also* believed that HIV could be transmitted by witchcraft and 61 per cent believed it could be transmitted by mosquito bites.

Correct information is, therefore, a prerequisite for the practice of safe behaviour, among members of this population at least.

Among injecting drug users, small media such as leaflets, buttons, calling cards and information packs have been used to promote HIV/AIDS-related risk reduction across a variety of settings. Audiovisual media have also been used both as a means of primary prevention, and to promote harm minimisation among those who inject. Several studies have reported on the successful use of videotaped recordings to educate injecting drug users on how to clean injection equipment with bleach (see, for example, Booth and Watters, 1994). Peers have also been used to provide information, generate peer support and utilise the culture of the target group in order to effect and sustain changes in behaviour (Burrows, 2001).

Empowerment approaches

While each of the above behaviour change approaches differs in its focus and approach, all share a commitment to bringing about reductions in risk-related behaviours. Each, moreover, posits a relatively straightforward link between what people know and feel about an issue and what they do. Empowerment approaches, on the other hand, question both the directness of this relationship, and the ease with which sustained changes in behaviour can be brought about.

Some of the best known-about empowerment approaches have utilised group work and couples counselling in order to assist individuals in making healthy life choices. Gay Men Fighting AIDS (GMFA) in the UK, for example, is one of several groups to run assertiveness training courses for gay men. (http://www.metromate.org.uk/frames.php/amm/gmfa/index.phtml). The emphasis is on improving individuals' abilities to communicate clearly, directly and honestly with one another. Workshops and activities also aim to strengthen relationships and enhance feelings of self-worth. In the US, the Mpowerment Project for young gay men in San Francisco has utilised similar approaches (Kegeles et al., 1996).

Couples counselling has been widely used to address the difficulties serodiscordant couples may face in communicating and negotiating for safer sex. It provides an opportunity for partners to clarify their feelings with one another. It can also lead to the identification of barriers to risk reduction. Couples counselling has also been used to explore the impact of gender norms and expectations in relationships and to allow women and men to speak more openly about their fears, desires and wishes.

In the US, the California Partner Study provided couples counselling in combination with social support to serodiscordant heterosexual couples where one partner is HIV positive and the other HIV negative. Condom use increased and no new HIV infections were reported among the couples (Padian et al., 1997).

Community-oriented approaches

A substantial number of HIV/AIDS health promotion programmes have sought to use community relationships and structures to promote safer practices. Using such an approach, *The Tribes* project in Australia has worked with many different groups of drug users. Fifteen separate projects were commenced between 1992 and 1995, targeting different communities of users, including over 35 year-olds, young people attending raves, workers in the sex industry, and prisoners. A different approach to safer sex and safer drug use was utilised with each group (Duckett, 1995).

Other community-oriented approaches include the work of the Sonagachi HIV/STD Intervention Project (SHIP) on Kolkata, India (http:// www.dfid. gov.uk/public/what/pdf/hpd_bengalstory.pdf). Working in the red-light districts of that city, the project sought to promote respect towards sex workers, reliance on them to run the programme, and recognition of their professional and human rights. Peer educators were trained to ensure that sex workers locally developed self-esteem and confidence, and had increased access to power so that they could articulate and advocate for their needs.

In Uganda, The AIDS Service Organisation (TASO) was founded in 1986 to address the needs of people living with AIDS (PWAs) and their families. TASO's work is guided by the notion of positive living. This philosophy calls on individuals, families and communities to uphold the rights and responsibilities of people affected by HIV/AIDS. At the individual level, TASO offers one-to-one counselling and support. At the family level, the organisation offers counselling to family members to dispel fears and anxieties, and nursing and nutritional materials to facilitate home care. At the community level, community counselling is offered to empower the community to offer an appropriate response.

Socially transformatory approaches

Socially transformatory models are committed to producing the fundamental changes necessary for the promotion of health and wellbeing. They may do this through challenges to the dominant economic, political and ideological order, by aiming to achieve that which is impossible at any one moment in time. Several examples of such approaches will be focused upon here.

Contrary to popular belief, safer sex was not identified by doctors, or by eminent scientists working in laboratories. In fact, communities of gay men discovered it at a time when such men were near universally vilified by politicians, the media and the church. Importantly, early descriptions of safer sex such as Callen and Berkowitz's (1983) *How to Have Sex in an Epidemic* were published before HIV had been identified. Nevertheless, they laid the foundations for what many people take for granted as being the fundamentals of safer sex today, the proper use of condoms and other rational precautions to make sex safer (http://members.aol.com/sigothinc/eking.htm). At a time when gay men were being publicly shunned, and were being told by some health authorities to give up having sex altogether, by stressing that it is an infection, not sex, that kills, this pamphlet transformed thinking about the epidemic.

Acción Ciudadana Contra el Sida (ACCSI) is a non-profit organisation founded in 1987 in Venezuela. To challenge the very limited access of people living with HIV/AIDS to treatment, ACCSI launched a series of lawsuits against the Ministries of Health, Defence and Social Security. The lawsuits were based on the rights of people with HIV/AIDS to non-discrimination, health, equality, access to science and technology, and access to social security, as guaranteed by the National Constitution, the American Convention on Human Rights, the International Pact on Economic, Social and Cultural Rights, and other conventions signed and ratified by the government of Venezuela.

Legal action by ACCSI over a number of years has resulted in the courts ordering the government to provide treatments for all people with HIV/AIDS in Venezuela. This has happened in stages. By August 1998, the social security system had established a programme of care and treatment for 2200 people with HIV/AIDS. Lawsuits filed against the Ministry of Health resulted in an additional 1500 women, children and men receiving anti-retroviral therapies. In January 1998, the court ruled in favour of the four military claimants and ordered the Ministry of Defence to provide anti-retroviral therapies and full medical services.

In South Africa, the Treatment Action Campaign (TAC) was launched in 1998 to campaign for greater access to treatment for all South Africans. More specifically, TAC has campaigned for AZT and Nevirapine to be made available to HIV positive pregnant women in the public healthcare system in order to prevent mother-to-child transmission (MTCT) of HIV/AIDS; for pharmaceutical companies to lower the cost of all HIV/AIDS medications; and for the import of cheap generic treatments drugs from countries such as Brazil and Thailand. Working in an extremely difficult context where, until recently, senior government officials have questioned whether HIV is the cause of AIDS, TAC has been responsible for securing wider access to treatment drugs than could have been imagined only a few years ago. Starting in 2004, four generic companies will sell triple drug anti-retroviral therapy to governments in sub-Saharan Africa at US $140 per patient per year.

In India, where stigma relating to HIV/AIDS is high, the HIV/AIDS Unit of the Lawyers Collective in New Delhi has successfully defended workers who have been discriminated against and lost their jobs on account of their HIV-positive status. A significant achievement has been the upholding of the suppression of identity clause, which allows a person with HIV/AIDS to file his or her case under a pseudonym. This is important, as people living with HIV and AIDS are often reluctant to proceed with litigation for fear that their positive status will be disclosed to the public at large, and that they will suffer discrimination. The Unit has also been active in the area of human rights of marginalised groups, including sex workers.

While the focus of action for transformation varies, all the above examples show how, through challenges to dominant economic, political and other forces, health can and has been promoted within the context of HIV/AIDS.

Some lessons learned

What can be learned from the different health promotion approaches to HIV/AIDS that have been reviewed? Is there any common ground between them, and what collectively do they add to our understanding of success in HIV/AIDS prevention and care? Five core principles emerge:

Taking into account the person

First, successful approaches engage with the person and their circumstances. Important differences between people exist with respect to gender, sexuality, ethnicity and culture. Interacting with these primary distinctions are socioeconomic, political and legal factors. Social inequality, social exclusion, migration and lack of access to health services are just a few of the contextual influences known to facilitate HIV transmission (Sweat and Denison, 1995). Other factors include sexism, racism, homelessness, homophobia and sexual coercion, together with actions that damage self-esteem, eliminate choices and make it harder for individuals to stand up for themselves (Harper and DiCarlo, 1999).

Some individuals, by virtue of their age, poverty, gender and prevailing political and economic realities are rendered more systematically vulnerable than others, young injecting drug users, and migrants and refugees, for example. Others may be more systematically protected, better-off and well-supported young people offered good quality education in sex and relationships, for example. Understanding and responding to systematic vulnerability is central to an effective public health response.

Promoting meaningful participation

Meaningful participation is central to success in HIV/AIDS health promotion. Involving people in programme design and development leads to greater acceptability and appropriateness. It can also result in programming that is inclusive rather than stigmatising and discriminating. Through meaningful participation, the members of heavily affected communities such as sex workers, injecting drug users, and gay and other homosexually active men, become a resource in addressing the global pandemic.

With respect to HIV/AIDS, social participation is vitally important to health. High levels of social capital, community trust, reciprocal help and support, a positive local identity, and high levels of civic engagement in a dense network of community associations, are positively associated with the health and wellbeing of children and young people (Rivers and Aggleton, 1998). One of the most important dimensions of health enhancing social capital is the perceived power to get things done (Campbell et al., 1999). This is present when people feel that their needs and views are respected and valued, and when they have channels to participate in decision making.

Commitment to rights

Promoting human rights within the context of HIV/AIDS is important, not only to tackle the structural factors that renders some groups systematically more vulnerable than others, but also to unleash the power of individuals and of communities to make a difference in their own lives (Mann et al., 1996).

There are numerous other international human rights instruments of public health relevance to health promotion and HIV/AIDS. These include the Universal Declaration on Human Rights; the International Covenant on Civil and Political Rights; the International Covenant on Economic Social and Cultural Rights; the Convention on Elimination of All Forms of Discrimination Against Women; the Convention on the Elimination of All Forms of Racial Discrimination, regional charters, and specific rights in relation to living with or being affected by HIV/AIDS.

Beyond these conventions, there are international agreements that offer a normative framework within which to organise and couch a response. These include ICPD+5 (http://www.unfpa.org/icpd5/icpd5.htm), the Beijing Declaration and Platform for Action and its five-year follow up (http://www.un.org/womenwatch/daw/beijing/platform/declar.htm), and the Millennium Development Goals (http://www.developmentgoals.org/).

Promoting gender equity

For many young women, first sexual experience takes place within the context of marriage, which is often construed as a safe and moral context. Girls, more than young men, are encouraged to wait until marriage before having sex. Yet, marriage for young women is often to older and more sexually experienced partners, and in contexts where marriage may not imply monogamy for many men. The result is both risk of infection at an age when young women are biologically most vulnerable, coupled with ill-conceived notions of security and safety.

All over the world, dominant images of femininity mean that young women have to negotiate between being knowledgeable, and appearing innocent, in order to protect their sexual and social reputations (Rivers and Aggleton, 1998). But it is not only young women that are made vulnerable to HIV/AIDS by existing gender norms. Dominant stereotypes and ideologies of masculinity and manliness can make it difficult for boys to seek sexual and reproductive health advice. Men are supposed to be knowledgeable and experienced about such issues, and to seek help is to risk being perceived as less of a man.

There is a pressing need to unpack the multiple ideologies of gender that exist, and the manner in which these are influenced by class, race and sexuality. While dominant forms of masculinity and femininity may be divisive and harmful, predisposing to greater vulnerability and risk, alternative and oppositional ways of living are possible. These should be made the starting point for future HIV/AIDS health promotion work (Mane and Aggleton, 2001).

Tackling risk and vulnerability

In the context of HIV/AIDS, *risk* can be defined as the probability that a person may acquire infection. Certain behaviours create, enhance and perpetuate risk. They include unprotected sex with an infected partner, multiple unprotected sexual partnerships, and injecting drug use where injecting equipment and drug preparations are shared.

Experience has shown, however, that HIV/AIDS health promotion should focus not only on risk taking behaviours, but also on environmental and societal factors. In many contexts, decisions relating to sex, for example, involve the family and community as well as the individual. Young women may be pressurised to remain ignorant about sexual matters, whereas young men may be encouraged to brag about sex while gaining experience through liaisons with girl friends and sex workers. Likewise, with respect to drug use, the peer group and social networks may be influential in determining whether or not a young person injects, and does so safely.

Political, economic and social inequalities influence *vulnerability* to HIV/AIDS. Important in affecting vulnerability are the social networks of which an individual is a part. Some people, for example, may find themselves at enhanced vulnerability for HIV infection by virtue of their membership of a group in which HIV infection is particularly prevalent, such as by being injectors or by being involved in sex work in contexts where levels of infection are high. Beyond this, however, vulnerability is also influenced by service and programme factors, including the cultural appropriateness or inappropriateness of HIV/AIDS prevention programmes, the accessibility or inaccessibility of services due to distance, cost and other factors, and the capacity of health systems to respond to growing demand.

Broader, societal and environmental factors influencing vulnerability include political decisions, economic inequalities, laws and cultural norms that act as barriers or facilitators to prevention. These may lead to the inclusion, neglect or social exclusion of individuals depending on their lifestyles and socio-cultural characteristics. Radical and transformatory action may be required to change these constraints.

Successful HIV/AIDS health promotion, therefore, consist of two principal components: the reduction of risk through specific prevention, care and impact-alleviation efforts; and the reduction of vulnerability through more broad-based social, cultural and economic change. These two components need to be present regardless of whether the focus of our work is on populations as a whole, or on specific groups.

HIV/AIDS poses one of the greatest threats to health and wellbeing that the world has ever known. Yet in a relatively short period of time, much has been learned about the most effective ways of organising prevention and care. The strengths and limitations of different models or frameworks for health promotion are becoming better understood, as indeed are the principles underpinning effective responses. The challenge for the future lies in scaling up existing efforts and enlisting input from a wider range of professionals than hitherto. Central among these are health promotion specialists who see HIV/AIDS not as an irrelevance or as a special cause, but as central to health promotion work.

References

Aggleton, P. (1989) Evaluating health education about AIDS. In Aggleton, P., Hart, G. and Davies, P. (eds) *AIDS: Social Representations, Social Practices*. Lewes: The Falmer Press.

Aggleton, P. (1993) Promoting whose health? models of health promotion and education about HIV disease. In Albrecht, G. and Zimmerman, R.S. (eds) *Advances in Medical Sociology*, Volume 3. Greenwich, CT: JAI Press.

Booth, R.E. and Watters, J.K. (1994) How effective are risk-reduction interventions targeting injecting drug users? *AIDS*, **8:** 1515–24.

Burrows, D. (2001) *A Best Practice Model of Harm Reduction in the Community and in Prisons in the Russian Federation*. Final project report to the World Bank, Washington/Moscow.

Callen, M. and Berkowitz, R. (1983) *How to Have Sex in an Epidemic*. New York: News From the Front Publications.

Campbell, C. with Wood, R. and Kelly, M. (1999) *Social Capital and Health*. London: Health Education Authority.

Centro Brasileiro de Estudos de Saude (2003) The Brazilian Response to HIV/AIDS: Assessing its transferability. *Divulgação em Saúde para Debate*. 27 August.

Centers for Disease Control (2003) Press Release, *New Study Shows Overall Increase in HIV Diagnoses*. 26 November. Available at http://www.cdc.gov/od/oc/media/pressrel/r031126.htm.

Duckett, M. (1995) *The TRIBES Evaluation Report*. Sydney, Australia: NSW Users & AIDS Association (NUAA).

Harper, G. and DiCarlo, P. (1999) *What are Adolescents' HIV Prevention Needs*. San Francisco, CAPS Project. http://www.caps.ucsf.edu/adolrev.html.

Homans, H. and Aggleton, P. (1987) *Educating About AIDS*. Bristol: National Health Service Training Authority.

Hughes, H., Pinel, A. and Svenson, G. (2001) Youth intervention programs. In Lamptey, P. and Gayle, J. (eds) *HIV/AIDS Prevention and Care in Resource*

Constrained Settings: A Handbook for the Design and Management of Programs. Washington, DC: Family Health International.

Kegeles, S.M., Hays, R.B. and Coates, T.J. (1996) The Mpowerment Project: a community-level HIV prevention intervention for young gay men. *American Journal of Public Health*, **86**: 1129–36.

Maluwa, M., Aggleton, P. and Parker, R. (2003) HIV/AIDS stigma, discrimination and human rights – a critical overview. *Health and Human Rights*, **6** (1): 1–15.

Mane, P. and Aggleton, P. (2001) Gender and HIV/AIDS. What do men have to do with it? *Current Sociology*, **49** (6): 23–37.

Mann, Jonathan (1987) Statement at an informal briefing on AIDS to the 42nd Session of the United Nations General Assembly, 20 October, New York.

Mann, J. and Tarantola, D. (eds) (1996) *AIDS in the World 2.* New York: Oxford University Press.

Padian, N.S., Shiboski, S.C. and Glass, S.O. (1997) Heterosexual transmission of human immunodeficiency virus (HIV) in northern California: results from a ten-year study. *American Journal of Epidemiology*, **146**: 350–57.

Parker, R. and Aggleton, P. (2003) HIV and AIDS-related stigma and discrimination – A conceptual framework and implications for action. *Social Science and Medicine*, **57** (1): 13–24.

Rivers, K. and Aggleton, P.J. (1998) *Adolescent Sexuality, Gender and the HIV Epidemic.* New York: United Nations Development Programme.

Sweat, M.D. and Denison, J. (1995) HIV incidence in developing countries with structural and environmental interventions, *AIDS*, **9**, Suppl A: S251–57.

UNAIDS and WHO (2003) *AIDS Epidemic Update, December 2003.* Geneva: UNAIDS and WHO.

Vuylsteke, B. and Jana, S. (2001) Reducing HIV risk in sex workers, their clients and partners. In Lamptey, P. and Gayle, J. (eds) *HIV/AIDS Prevention and Care in Resource Constrained Settings: A Handbook for the Design and Management of Programs.* Washington, DC: Family Health International.

CHAPTER 10

Global Environmental Change and Health

PAUL WILKINSON

Population growth and consumption-based economic activity pose serious threats to the environment and new risks to human health. Human activity is disrupting at global level some of the critical support systems that provide environmental stabilisation and replenishment. Through our demand for energy and resources and production of waste we are now changing the gaseous composition of the atmospheres, reducing the productivity of land, depleting ocean fisheries, over-exploiting many of the great aquifers upon which irrigated agriculture depends, and causing an unprecedented rate of species loss. These unsustainable changes pose long-term risks to population health. At the same time, more traditional local environmental concerns, such as those relating to pollution of the air, poor sanitation and land degradation, remain prominent concerns for many populations, especially those in lower and middle income countries undergoing rapid urbanisation and industrialisation. This chapter discusses the health risks associated with these global trends, and the needed public health responses to them.

Human activity is disrupting some of the earth's life support systems at a global level. This disruption carries risks to our health (McMichael, 2002) and without corrective action, those risks seem set to increase over coming decades as the consequences of global environmental change take hold. Public health therefore faces a set of new and unfamiliar challenges. In the past, environment and health concerns were largely focused on local risks arising from chemical and biological contamination of the air, water and soil. The new threats arise through more complex and extended pathways that have global reach. They endanger the very processes that provide stability to ecological systems, and the replenishment and recycling of natural resources. The combination of population growth and increasing demand for energy and materials arising from consumption-based economic growth is having far-reaching consequences. We are exploiting the earth's resources at a rate far greater than can be sustained in the medium term, and causing the progressive build up of environmental contaminants. The resulting disruption to global life support systems threatens both human and non-human populations, changing the composition of the atmosphere, reducing the productive potential of land and sea, depleting the great aquifers, and contributing to an unprecedented rate of

129

species loss (UNEP, 2002; World Resources Institute, 2003). Although the long-term consequences are not accurately predictable, we have sufficient evidence to understand the importance to the promotion of health of trying to slow, and in time reverse, these global changes, and of developing strategies to adapt to the kinds of environmental disruption that now appear inevitable.

Global climate change

Majority scientific view now holds that we are in a period of global warming driven in part by anthropogenic emissions of greenhouse gases. The 2001 report from the UN's Intergovernmental Panel on Climate Change (IPCC) (IPCC, 2001) estimates that global average land and sea surface temperature has increased by $0.6 \pm 0.2°C$ since the mid-nineteenth century (see Figure 10.1). Projections suggest that global temperatures may rise by a further 1.4–5.8°C by 2100 compared with a 1990 baseline, which represents a faster rise than at any stage since the beginning of agriculture around 10,000 years ago. It is thought that these projected temperature changes will be accompanied by altered patterns of precipitation, with probable drying of some arid and semi-arid regions, while other areas, especially at mid to high latitudes, become wetter, with a disproportionate increase in the frequency of heavy precipitation events. The nature and degree of climate change will have regional variations, but populations in low income countries are likely to be particularly vulnerable to its health impacts because climate-sensitive diseases are more common in such populations and their capacity to adapt is limited (McMichael et al., 2003).

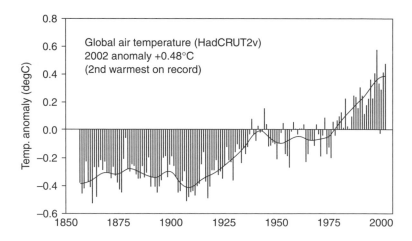

Figure 10.1   Combined global land and marine surface temperature record, 1856–2002

Source: Jones et al., 1999, Jones and Moberg, 2003. Climate Research Unit, University of East Anglia

Climate-related health impacts include those relating to the direct effects of exposure to high and also low temperatures; the impacts of extreme weather events, including floods, high winds and droughts; increased frequency of food- and water-borne disease; and changes in the spatial and temporal distribution of vector-borne disease. Other impacts include the indirect effects on food productivity, changes in air pollution, and social, economic and demographic dislocations due to effects on infrastructure and resources. The relative importance of these impacts depends on the prevailing climate, level of socioeconomic development and disease spectrum in the local populations

Direct effects of thermal extremes

Seasonal variation in mortality and morbidity has been found in all populations that have been studied in detail (see for example Curriero et al., 2002 and ISOTHURM Study Group, 2004). The main evidence of temperature dependence comes from daily time-series studies. The example of Delhi is shown in Figure 10.2. Here, as in other populations, all cause mortality increases at higher temperatures. This increase may reflect a range of patho-physiological mechanisms. Any rightward shift in the ambient temperature distribution under climate change is likely to increase the burden of heat-related deaths.

In higher income countries, the mortality rise is mainly accounted for by an increase in deaths from cardiovascular and respiratory illness, especially in the elderly population, presumably reflecting direct patho-physiological effects of rapid dehydration and thermal stress. But the more limited evidence from lower income countries suggests that heat may be accompanied by

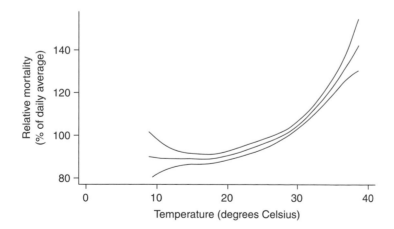

Figure 10.2 Mortality, Delhi, India, 1993–94: relationship between mortality and daily temperature (average of the same- and preceding-day temperature). Outer lines indicate 95 per cent confidence limits

comparatively large mortality rises in younger age groups as well, with infectious diseases being a substantial contributor to the mortality burden. Although populations may adapt to increasing temperatures, the observed mortality patterns suggest that populations in many countries are likely to have substantial vulnerability to forecast patterns of climate change. Vulnerability will depend on factors that are intrinsic to the population itself, such as its age structure, and underlying disease prevalence, as well as on the level of economic development and capacity to adapt. However, much heat-related mortality and morbidity is theoretically avoidable through public health and other interventions, and this will need to be an increasing focus of attention.

Flooding, storms and droughts

Through increases in the intensity of the hydrological cycle, it is predicted that climate change will also increase the occurrence of extreme precipitation and the frequency of riverine and coastal flooding. The frequency of droughts is also likely to rise, in part because of altered precipitation patterns in some regions, but also because of over-utilisation of water resources and land use changes.

Across the twentieth century as a whole, over 2000 flood and 2300 storm/hurricane disasters were recorded, and some 8.7 million deaths attributed to them. Most of the worst impacts have been in populations in low to middle income countries, see Figure 10.3. There have been many recent examples: Hurricane

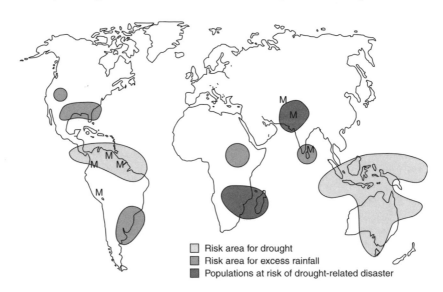

Figure 10.3   Risk areas for drought and rainfall based on 'teleconnections' with El Niño Southern Oscillation (ENSO)

Note: M = areas where there is risk of epidemic malaria after an ENSO event.

Source: Kovats et al. (2003) *Lancet* **362**: 1481–89

Mitch in central America, the Orissa cyclone in India, the giant mudslides in Venezuela, and the severe food shortages from drought in the Horn of Africa and Sudan, and the floods in Mozambique. There is statistical evidence that long-term weather cycles such as the El Niño Southern Oscillation (ENSO) quasi-periodic cycle are correlated with the incidence of such natural disasters and hence with the deaths and injuries attributable to them (Kovats et al., 2003).

There is an obvious causal chain between increasing variability in precipitation, droughts and their associated health impacts, particularly food shortages and, if not appropriately managed, famine (see Chapter 7 in this section for a further examination of the causes of famine). The health impacts of these weather events are modulated by multiple aspects of population vulnerability, local topography, housing quality, weather warning systems, disaster preparedness and economic resources. Populations that are most vulnerable are often made so through a combination of factors.

Good warning and preparedness for severe weather events can do much to alleviate their immediate effects on health. Hurricane Michelle, which struck Cuba in November 2001, led to wide devastation but only a handful of deaths, thanks in large part to the effective warning and civil defence measures, which entailed evacuation of more than six hundred thousand people from vulnerable areas. However, the health impacts of such disasters extend beyond the immediate risks of trauma and drowning, and these present their own challenges to public health.

Food and water-borne disease

As a broad generalisation, the infectious diseases that appear most sensitive to weather conditions are those where the pathogen or its vector replicates outside the human host: bacteria and other enteric pathogens in water or food, enteroviruses in the environment. Diarrhoeal disease shows strong seasonality in numerous regions and the temperature dependence may in part explain the observation that populations without access to adequate clean water and sanitation have higher rates of diarrhoea during summer months, particularly on hotter days and during strong El Niño events. Climate also affects the rate at which water-borne pathogens come into contact with humans, rates often being higher when rainfall is either unusually high, leading to flooding, or unusually low, leading to prolonged water storage and concentration of pathogens. The relative importance of different pathogens and modes of transmission, such as via water, food, insects or human to human contact, varies between areas, and is influenced by level of sanitation. As pathogens are known to vary in their response to climate, this is likely to cause geographical variation in temperature relationships, depending on level of development.

An example of the relationship between daily hospital admissions and climatic conditions is shown in Figure 10.4 (Checkley et al., 2000). These data, from a single paediatric diarrhoeal disease clinic in Lima, Peru, show

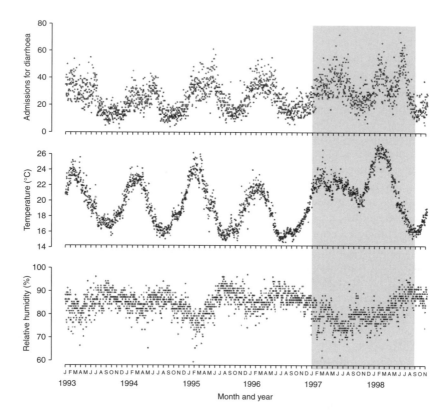

Figure 10.4   Daily time-series between 1 January 1993, and
15 November 1998, for admissions for diarrhoea, mean ambient
temperature, and relative humidity in Lima, Peru

Source: Checkley et al. *Lancet* **355**: 442–50

hospital admissions over a period of six years. In quantitative terms, each
degree Celsius increase in temperature was associated with a 4 per cent
increase in admissions during the hotter months and a 12 per cent increase per
degree Celcius in the cooler months. During the 1997–98 El Niño period,
there was an additional increase in admissions above that expected on the basis
of pre-El Niño temperature relationships. Others have reported a relationship
between the El Nino and Southern Oscillation (ENSO) and cholera prevalence in Bangladesh (Rodo et al., 2002).

Diarrhoeal illness is already of major importance because of its large contribution to the burden of ill health (Ezzati et al., 2002). Although that burden
is much more a consequence of poor sanitation and nutrition than of climatic
conditions, the demonstration of climate sensitivity suggests that climate
change is likely to contribute to an increase in morbidity unless counteracted
by increasing standards of living and improved public health.

Vector-borne disease

Many vector-borne diseases, that is diseases in which viruses, bacteria, proto-zoa or helminths are transmitted by biting insects or other intermediate hosts, are known to be sensitive to the ambient conditions of temperature, humidity and rainfall. Quantitative evidence of such dependence has been obtained through studies of vector and pathogen population biology in the laboratory and through studies of geographical and seasonal patterns of transmission intensity in the field. The prediction is that the geographic distribution of vectors and associated diseases will change as a consequence of changing climate patterns. The degree to which this is true will depend on the relative importance for vector borne disease of climatic influences from the non-climatic, such as population movement, changes in land use, changes in surface configurations of freshwater, human population density, control programmes, and the population density of insectivorous predators.

Several groups have tried to quantify likely changes in future disease distri-butions using spatial models. One such study suggests that the geographical distribution of dengue is likely to expand, as indicted in Figure 10.5 (Hales et al., 2002). Whether such changes occur in practice will depend on the

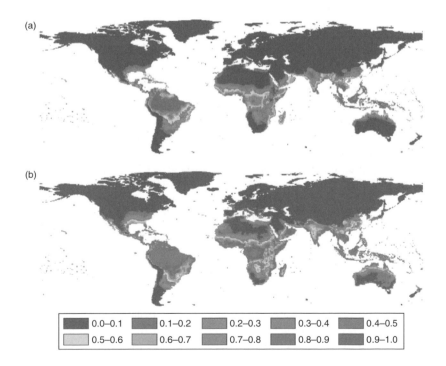

Figure 10.5 Estimated population at risk of dengue fever: (A) 1990, (B) 2085

Sources: Hales, S. et al. (2002) *Lancet* **360** (9336): 830–34

accuracy of current models and the modifying influences of future environmental and population factors. There is clearly much uncertainty in attempt-
ing to predict how disease such as malaria and dengue will respond to the
much larger climatic changes that are expected to occur over the twenty-first
century. However, having reviewed the evidence, the Inter-governmental
Panel on Climate Change concluded that climate change is likely to expand
the geographic distribution of several vector-borne diseases to higher altitudes
and to extend the transmission seasons in some locations. It was less confident
that these diseases will expand into higher latitudes and suggests that such an
expansion is possible only where public health defences are limited, or that
decreases in transmission may occur by reductions in rainfall or temperatures
too high for transmission.

Water and health

Although water is a widespread and renewable resource, growing demand for
it, together with pollution of water courses, is leading to a global water crisis.
The 2003 World Water Development Report identifies the problem as a crisis
of water governance (United Nations/World Water Assessment Programme
[UN/WWAP], 2003). Population growth and improvement in living standards, with consequent increase in per capita consumption, are the main
causes of a relentlessly growing demand. We currently abstract for human use
8 per cent of the total annual renewable freshwater, 26 per cent of annual
evapo-transpiration and 54 per cent of accessible run-off. Within these global
figures there are important regional variations, and many areas of water
shortage and scarcity. It is estimated that approximately 40 per cent of the
world's population face some level of water shortage. Underground water
reserves in many countries are being used faster than they are replenished
(UN/WWAP, 2003).

In the north China plain, which produces nearly 40 per cent of the Chinese
grain harvest, the fall in the water table averages 1.5 metres a year. Regions
under the most water pressure include China's Yellow River basin, the Middle
East and the Aral Sea region of Central Asia. Most of the water from these
sources is used for irrigation and industry rather than household use. In this
context, the inefficiency in water use is a key factor, especially in the area of
food production. Approximately 70 per cent of the world's exploited freshwater resource base is diverted to agriculture, and yet crops and plants use only
30 per cent of this diverted water.

The availability of freshwater relative to water withdrawals can be an important constraint on development. Unless changes are made, it is estimated that,
within the next two decades, the use of water by humans will increase by about
40 per cent and demand will outstrip available supplies. The proportion of the
world's population that will be subject to water stress, that is where
withdrawals of water are more than 20 per cent of the renewable supply, is

projected to increase to two-thirds by 2025. Climate change contributes to this increase, as rainfall within many tropical and subtropical regions is expected to decline and to be more erratic, climate change may account for 20 per cent of the increase in water scarcity.

The growing problem of water scarcity adds to the continuing blight of inadequate access to clean water for much of the world's population. There are estimated to be 1.1 billion people who do not have access to an improved water supply and 2.4 billion who do not have adequate sanitation. A lack of access to clean water remains one of the greatest threats to global health, and arguably the largest of the environmental risks to health (Ezzati et al., 2002). A Ministerial Declaration at the second World Water Forum in the Hague in March 2000 set out a number of challenges as the basis of future action on water (UN/WWAPP, 2003) as follows:

World Water Development: Challenges for Future Action

1. Meeting basic needs – for safe and sufficient water and sanitation
2. Securing the food supply – especially for the poor and vulnerable through the more effective use of water
3. Protecting ecosystems – ensuring their integrity via sustainable water resource management
4. Sharing water resources – promoting peaceful cooperation between different uses of water and between concerned states, through approaches such as sustainable river basin management
5. Managing risks – to provide security from a range of water-related hazards
6. Valuing water – to manage water in the light of its different values (economic, social, environmental, cultural) and to move towards pricing water to recover the costs of service provision, taking account of equity and the needs of the poor and vulnerable
7. Governing water wisely – involving the public and the interests of all stakeholders.

To these were added a further four:

8. Water and industry – promoting cleaner industry with respect to water quality and the needs of other users
9. Water and energy – assessing water's key role in energy production to meet rising energy demands
10. Ensuring the knowledge-base – so that water knowledge becomes more universally available
11. Water and cities – recognising the distinctive challenges of an increasingly urbanised world.

There is sufficient understanding of how these challenges could be met given sufficient will and political leadership, but progress to date has been very disappointing.

Environmental change and infectious disease

Environmental changes, and the trends of a globalising world, have also contributed to the emergence and rapid transmission of infectious disease (Aron and Patz, 2001). Changes in ecosystems, the intensification of agriculture, the mixing of human and animal populations, and the enormous increase in human mobility have all played a part in this. An unusually large number of new or newly discovered infectious diseases have been recorded in the past 25 years, including HIV/AIDS (see Chapter 9 in this part of the book) the Ebola virus, Lyme disease, cryptosporidiosis, legionellosis, hepatitis C, Hantavirus pulmonary syndrome, *E. coli* 0157and others.

International travel and long distance trade have contributed to the geographical redistribution of pests and pathogens. This has been well illustrated by the HIV pandemic, the worldwide dispersal of rodent borne hantaviruses, and the rapid dissemination of a new epidemic strain of bacterial meningitis along routes of travel and trade. More recently, the 2003 epidemic of severe acute respiratory syndrome (SARS), caused by a coronavirus, has demonstrated the potential rapidity of global spread (WHO, 2003 and Part III, Chapter 14 of this book). More recently, the cases of avian influenza, caused in large part by the close contact been humans and farmed poultry, has raised the spectre of a worldwide epidemic.

Intensification of food production and processing methods appears to have been a critical factor in the emergence of Bovine Spongiform Encephalopathy in Britain, and the subsequent spread of variant CJD to humans (Collinge, 1999). Industrial farming is also a likely factor in the increases in reported rates of food poisoning in many countries, and the potentially fatal toxin producing *E. coli* 0157 in North America and Europe in the mid 90s appears to have accompanied beef imported from infected cattle in Argentina where the rates of human infection with *E.coli* 0157 are reportedly higher than in western countries.

Changes to the natural environment have also adversely affected infectious disease patterns. Deforestation, irrigation schemes, land reclamation, road construction and population resettlement programmes have often potentiated the spread of malaria, dengue fever, schistosomiasis and trypanosomiasis. Patterns of infectious diseases are widely influenced by land clearance activities in populous regions of the developing world and by the extension of irrigation. Various viral haemorrhagic fevers have emerged over the past several decades as intensified land clearance and habitat disruption, especially in South America, have exposed human populations to new viruses that previously circulated exclusively within wilderness ecosystems.

Policy response

The challenges presented by global environmental change are substantial, given their origin in consumption-based economic development and the growth of the world's population. Slowing and, in time, reversing global environmental changes will therefore require decisive action, but such action that is likely to be resisted by those on whom the associated costs and needed restraints fall. One of the difficulties is the lack of awareness of global environmental change as an immediate threat. Each individual's contribution to global environmental change is small, and the lead time to future adverse effects long. As a result, it is easy to disregard the urgency for remedial action, and to place hope in a future generation's ability to find technological solutions.

From the perspective of health protection, actions can be taken on two fronts: first, to contribute to efforts to limit the extent and rapidity of environmental change, and second to adapt to the changes that occur. To date, progress on both fronts has been limited. With respect to climate change, we now have good scientific understanding and fairly broad acceptance of it as a global threat. Encouragingly, the 1992 Rio Framework Convention on Climate Change committed high income countries to return emissions of greenhouse gases to 1990 levels by the year 2000 (United Nations, 1992). In December 1997, further agreement was reached in Kyoto to cut emissions of the six main greenhouse gases by 6 per cent below 1990 levels between 2008 and 2012. Eighty four parties have signed the Kyoto Protocol. But even though the limits set by these agreements is modest, the Kyoto Protocol has yet to be formally ratified. Most disappointingly, the US and some other large emitters of greenhouse gases have not signed the Kyoto protocol. Industrial and economic interests and political constraints have proved substantial barriers. There is, moreover, no clear agreement on the penalties for nations that do not meet their pollution targets, and no systematic framework for assisting the transfer of the needed technology and investment from high income to the low income parts of the world. Nonetheless, some countries are making firm commitments to emission reductions and some progress in limiting the rise in emissions of carbon dioxide, the main greenhouse gas produced by human activity, achieved by energy efficiency gains, shifts towards low energy industries and falling coal use.

In this, as in many areas, there is enormous inequity between the wealthiest and poorest countries, there being the more than ten-fold variation in per capita carbon dioxide emissions. If, in coming decades, all countries come to achieve a level of economic development and resource consumption already found in the highest income countries that considerations of equity would allow, the stresses on the environment would be very great indeed. There is need for technological and social solutions that reduce our collective resource consumption in all countries to more sustainable patterns.

A more optimistic example is the case of stratospheric ozone depletion, first observed in the 1970s over Antarctica. This was perhaps the first clearly recognised form of global environmental change presenting hazards to human health as well as to other systems. Its link to atmospheric emission of chlorofluorocarbons (CFCs) and other related halogenated compounds used as refrigerants, aerosol sprays, solvents, foam blowing agents, fire extinguishers, and nitrogen oxides (by products of combustion processes) was quickly established, as were its consequences: a rise in ultra violet radiation (< 290 nm wavelength) reaching the Earth's surface, increasing the potential for damage to DNA, skin cancers, cataracts and immunological disturbance.

The first global agreement to restrict CFCs was the 1987 Montreal Protocol, whose goal was to reduce CFC emissions by half by the year 2000. Several amendments tightening these restrictions have followed in the light of improved scientific understanding. But despite these generally successful efforts, the return to previous ozone levels will take many years to achieve. Initial projections suggested that if international agreements were fully implemented, full recovery of the ozone layer would not occur until the middle of the century. Nonetheless, this must be viewed as a success story of international collaboration and action.

There is now wide recognition that we must base future action on the principle of environmental sustainability, as outlined in 1987 by the World Commission on Environment and Development in its report, *Our Common Future*. Sustainability, and the protection of biodiversity, is seen as essential to the long-term health of the planet as a whole, and to the human population in particular. Achieving it will require much wider consideration of environment and health in all areas of national and local decision making, perhaps through promoting the principles of Environment and Health Impact Assessment to identify, predict and evaluate the likely changes in health risk, both positive and negative, associated with the environmental consequences of policies and programmes. In a wider sense, it is hoped that such assessments will be useful not just to help minimise environmental risks to health, but also to support the positive enhancement of health in all aspects of national and local action.

Many of the consequences of global environmental change are unknown, and some may occur not as gradual processes, but as non-linear shifts in which critical destabilisation of habitats occur rapidly and irreversibly once a certain point is reached. Examples might be where changes in rainfall is reduced to the point where the land can no longer support human needs, or where food chains break down because of critical depletion of one species within it. We cannot therefore afford to wait for the adverse effects to occur, but need to ensure the wide adoption of the principles of development that are consonant with sustainability and the promotion of healthy living. At the same time, we must be prepared to adapt to the environmental changes that are already certain to occur.

There are serious threats to global systems posed by population growth, unsustainable consumption and bio-diversity loss, issues that were brought into focus at the 1992 Rio Conference with recognition of the health impacts of stratospheric ozone depletion, human-induced climate change and various other large-scale environmental impacts. Meeting the needs of the current total world population, with its high levels of consumption and waste generation, now depends substantially on depleting global stocks of resources and on overloading environmental sinks, as is happening with greenhouse gas accumulation in the lower atmosphere. This situation presents us with many challenges for the future health of human populations.

At the time of the 2003 World Summit on Sustainable Development, it was recognised that progress in implementing sustainable development has been disappointing, with poverty deepening and environmental degradation worsening. The Johannesburg meeting did not produce decisive agreement in many areas, though some important new targets were established, including the goal to halve the proportion of people without access to basic sanitation by 2015; to use and produce chemicals by 2020 in ways that do not lead to significant adverse effects on human health and the environment; and to achieve by 2010 a significant reduction in the current rate of loss of biological diversity. But if we are to limit global environmental change and its associated impacts on health, we will need a level of political commitment that so far has proved difficult to obtain.

References

Aron, J. and Patz, J. (2001) *Ecosystem Change and Public Health. A Global Perspective.* Baltimore and London: The Johns Hopkins University Press.

Checkley, W., Epstein, L.D., Gilman, R.H., Figueroa, D., Cama, R.I., Patz J.A., et al. (2000) Effects of El Nino and ambient temperature on hospital admissions for diarrhoeal diseases in Peruvian children. *Lancet,* **355**: 442–50.

Collinge, J. (1999) Variant Creutzfeldt–Jakob disease. *Lancet,* **354**: 317–23.

Curriero, F.C., Heiner, K.S., Samet, J.M., Zeger, S.L., Strug, L. and Patz, J.A. (2002) Temperature and mortality in 11 cities of the eastern United States. *American Journal of Epidemiology,* **155**(1): 80–8.

Ezzati, M., Lopez, A.D., Rodgers, A., Vander Hoorn, S. and Murray, C.J. (2002) Selected major risk factors and global and regional burden of disease. *Lancet,* **360**: 1347–60.

Hales, S., de Wet, N., Maindonald, J. and Woodward, A. (2002) Potential effect of population and climate changes on global distribution of dengue fever: an empirical model. *Lancet,* **360**: 830–34.

Intergovernmental Panel on Climate Change (IPCC) (2001) Climate change 2001: the scientific basis. The contribution of Working Group 1 to the Third Assessment Report of the Intergovernmental Panel on Climate Change. New York: Cambridge University Press.

ISOTHURM Study Group (2002) International study of temperature and heatwaves on urban mortality in low and middle income countries. *Epidemiology,* S81.

Jones, P., New, M., Parker, D., Martin, S. and Rigor, I. (1999) Surface air temperature and its changes over the past 150 years. *Reviews of Geophysics,* **37**: 173–99.

Jones, P. and Moberg, A. (2003) Hemispheric and large scale surface air temperature variations: An extensive revision and an update to 2001. *Journal of Climate,* **16**: 206–23.

Kovats, R.S., Bouma, M.J., Hajat, S., Worrall, E. and Haines, A. (2003) El Nino and health. *Lancet,* **362**(9394): 1481–89.

McMichael, A. (2002) *Human Frontiers, Environments and Disease. Past Patterns, Uncertain Futures.* Cambridge: Cambridge University Press.

McMichael, A., Cambell-Lendrum, D., Corvalan, C., Ebi, K., Githeko, A., Scheraga, J., et al. (2003) *Climate Change and Human Health. Risks and Responses.* Geneva: World Health Organisation.

Rodo, X., Pascual, M., Fuchs, G. and Faruque, A.S. (2002) ENSO and cholera: a non stationary link related to climate change? *Proceedings of the National Academy of Science*, USA: **99**(20): 12901–06.

United Nations Environment Programme (2002). Global Environment Outlook 3 (GEO-3). *Past, Present and Future Perspectives.* London: Earthscan.

United Nations (1992) *Earth Summit. Agenda 21: the United Nation Programme of Action from Rio.* New York: UN Department of Information.

United Nations/World Water Assessment Programme (UNWWAP) (2003) *UN World Water Development Report: Water for People, Water for Life.* Paris, New York and Oxford: UNESCO (United Nations Educational, Scientific and Cultural Organisation) and Berghahn Books.

World Health Organisation (2003) *Consensus Document on the Epidemiology of Severe Acute Respiratory Syndrome (SARS).* Geneva: World Health Organisation.

World Resources Institute (2003) *Ecosystems and Human Well-being. A Framework for Assessment.* Washington DC: Island Press.

PART III

STRATEGIES FOR PROMOTING HEALTH IN THE GLOBAL CONTEXT: AN OVERVIEW

ANGELA SCRIVEN

The relevance of health promotion as an international concept has been questioned in the past, with some suggesting that it is a phenomenon of wealthy nations. The importance of this section of the book is that chapters are devoted to the examination of health promotion in countries and regions spread worldwide, with the contributions forming critical case studies. Approaches to the promotion of health are explored and it is possible to judge whether there is universal meaning to the terms applied to the methods used to promote health or whether there is disparity. The case studies and the examples discussed can also be judged in the context of the issues and the challenges set out in the earlier sections of the book.

Many parts of the world are covered in this section, which begins with a generic contribution exploring health promotion action in low and middle income countries. There are then chapters presenting case studies on Africa, Latin America, the Greater China Region and the Former Soviet Union and high income parts of the world, including Australia and New Zealand, Europe, Canada and the USA.

A number of comparisons can be drawn from these case studies. There are many vibrant and established ideas about the role of health promotion in the wider context of public health, but there are clearly discrepancies in how health promotion is conceived, valued and approached in different regions of the world. Similar health priorities are being addressed within countries and these reflect the issues and challenges discussed in earlier sections. Inequalities emerge as a serious issue; with lifestyle-induced noncommunicable diseases and HIV/AIDS included in public health targets in most countries.

The Ottawa Charter (see Chapter 1 for an overview of Ottawa) and other WHO declarations have been a significant influence on many of the developments discussed in the chapters. The language of Ottawa permeates the debates that take place and the principles of Ottawa have clearly informed national policies and frameworks for health promotion. National directives are however different and reflect not only local and national priorities, but also

143

political, cultural and economic differences between countries. In Africa, for example, community development approaches are more common whilst in the Former Soviet Union the use of more legislative, top-down approaches appears to be a strong influence, whilst the settings approach has dominated the promotion of health in many European countries.

On a similar point, many countries have published national strategies or are in the process of developing a national framework. Nonetheless, what is made clear from the contributions is that to move outside national boundaries and to have regional strategies in place has proved very difficult. The European, Latin American and US case studies are three examples that demonstrate not only the diversity of perceptions, priorities and practice across national or state boundaries in the same region, but also the problems that have been experienced by those working at a strategic level to develop regional or federal strategies. This is an important issue and reflects the complexity of promoting health globally, where international agreement and action is required.

There are variations in the amount of development that has taken place. Countries such as Canada, with its long history of health promotion, have an evolved and sophisticated framework compared to some of the counties in the Former Soviet Union, which are less advanced in terms of both their ideas and approaches. Health promotion is still a relatively new area of practice (see Chapter 1 for a further discussion of the history of health promotion) but changing perspectives are evident, with the African case study for example, covering 30 years of development and the Canadian case study showing the evolution of ideas resulting in a moving away from and then a return to more traditional principles.

As to the future, there are many predictions, recommendations and identified trends contained within these chapters. There is clearly a move in some countries to a more scientific, research-led and evidence-based approach to practice and there is also a recognition that workforce development is a necessary investment if public health targets are going to be effectively met.

Concluding remarks

What is common about the analysis presented in this section is that the direction of health promotion in all regions and countries is influenced by socioeconomic conditions and as in other sections of this book, there is a universal call for strong intersectoral partnerships and networking at local, national and international levels in order that global health can be promoted effectively through the wider context of social reforms and investments. This has dominated the analysis by all authors in the book and must therefore stand as a significant presumption from the debates that have taken place.

What the chapters in this section demonstrate is that health promoters have a vital contribution to make in advocating for sustained international investment in health and for influencing local and global policies so that they are directed at effective action for health. As part of this, evidence-based practice is regarded as crucial, but needs to be accommodated in the complex dynamics of politics, priorities and international and national policy development.

One of the conclusions drawn from Parts I and II of the book is that there is much to be done that requires innovatory, properly resourced health promotion action. What the case studies in this Part point to is a chronic shortage of resources, including difficulty associated with workforce capacity and capability. There is urgent need therefore to increase capacity and to develop the skills necessary to make an impact on global health and to achieve the real possibilities that authors have set out for health promotion in this text.

CHAPTER 11

Promoting Health in Low and Middle Income Countries: Achievements and Challenges

JOHN HUBLEY

While health promotion has become the unifying term in high income countries, this is by no means the case in most of the world where health education, information education and communication (IEC), health communication, social marketing and, most recently, behaviour change communication are used often interchangeably and without clear definition. This review draws on work carried out using all of these terms. It will use the Health Education, Service Improvement and Advocacy (HESIAD) framework (Figure 11.1) to show their relation to health promotion.

This framework was developed while working with WHO on an intervention planning manual and is described elsewhere (Hubley, 2001, 2004). It is based on the Ottawa Charter and sees health promotion as involving the three components of health education, service improvement and advocacy. The emphasis of this review is on health promotion in low income and middle income countries that share the characteristics shown in Table 11.1 (for further discussion of the significance of the Ottawa Charter for global health promotion, see Chapter 1).

Leeds Health Education Database

It was a need to establish the evidence base for health promotion in low and middle income countries that led to the establishment of the Leeds Health Education Database project in 1998. This involved an extensive search for reports on heath promotion interventions including advocacy for changes in health policies and health education directed at communities. Criteria used for selection included the following: the report should be published in an accessible source, preferably a peer-reviewed journal, the intervention should be adequately described, there should be valid evidence of impact on the community from either quantitative or qualitative data and the research design should be sufficiently strong to attribute impact to the intervention. In the process some

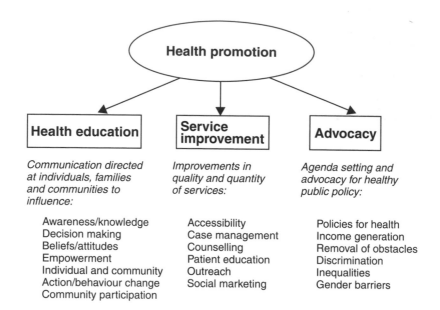

Figure 11.1   The contribution of health education, service improvement and
advocacy (HESIAD) to health promotion

700 studies were reviewed and 350 were entered in the database that are listed in full on an Internet website (http://www.hubley.co.uk) and form the basis for this review.

Table 11.1   Some key health related features of low income and
middle income countries

A young population, as much as half the population < 15 years;
A higher level of infectious than chronic disease;
Low income and poverty as underlying cause of many health problems;
Inequalities in health a reflection of inequalities in income, land ownership, housing, education and gender;
Lack of access to adequate amounts of clean water;
Large sections of the population without access to adequate healthcare;
Large sections of the public without access to schooling and low levels of literacy among adults;
A population mainly living in rural areas lacking in facilities and amenities of towns;
Rapid migration to cities with growing numbers of marginalised people living in urban poverty;
An extensive network of alternative non-western systems of medicines that are often part of traditional belief systems.

Not surprisingly, given the prevailing patterns of health and disease in the developing world, most evaluated health promotion activities have been directed against infectious diseases and malnutrition. However, many countries are experiencing a health transition and alongside the traditional patterns of health have been experiencing an increase in the so-called diseases of westernisation, such as cancers, heart disease, hypertension, diabetes, traffic accidents and addictions including tobacco, alcohol and drugs. This is a reflection of ageing populations, changing lifestyles, and the adoption of western patterns of living including those of diet and exercise. The Leeds Health Education Database has strong representation in the area of HIV/AIDS, family planning, maternal health, child health and infectious disease control. It also contains useful material on education, particularly in the fields of water, sanitation and hygiene. In contrast it records few published interventions on chronic diseases such as heart disease (Dowse et al., 1995), hypertension (Jinxiang et al., 1998) or injury prevention (Krug et al., 1994; Swaddiwudhipong et al., 1998). These neglected areas require more attention.

Addressing the complexity of human behaviour

Much early health education was based on simplistic notions that merely providing knowledge would lead to changes in attitudes and practices. It became evident that human behaviour was influenced by factors that can operate at the community, district, regional, national and even international level. These include beliefs, norms, social pressure from others in the network, access to services and economic factors such as income. These are usually underpinned by cultural and traditional factors as well as external influences from an increasingly globalised world.

A range of theoretical models has evolved in an attempt to explain influences on human decision making (Glanz and Rimer, 1997). The use of theory to plan interventions by the studies in the Leeds Health Education Database is disappointingly low. The two most popular models are the Health Belief Model (Ford et al., 1996; Visser, 1996; Attia et al., 1997; Glik et al., 1998; Rubabt et al., 1999; Agha, 2003) and the Theory of Reasoned Action (Klepp et al., 1994; Middlestadt et al., 1995; Visser, 1996; Wong et al., 1996, 1998; Kane et al., 1998; Kinsman et al., 2001). Other models used include social learning theory (Dick and Lombard, 1997; Martiniuk et al., 2003), social construction theory (Nastasi et al., 1998), social cognitive theory (Hunter et al., 1991; Ford et al., 1996), communication of innovations theory (Glik et al., 1998) and the Transtheoretical Model (Thevos et al., 2000). It is not possible to draw any conclusions on the relative merits of the different models from the database (see Part I, Chapter 4 for a further discussion of models).

Some interventions sought to identify and target influential persons in the family or community. Examples include a programme that involved Buddhist monks in Thailand to support education on tobacco smoking (Swaddiwudhipong et al., 1993), the involvement of Islamic leaders in AIDS education in Uganda (Kagimu et al., 1998) and traditional healers to promote oral rehydration in Brazil (Wilson et al., 1989). In Ethiopia (Terefe and Larson, 1993) a family planning programme targeted husbands to gain their approval. In Guatemala a programme using volunteers to promote family planning found it beneficial to provide training for the spouses of the volunteers to engage their support (Pineda et al., 1983).

A critical decision in any intervention is whether to seek to change a belief or to work around it. For example an evaluation of a hygiene education intervention in Bangladesh found that it was necessary to develop the concept of the germ theory in their community (Ahmed and Zeitlin, 1993). This contrasts with the experience of a programme in North East Brazil that found that they were able to involve popular healers in the promotion of oral rehydration while still working within their traditional beliefs on diarrhoea.

Some kind of needs assessment is vital to understand the influences on behaviour. Most reports in the database had conducted a baseline study of some kind, usually a KAP (Knowledge, Attitude and Practice) study. Recognising the importance of cultural barriers, some studies based their interventions on data from ethnographic research for example hygiene education in Bangladesh (Ahmed et al., 1991, 1993, 1994; Ahmed and Zeitlin 1993), pregnancy in Latin America (Belizan et al., 1995; Langer et al., 1996), control of onchocerciasis in Nigeria (Brieger et al., 1988) and schistosomiasis in Brazil (Uchoa et al., 2000), uptake of malaria prophylaxis by pregnant women in Malawi (Helitzer-Allen et al., 1993, 1994), and weaning foods in Brazil (Monte et al., 1997).

One of the most interesting recent developments in community based health promotion has been the movement for participatory rural appraisal methodology (PRA) that has also been called participatory learning and action (PLA) and health analysis and action cycle. PRA uses a range of methods to help communities to identify their needs and develop solutions to their problems including, mapping, construction of seasonable calendars, problem ranking, body mapping. PRA has been used both for general community based work, for example with women in Nepal, (Gibbon and Cazottes, 2001) and for specific health topics including sexual health in Nepal (Butcher and Kievelitz, 1997) and Uganda (Ssembatya et al., 1995) and hygiene education (Young, 1998). Exciting though PRA certainly is, it is a process that requires skilled field staff, has to be repeated with each separate community and is therefore labour intensive. Unfortunately, many accounts of PRA tend to be descriptive reports, rich in anecdotes but with little data on impact to justify such an investment in human resources.

Community based health promotion

Community participation was a focus of the Primary Health Care Movement that followed on from the Alma Ata Declaration of 1976. The 1970s and 1980s were decades of widespread experimentation especially in selection, training and support of village health workers. Subsequent evaluations showed that success of these programmes depended heavily on initial selection and training, on-going supervision and support and the need for constant vigilance to monitor and allow for the turnover of volunteers in the community for working with local communities and developing local capacity. These lessons were subsequently applied to other groups in the training of traditional birth attendants (Rashid et al., 1999), volunteers in women's health programmes (Bentley, 1989; Matomora, 1989; Akram and Agboatwalla, 1992; Quigley and Ebrahim, 1994; Agboatwalla and Akram, 1995; Chongsuvivatwong et al., 1996; Kidane and Morrow, 2000), nutrition educators (Brown et al., 1992, 1994) and traditional healers (Nations et al., 1996; Nations and de Souza, 1997). The lessons were also relevant to other less well documented training programmes as with volunteers as water-facility minders, guinea-worm control and the community based distribution of mectizan for onchocerciasis control.

A further extension of these ideas, especially in the field of sexual health, is the concept of peer education which has been applied to diverse groups such as sex workers (Visrutaratna et al., 1995; Walden et al., 1999), truck drivers (Laukamm-Josten et al., 2000), persons in prisons (Simooya and Sanjobon, 2001) and young people in the community (Brieger et al., 2001; Speizer et al., 2001; Agha, 2003). Unfortunately the valuable lessons from the early primary healthcare projects were often ignored in peer education programmes, especially about the high turnover and the need for support. Many of the evaluations of peer education programmes, while demonstrating effectiveness, indicate the need for continued support, raising issues about their long-term sustainability.

While early health education put a great deal of emphasis on the use of visual aids, more recent work has built on the rich oral traditions of drama, music, songs and storytelling that exist in large parts of the world. Most of the evaluated reports of the use of drama in communities have been for the promotion of family planning and prevention of AIDS. Examples include the use of street theatre in Peru (Valente et al., 1994), songs and drama for AIDS education in Ghana (Bosompra, 1992), puppets and street theatre in the streets of South Africa (Skinner et al., 1991), community drama in Sri Lanka (McGill and Joseph, 1997) and India (Valente and Bharath, 1999), and education at cattle markets and festivals in rural northeast Thailand (Dole et al., 1998). A weakness with many of these evaluations is that few carried out data collection before and after performances, used controls and, with the notable exception of Bosompra (1992), rarely measured longer term impact. Given these limitations, folk media can attract large numbers and can spread awareness and knowledge. The main problem appears to be that of the cost of sustaining performers.

The concept of empowerment has its roots in the work of Paulo Freire in Brazil. His ideas were taken up in the nonformal and adult education movements and organisations such as World Education, Save the Children, and

United Nations Development Programme and Training for Transformation (Hope and Timmel, 1984). They produced excellent manuals with a range of participatory group exercises that could be used to encourage communities to reflect on their situations and how they might be improved.

Evaluations of these community based participatory methods are rare (Clark and Gakuru, 1982; Zimmerman et al., 1997). A study in Ghana (Laverack et al., 1997) described how it followed a process of developing participatory materials for use by teachers and health workers that were developed with full involvement of the intended users and carefully pre-tested by the community. Despite this, their follow-up showed that the materials produced were not used by the field staff and highlighted the problems of developing participatory approaches within existing health and education services.

Empowerment has been proposed as one of the main aims of health promotion, yet despite a growing literature on the topic, evidence for the impact of empowerment programmes on health remains elusive. Most of the published reports of empowerment approaches in developing countries consist mainly of anecdotal descriptions of activities with little systematic documentation of impact using either quantitative or qualitative evaluation methods (for the political difficulties in effecting empowerment strategies in low income countries see Part III, particularly Chapters 12 and 18).

Mass media

The orthodoxy in early discussions has been that mass media is suitable for promoting knowledge and awareness but that changing behaviour requires the use of face-to-face approaches (Rogers and Shoemaker, 1971). However, there is now ample evidence (Hornik, 1989) that well-designed and executed mass media can bring about changes in some behaviour. Moreover, in countries with fragile primary healthcare infrastructures and few trained field staff on the ground there are no alternatives to mass media use.

In reality, the debate between the use of the mass media and face-to-face interactions has been carried out in simplistic terms. Comparisons need to take into account both issues of behaviour change effectiveness and cost-effectiveness. The mass media has been poorly used in many countries with outputs that were both boring and low quality, with messages that were too generalised, culturally inappropriate and complex in language. There has been a tendency to discuss mass media in general terms rather than to assess the impact of different formats as, for example, those of advertising, news broadcasts and entertainment.

In recent years there have been a series of studies from low and middle income countries that demonstrate that well-planned mass media interventions can be effective in bringing about changes in behaviour, especially the uptake of family planning services and immunisation. These include both general mass media programmes (Cerqueira et al., 1979; Foreit et al., 1989;

Piotrow et al., 1990; Kincaid et al., 1993; Lettenmaier et al., 1993; Westoff and Rodriguez, 1995; Kane et al., 1998; Reeta and Rajeev, 1998; Storey et al., 1999; Vaughan et al., 2000a, 2000b; Mohammed, 2001; Tambashe et al., 2003) as well as those which explicitly take the social marketing approach described below.

Some effective mass media interventions have applied a social marketing approach. Examples include the promotion of condoms (Black and Harvey, 1976; Agha and Rossem, 2002), oral rehydration solution (Kenya et al., 1990; Koul et al., 1991; Miller and Hirschhorn, 1995) and mosquito nets (Schellenberg et al., 1999). This approach places emphasis on pricing and packaging, the mobilisation of sales and distribution outlets and promotion through mass media use with additional interpersonal support.

Another promising approach is to embed health education messages into entertainment such as in Turkey (Kincaid et al., 1993), Tanzania (Rogers et al., 1999; Vaughan and Rogers, 2000) and St Lucia (Vaughan et al., 2000b). The Johns Hopkins Population Communications Institute has played a leading role in this approach with programmes in Mexico, Philippines and Turkey. This has led to a movement for enter-education. A well known product of this movement is the Soul City programme in South Africa, which used a television soap opera format supported by printed media such as booklets. A note of caution is that a high entertainment level alone does not ensure an impact. An evaluation of the use of songs for education on AIDS in Ghana found that people enjoyed dancing to the music but did not pay attention to the words (Bosompra, 1992).

Evaluation of mass media poses methodological issues. It is difficult to set controls in the evaluation of mass media interventions except in rare cases such as the *Twende na Wakati* radio soap opera in Tanzania where it was possible to take advantage of regional broadcasting services (Vaughan et al., 2000a). In the absence of controls, a widely used method to attribute a programme's impact has been to carry out a survey and demonstrate that the people who changed were those who saw, heard and remembered the specific input. Such an approach, as used in Zambia (Yoder et al., 1996), can be criticised because it is always possible that the section of the community who were motivated and predisposed to accept the change might also be the ones who were motivated to see and remember the advertisement. In some cases additional qualitative research is used to strengthen evidence for a case effect. The existence of a dose response effect, a surge in family planning clinic attendance immediately after broadcasts, has also been used to infer a causal relationship (Bailey and Cabrera, 1980).

Despite the low cost per person reached, mass media does involve considerable initial expense. While a decade ago national mass media services were willing to offer air time free or at low cost for public service use, this seems less the case now. Many of the high profile mass media health promotion initiatives are dependent on funding by international donors raising concerns about long-term sustainability (for further discussion of the mass media, see Part I, Chapter 5).

Little media

Little media include educational materials such as leaflets (Hira et al., 1990), posters, audiocassettes, video (Mathews et al., 1999) and films (Attia et al., 1997). Improved printing technologies have allowed an increasingly imaginative range of materials including stickers (Berhane and Pickering, 1993), messages on balloons, T shirts, and key rings. These can be used on their own or learning aids to support face-to-face communication in community settings, such as clinics and schools.

Much of the early discourse on the use of such materials focused on the problem of comprehension of written and pictorial instructions (see reviews by McBean, 1988; UNICEF, 1976; Cripwell, 1989). The term visual literacy was introduced to describe the problems faced by illiterate or newly literate communities in understanding the graphics conventions in pictures.

Media have been effectively used to reinforce patient education and support a range of mass media and community based health promotion activities including peer education and home visits. A technical problem faced in the evaluation of media is that it can be quite difficult to separate the contribution of specific media in multimedia campaigns. Another problem is that, while some media are designed to communicate specific messages, others are intended to provide triggers for discussion and participatory learning and therefore require a different approach to evaluation.

Increased community exposure to pictures, greater availability of colour printing and more widespread acceptance of the concept of pre-testing (Linney, 1985, Hugo and Skibbe, 1991; Hugo, 1994; 1995; Röhr-Rouendaal, 1997) have all played a part increasing the potential of printed materials. However, as communities in traditional societies become more exposed to media, they will also become more sophisticated and discriminating in their response to media. Health promoters will need to pay more attention to quality and creativity to gain attention and communicate their messages.

School based interventions

Attempts to improve the quality of health promotion in schools face formidable obstacles such as large classes, shortages of trained teachers, lack of books and inadequate facilities including buildings, water supply, toilets and safe play areas. High levels of dropouts from poor children, especially girls (Hyde, 2001), means that the groups who might benefit most from health education are not able to receive it. School based interventions in low and middle income countries need to take into account the realities facing children, teachers and communities. Health education in the classroom needs to be supplemented by improvements in the school environment and the development of school health services.

There is now good evidence that schools based interventions can be effective in a range of areas including oral health (Albandar et al., 1994; Axelsson et al., 1994; Reis, 1994; Nyandindi et al., 1996), worms (Lefroy et al., 1995; Lansdown et al., 2002), screening for eyesight (Murthy et al., 1994; Ajuwon et al., 1997), malaria (Marsh et al., 1996), schistosomiasis (Yuan et al., 2000) and mental health promotion (Froozani et al., 1999). Concerns about AIDS, teenage pregnancy and reproductive health in general has resulted in a wide range of well documented programmes showing the value of sex education on knowledge and in some cases behaviour (Russel-Browne et al., 1992; Caceres et al., 1994; Klepp et al., 1994; Kuhn et al., 1994; Aplasca et al., 1995; MacLachlan et al., 1997; Mbizvo et al., 1997; Rusakaniko et al., 1997; Shuey et al., 1999; Eggleston et al., 2000; Martiniuk et al., 2003) Most of the evaluated examples of school health promotion tend to be small-scale interventions on single issues where health education is supplemented with programmes to train and support teachers, upgrade the school surroundings and provide school services, such as screening.

A barrier to the effective development of school health education has been the widespread use of formal didactic teaching underpinned by a system of examinations. The most progressive movement for change has been the Child-to-Child programme. Launched at the international year of the child in 1979, and using activity-based learning methods advocated by the visionary Hugh Hawes, it has become justly famous for its child-centred approach (Hawes, 1988; Bonati and Hawes, 1992; Hawes and Scotchmer, 1993). More recently the same package of methods has re-emerged and been branded as the 'life skills' approach.

While the small-scale studies in the Leeds Database clearly demonstrate that school based interventions can be effective, incorporating these innovative methods into existing structures is not easy. A good discussion of the problems (Kinsman et al., 1999, 2001) also explores reasons why a school health education programme in Uganda failed to replicate the impact on increased sexual abstinence achieved by an earlier programme in the same country (Shuey et al., 1999). In contrast with apparently successful school based activities, his programme placed great emphasis on working through existing structures to provide a replicable model.

Given the importance of school based health promotion, there is an urgent need for effective international advocacy and action. The recent extension, with the support of WHO, of the Health Promoting Schools Initiative to the developing world is a welcome step. It is still not clear how this mainly European model will adapt to the harsh realities that children face in their daily lives in much of the world (for a discussion of this initiative in Africa, see Part III, Chapter 12).

Advocacy

Advocacy includes any activity directed at influencing policies and laws that promote health. Despite widespread use of the term, there is no consensus on what advocacy methods involve. Recent manuals on advocacy for tuberculosis (WHO, 1999), polio programmes and AIDS and reproductive rights mainly deal with issues such as use of media, writing press releases, and staging media events.

Within pluralistic societies advocacy and lobbying of government is a recognised activity carried out by pressure groups, special interest groups, such as trade unions and a strong and independent media. However many countries are still in the process of democratisation and establishing a civil society. Opportunities for effective advocacy are less developed and in some cases even dangerous to organise. Strong controls on activities of NGOs and newspapers can make it difficult to openly criticise national policy. Vested interests in the private sector such as tobacco, drugs and oil companies can be very powerfully established. However, there are examples of developing countries where a tradition of political activism has lead to the emergence of pressure groups carrying out advocacy for change. Good examples are the AIDS action groups in South Africa lobbying for access to anti-retroviral drugs and breast feeding pressure groups such as BUNSO in the Philippines (for a discussion of the difficulties of advocacy in some low income countries, see Chapter 12).

Advocacy at the international level has played an important role in health promotion with the increasing realisation that problems of globalisation require globalised responses. An early example of effective advocacy was that of the establishment of the International Code for Marketing of Breast Milk Substitutes. Another example has been the success of UNICEF in convincing a range of governments in Asia and Africa to run high profile national immunisation days and issue stamps showing key components of its child survival strategy. WHO's role in advocacy is most obvious in the annual World Health Assembly. A recent example was the adoption in 2003 of the Framework Convention for Control of Tobacco, which has the force of a national treaty (see also Part II, particularly Chapters 6 and 8).

Many international agencies and pressure groups are now taking a rights-based approach which places health goals within a framework of human rights legislation. A good example of this has been the work of UNICEF to secure international agreement to the International Charter for the Rights of the Child and subsequent pressure at a national level for governments to recognise the charter. Another example is the reproductive rights movement spearheaded by a range of international agencies and pressure groups. They often work through international conferences such as that on population at Cairo (1994) and on women in Beijing (1995).

The issue of advocacy raises ethical issues. A particular health topic or policy might be adopted because of successful advocacy effort by a well organised pressure group and other equally pressing health topics may be neglected because they do not have effective groups to champion them. Since many countries can rely heavily on foreign aid their health policies can be donor driven. A recent global phenomenon is the emergence of powerful foundations, such as that of Bill and Melinda Gates, that are playing an increasing role in funding health promotion activities (see also, Chapters 5 and 6).

Most advocacy activities in developing countries have been poorly documented or researched. Accounts in the literature rarely go beyond simple description to include reflective and analytical descriptions of the process of promoting change. The reasons for this neglect are not clear. It may be that the persons involved in such advocacy activities are not part of a research culture of writing and publishing. Another reason may be that, while donor agencies are willing to fund evaluation research on the impact of projects, the topic of evaluation of advocacy is less attractive. There is an urgent need for good quality research that documents and evaluates different approaches by pressure groups at community and national level that have been used in advocacy for policy change in low and middle income countries. Such research would be invaluable for providing evidence-based guidelines for future advocacy (for a further discussion of advocacy and alliances see Chapters 4 and 6).

Challenges for the future

It was disappointing that so many interesting and challenging activities could not be included in the Leeds Database because insufficient evidence of impact was provided or they were poorly documented. Inevitably such a database shows a publication bias because much good work is probably not published and shared. A challenge is to improve the quality of evaluation, especially of community based empowerment programmes and to encourage the sharing of experiences through the publication of evaluations.

Few of the studies in the database measure the long-term impact and sustainability of interventions or provide data on cost-effectiveness of the methods used. Another problem is that much evidence of effectiveness of health education and health promotion in the database comes from small-scale pilot programmes that are often not sustained beyond the lifetime of the project. Scaling up and integrating these improved practices within routine services is vital to have a meaningful impact on the health of communities.

Scaling up inevitably involves working through the existing infrastructure of field staff in health and other services which is already stretched and working under difficult conditions. Often the key responsibilities for planning at a national level are carried out by medically trained personnel with little training in health promotion. The result is often poorly conceived health promotion programmes, lacking clear focus and coordination, based on inappropriate and untested messages delivered by inadequately trained field staff (see Part III, particularly Chapters 12 and 13 for further discussion of this potential difficulty).

The role of a specialist service should to be to act as a focal point for the planning, coordination and strengthening of health promotion activities within local services. Where such services exist they usually retain the name of health education, IEC or behaviour change communication and not health promotion. Their role is poorly understood and often seen to be that of production of posters and educational materials with staff of a junior status without training or authority to influence national policy.

The role of health promotion services in low and middle income countries has only received a little attention in the literature (Dehne and Hubley, 1993; Hubley, 1986). There have been a number of initiatives to strengthen health education in these that have come to the author's attention, but they have gone largely undocumented. A welcome exception is a recent report from Mali (Barker, 2003) that uses an organisational approach to present a case study of an initiative to strengthen a national IEC centre. Critical to the success of this initiative was a strong commitment by government and donors to strengthening IEC services. There is an urgent need for advocacy for health promotion and the development of guidelines for the organisation and delivery of health promotion.

We are only just beginning to see the impact the Internet can have in a globalised world. The Internet opens up new channels of interactive communication with communities as well as providing a means of support and training for health promoters throughout the world. Many organisations now post manuals, research papers and databases on web sites and there is a global movement to free up information and make academic journals available at no cost to persons from developing countries. Through email and news groups and discussion groups, opportunities are opening up for dialogue, sharing, coordinating and advocacy at an unprecedented level. For some developing countries the Internet is becoming increasingly available. However, for many countries especially in Africa, the digital divide persists with Internet access still beyond the reach of many (Berhardt and Hubley, 2001).

With more than 350 entries and still growing the Leeds Health Education Database project now provides clear evidence that effective health promotion can be carried out within the demanding conditions found in low and middle income countries. The challenge is to put this into practice.

References

Agboatwalla, M. and Akram, D.S. (1995) An experiment in primary health care in Karachi, Pakistan. *Community Development Journal*, **30**: 384–91.

Agha, S. (2003) A quasi-experimental study to assess the impact of four adolescent sexual health interventions in sub-Saharan Africa. *International Family Planning Perspectives*, **28**: 67–117.

Agha, S. and Rossem, R.V. (2002) Impact of mass media campaigns on intentions to use the female condom in Tanzania. *International Family Planning Perspectives*, **28**: 151–57.

Ahmed, N.U. and Zeitlin, M.F. (1993) Assessment of the effects of teaching germ theory on changes in hygiene behaviours, cleanliness and diarhoeal incidence in rural Bangladesh. *International Quarterly of Community Health Education*, **14**: 283–97.

Ahmed, N.U., Zeitlin, M.F., Beiser, A.S., Super, C.M. et al. (1991) Community-based trial and ethnographic techniques for the development of hygiene intervention in rural Bangladesh. *International Quarterly of Community Health Education*, **12**: 183–202.

Ahmed, N.U., Zeitlin, M.F., Beiser, A.S., Super, C.M. and Gershoff, S.N. (1993) A longitudinal study of the impact of behavioural change intervention on cleanliness, diarrhoeal morbidity and growth of children in rural Bangladesh. *Social Science and Medicine*, **37**: 159–71.

Ahmed, N.U., Zeitlin, M.F., Beiser, A.S., Super, C.M., Gershoff, S.N. and Ahmed, M.A. (1994) Assessment of the impact of a hygiene intervention on environmental sanitation, childhood diarrhoea, and the growth of children in rural Bangladesh. *Food and Nutrition Bulletin*, **15**: 40–52.

Ajuwon, A.J., Oladepo, O.O., Sati, B. and Otoide, P. (1997) Improving primary school teachers' ability to promote visual health in Ibadan, Nigeria. *International Quarterly of Community Health Education*, **16**: 219–27.

Akram, D.S. and Agboatwalla, M. (1992) A model for health intervention. *Journal of Tropical Paediatrics*, **38**: 85–87.

Albandar, J.M., Buischi, Y.A., Mayer, M.P. and Axelsson, P. (1994) Long-term effect of two preventive programs on the incidence of plaque and gingivitis in adolescents. *Journal of Periodontology*, **65**: 605–10.

Aplasca, M.R., Siegel, D., Mandel, J.S., Santana-Arciaga, R.T., Paul, J., Hudes, E.S., Monzon, O.T. and Hearst, N. (1995) Results of a model AIDS prevention program for high school students in the Philippines. *AIDS*, **9** Suppl 1: S7–13.

Attia, A.K., Rahman, D.A.M.A. and Kamel, L.I. (1997) Effect of an educational film on the Health Belief Model and breast self-examination practice. *Eastern Mediterranean Health Journal*, **3**: 435–43.

Axelsson, P., Buischi, Y.A., Barbosa, M.F., Karlsson, R. and Prado, M.C. (1994) The effect of a new oral hygiene training program on approximal caries in 12–15-year-old Brazilian children: results after three years. *Advances in Dental Research*, **8**: 278–84.

Bailey, J. and Cabrera, E. (1980) Radio campaigns and family planning in Columbia (1971–1974). *Bulletin of the Pan American Health Organisation*, **14**: 126–34.

Barker, K. (2003) Order from chaos: organisational aspects of information, education and communication (a case study from Mali). *Journal of Health Communication*, **8**: 383–94.

Belizan, J.M., Barros, F., Langer, A., Farnot, U., Victora, C. and Villar, J. (1995) Impact of health education during pregnancy on behavior and utilisation of health resources. Latin American Network for Perinatal and Reproductive Research. *American Journal of Obstetrics and Gynecology*, **173**: 894–99.

Bentley, C. (1989) Primary healthcare in northwestern Somalia: a case study. *Social Science and Medicine*, **28**: 1019–30.

Berhane, Y. and Pickering, J. (1993) Are reminder stickers effective in reducing immunisation dropout rates in Addis Ababa, Ethiopia? *Journal of Tropical Medicine and Hygiene*, **96**: 139–45.

Berhardt, J.M. and Hubley, J.H. (2001) Health education and the internet: the beginning of a revolution (editorial.) *Health Education Research: Theory and Practice*, **16**: 643–45.

Black, T.R.L. and Harvey, P.D. (1976) A report on a contraceptive social marketing experiment in rural Kenya. *Studies in Family Planning*, **7**: 101–08.

Bonati, G. and Hawes, H. (1992) *Child-to-Child: a resource book*. London: Child to Child Trust.

Bosompra, K. (1992) The potential of drama and songs as channels for AIDS education in Africa: a report on focus group findings from Ghana. *International Quarterly of Community Health Education*, **12**: 317–42.

Brieger, W.R., Delano, G.E., Lane , C.G., Oladepo, O. and Oyediran, K.A. (2001) West African Youth Initiative: outcome of a reproductive health education program. *Journal of Adolescent Health*, **29**: 436–46.

Brieger, W.R., Ramakrishna, J., Adeniyi, J.D. and Kale, O.O. (1988) Health education interventions to control onchocerciasis in the context of primary healthcare. In Carlaw, R. and Ward, B. (Eds) *Primary healthcare: the African experience*. Oakland, CA: Third Party Publishing Company

Brown, L.V., Zeitlin, M.F., Peterson, K.E., Chowdhury, A.M., Rogers, B.L., Weld, L.H. and Gershoff, S.N. (1992) Evaluation of the impact of weaning food messages on infant feeding practices and child growth in rural Bangladesh. *American Journal of Clinical Nutrition*, **56**: 994–1003.

Brown, L.V., Zeitlin, M.F., Weld, L.H., Rogers, B.L., Peterson, K.E., Huq, N. and Gershoff, S.N. (1994) Evaluation of the impact of messages to improve the diets of lactating rural Bangladeshi women on their dietary practices and the growth of their breast-fed infants. *Food and Nutrition Bulletin*, **15**: 320–34.

Butcher, K. and Kievelitz, U. (1997) Planning with PRA: HIV and STD in a Nepalese mountain community. *Health Policy and Planning*, **12**: 253–61.

Caceres, C.F., Rosasco, A.M., Mandel, J.S. and Hearst, N. (1994) Evaluating a school-based intervention for STD/AIDS prevention in Peru. *Journal of Adolescent Health*, **15**: 582–91.

Cerqueira, M.T., Casanueva, E., Ferrer, A.M., Chávez, A. and Flores, R. (1979) A comparison of mass media techniques and a direct method for nutrition education in rural Mexico. *Journal of Nutrition Education*, **11**: 133–37.

Chongsuvivatwong, V., Mo-suwan, L., Tayakkanonta, K., Vitsupakorn, K. and McNeil, R. (1996) Impacts of training of village health volunteers in reduction of morbidity from acute respiratory infections in childhood in southern Thailand. *Southeast Asian Journal of Tropical Medicine and Public Health*, **27**: 333–38.

Clark, N.M. and Gakuru, O.N. (1982) The effect on health and self-confidence of participation in collaborative learning activities. *Hygie*, **1**: 47–56.

Cripwell, K.R. (1989) Non-picture visuals for communication in health learning manuals. *Health Education Research: Theory and Practice*, **4**: 297–304.

Dehne, K.L. and Hubley, J. (1993) Health education services in developing countries: the case of Zimbabwe. *Health Education Research: Theory and Practice*, **8**: 525–36.

Dick, J. and Lombard, C. (1997) Shared vision – a health education project designed to enhance adherence to anti-tuberculosis treatment. *International Journal of Tuberculosis and Lung Disease*, **1**: 181–86.

Dole, L.R., Elkins, D.B., Boonjear, K., Phiensrithom, S. and Maticka-Tyndale, E. (1998) Cattle markets and local festivals: development of HIV/AIDS prevention interventions for specific risk situations in rural northeast Thailand. *Health and Place*, **4**: 265–72.

Dowse, G.K., Gareeboo, H., Alberti, K.G.M.M., Zimmet, P., Tuomilehto, J., Purran, A., Fareed, D., Chitson, P., Collins, V.R. and Hemraj, F. (1995) Changes in population cholesterol concentrations and other cardiovascular risk factor levels after five years of the non-communicable disease intervention programme in Mauritius. *British Medical Journal Clinical Research Edition*, **311**: 1255–59.

Eggleston, E., Jackson, J., Rountree, W. and Pan, Z. (2000) Evaluation of a sexuality education program for young adolescents in Jamaica. *Revista Panamerica de Salud Publica*, **7**: 102–12.

Ford, K., Wirawan, D.N., Fajans, P., Meliawan, P., MacDonald, K. and Thorpe, L. (1996) Behavioral interventions for reduction of sexually transmitted disease/HIV transmission among female commercial sex workers and clients in Bali, Indonesia. *AIDS*, **10**: 213–22.

Foreit, K.G., de Castro, M.P.P. and Franco, E.F.D. (1989) The impact of mass media advertising on a voluntary sterilisation program in Brazil. *Studies in Family Planning*, **20**: 107–16.

Froozani, M.D., Permehzadeh, K., Dorosty Motlagh, A.R. and Golestan, B. (1999) Effect of breastfeeding education on the feeding pattern and health of infants in their first 4 months in the Islamic Republic of Iran. *Bulletin of the World Health Organisation*, **5**: 381–85

Gibbon, M. and Cazottes, I. (2001) Working with women's groups to promote health in the community using the health analysis and action cycle within Nepal. *Qualitative Health Research*, **11**: 728–49.

Glanz, K. and Rimer, B.K. (1997) *Theory at a glance – a guide for health promotion practice.* Bethesda, MD: US Department of Health and Human Services, Public Health Service, National Institutes of Health, National Cancer Institute.

Glik, D.C., Rubardt, M., Nwanyanwu, O., Jere, S., Chikoko, A. and Zhang.W. (1998) Cognitive and behavioural factors in community-based malaria control in Malawi. *International Quarterly of Community Health Education*, **18**: 391–413.

Hawes, H. (1988) *Child-to-child another path to learning.* Hamburg: Unesco Institute for Education.

Hawes, H. and Scotchmer, C. (1993) *Children for health.* London, New York: Child-to-Child Trust/UNICEF.

Helitzer-Allen, D.L., Macheso, A.P., Wirima, J.J. and Kendall, C. (1994) Testing strategies to increase use of chloroquine chemoprophylaxis during pregnancy in Malawi. *Acta Tropica*, **58**: 255–66.

Helitzer-Allen, D.L., McFarland, D.A., Wirima, J.J. and Macheso, A.P. (1993) Malaria chemoprophylaxis compliance in pregnant women: a cost-effectiveness analysis of alternative interventions. *Social Science and Medicine*, **36**: 403–07.

Hira, S.K., Bhat, G.J., Chikamata, D.M., Nkowane, B., Tembo, G., Perine, P.L. and Meheus, A. (1990) Syphilis intervention in pregnancy: Zambian demonstration project. *Genitourinary Medicine*, **66**: 159–64.

Hope, A. and Timmel, S. (1984) *Training for Transformation – A Handbook for Community Workers (3 volumes).* P.O. Box 779, Gweru, Tanzania: Mambo Press.

Hornik, R. (1989) *Channel Effectiveness in Development Communication Programs.* University of Pennsylvania: Centre for International Health and Development Communication.

Hubley, J. (1986) Barriers to health education in developing countries. *Health Education Research: Theory and Practice*, **1**: 233–45.

Hubley, J.(2001) Health promotion. In Walley, J., Wright, J. and Hubley, J. (eds) *Public Health – An Action Guide to Improving Health in Developing Countries.* Oxford: Oxford University Press.

Hubley, J. (2004) *Communicating health – An Action Guide to Health Education and Health Promotion*, 2nd Ed. Oxford: Macmillan.

Hugo, J. (1994) Ethnic-based learner response to child accident prevention illustrations.*Media in Medicine*, **17**: 169–73.

Hugo, J. and Skibbe, A. (1991) Facing visual illiteracy in South African health education: a pilot study. *Journal of Audiovisual Media in Medicine*, **14**: 47–50.

Hunter, S.M., Steyn, K., Yach, D. and Sipamla, N. (1991) Smoking prevention in black schools: a feasibility study. *South African Journal of Education*, **11**: 137–41.

Hyde, A.L. (2001) *Girls' Education: Thematic Studies Document Produced for the World Education Forum, Dakar, 2000.* Paris: UNESCO.

Jinxiang, X., Jiguang, W. and Husheng, Y. (1998) Hypertension control improved through patient education. *Chinese Medical Journal*, 111: 581–84.

Kagimu, M., Marum, E., Nakyanjo, N., Walakira, Y. and Hogle, J. (1998) Evaluation of the effectiveness of AIDS health education interventions in the Muslim community in Uganda. *AIDS Education and Prevention*, 10: 215–28.

Kane, T.T., Gueye, M., Speizer, I., Pacque-Margolis, S. and Baron, D. (1998) The impact of a family planning multimedia campaign in Bamako, Mali. *Studies in Family Planning*, 29: 309–23.

Kenya, P.R., Gatiti, S., Muthami, L.N., Agwanda, R., Mwenesi, H.A., Katsivo, M.N., Omondi-Odhiambo, J., Surrow, A., Juma, R., Ellison, R.H. et al. (1990) Oral rehydration therapy and social marketing in rural Kenya. *Social Science and Medicine*, 31: 979–87.

Kidane, G. and Morrow, R.H. (2000) Teaching mothers to provide home treatment of malaria in Tigray, Ethiopia: a randomised trial. *Lancet*, 356: 550–55.

Kincaid, D.L., Yun, S.H., Piotrow, P.P.T. and Yaser, Y. (1993) Turkey's mass media family planning campaign. In Backer, T.E. and Rogers, E.M. (eds) *Organisational Aspects of Health Communication Campaigns: What Works?* London, New Delhi: Sage Publications.

Kinsman, J., Harrison, S., Kengeya-Kayondo, J., Kanyesigye, E., Musoke, S. and Whitworth, J. (1999) Implementation of a comprehensive AIDS education programme for schools in Masaka District, Uganda. *AIDS Care*, 11: 591–601.

Kinsman, J., Nakiyingi, J.K.A., Carpenter, L.Q.M.P.R. and Whitworth, J. (2001) Evaluation of a comprehensive school-based AIDS education programme in rural Masaka, Uganda. *Health Education Research: Theory and Practice*, 16: 85–100.

Klepp, K.I., Ndeki, S.S., Seha, A.M., Hannan, P., Lyimo, B.A., Msuya, M.H., Irema, M.N. and Schreiner, A. (1994) AIDS education for primary school children in Tanzania: an evaluation study. *AIDS*, 8: 1157–62.

Koul, P.B., Murali, M.V., Gupta, P. and Sharma, P.P. (1991) Evaluation of social marketing of oral rehydration therapy. *Indian Pediatrics*, 28: 1013–16.

Krug, A., Ellis, J.B., Hay, I.T., Mokgabudi, N.F. and Robertson, J. (1994) The impact of child-resistant containers on the incidence of paraffin (kerosene) ingestion in children. *South African Medical Journal*, 84: 730–34.

Kuhn, L., Steinberg, M. and Mathews, C. (1994) Participation of the school community in AIDS education: an evaluation of a high school programme in South Africa. *AIDS Care*, 6: 161–71.

Langer, A., Farnot, U., Garcia, C., Barros, F., Victora, C., Belizan, J.M. and Villar, J. (1996) The Latin American trial of psychosocial support during pregnancy: effects on mother's well-being and satisfaction. *Social Science and Medicine*, 42: 1589–97.

Lansdown, R., Ledward, A., Hall, A., Issae, W., Yona, E., Matulu, J., Mweta, M., Kihamia, C., Nyandindi, U. and Bundy, D. (2002) Schistosomiasis, helminth infection and health education in Tanzania: achieving behaviour change in primary schools. *Health Education Research*, 17: 425–33.

Laukamm-Josten, U., Mwizarubi, B.K., Outwater, A., Mwaijonga, C.L., Valadez, J.J., Nyamwaya, D., Swai, R., Saidel, T. and Nyamuryekunge'e, K. (2000) Preventing HIV infection through peer education and condom promotion among truck drivers and their sexual partners in Tanzania, 1990–1993. *AIDS Care*, 12: 27–40.

Laverack, G., Esi Sakyi, B. and Hubley, J. (1997) Participatory learning materials for health promotion in Ghana – a case study. *Health Promotion International*, 12: 21–26.

Lefroy, J.E., Swai, S., Hoopman, R. and van Hell, L. (1995) How effective is community health education in preventing worm infestation? *Tropical Doctor*, 25: 194

Lettenmaier, C., Krenn, S., Morgan, W., Kols, A. and Piotrow, P. (1993) Africa: using radio soap operas to promote family planning. *Hygie*, **12**: 5–10.

Linney, B. (1985) Pre-testing posters for communicating about water and sanitation. *Waterlines*, **4**: 2–4.

Linney, B. (1995) *Pictures, People and Power – People-centred Visual Aids for Development*. London and Basingstoke: Macmillan Education Ltd.

McBean, G. (1988) Rethinking visual literacy: research in progress. *Health Education Research: Theory and Practice*, **3**: 393–98.

McGill, D. and Joseph, W.D. (1997) An HIV/AIDS awareness prevention project in Sri Lanka: evaluation of drama and flyer distribution interventions. *International Quarterly of Community Health Education*, **16**: 237–55.

MacLachlan, M., Chimombo, M. and Mpemba, N. (1997) AIDS education for youth through active learning: a school-based approach from Malawi. *International Journal Of Educational Development*, **17**: 41–50.

Marsh, V.M., Mutemi, W., Some, E.S., Haaland, A. and Snow, R.W. (1996) Evaluating the community education programme of an insecticide-treated bed net trial on the Kenyan coast. *Health Policy and Planning*, **11**: 280–91.

Martiniuk, A.L., O'Connor, K.S. and King, W.D. (2003) A cluster randomised trial of a sex education programme in Belize, Central America. *International Journal of Epidemiology*, **32**: 131–36.

Mathews, C., Ellison, G., Guttmacher, S., Reisch, N. and Goldstein, S. (1999) Can audiovisual presentations be used to provide health education at primary care facilities in South Africa? *Health Education Journal*, **58**: 146–56.

Matomora, M.K. (1989) A people-centered approach to primary healthcare implementation in Mvumi, Tanzania. *Social Science and Medicine*, **28**: 1031–37.

Mbizvo, M.T., Kasule, J., Gupta, V., Rusakaniko, S., Kinoti, S.N., Mpanju-Shumbushu, W., Sebina-Zziwa, A.J., Mwateba, R. and Padayachy, J. (1997) Effects of a randomised health education intervention on aspects of reproductive health knowledge and reported behaviour among adolescents in Zimbabwe. *Social Science and Medicine*, **44**: 573–77.

Middlestadt, S., Fishbein, M., Albarracin, D., Francis, C., Eustace, M.A., Helquist, M. and Schneider, A. (1995) Evaluating the impact of a national AIDS prevention radio campaign in St Vincent and the Grenadines. *Journal of Applied Social Psychology*, **25**: 21–34.

Miller, P. and Hirschhorn, N. (1995) The effect of a national control of diarrheal diseases program on mortality: the case of Egypt. *Social Science and Medicine*, **40**: S1–S30

Mohammed, S. (2001) Personal communication networks and the effects of an entertainment-education radio soap opera in Tanzania. *Journal of Health Communication*, **6**: 137–54.

Monte, C.M.G., Ashworth, A., Nations, M.K., Lima, A.A., Barreto, A. and Huttly, S.R.A. (1997) Designing educational messages to improve weaning food hygiene practices of families living in poverty. *Social Science and Medicine*, **44**: 1453–64.

Murthy, G.V., Verma, L. and Ahuja, S. (1994) Evaluation of an innovative school eye health educational mode. *Indian Pediatrics*, **31**: 553–57.

Nastasi, B., Schensul, J.J., Amarasiri de Silfa, M.W., Varjas, K., Silva, K.T., Ratnayake, P. and Schensul, S. (1998) Community-based sexual risk prevention programme for Sri Lankan youth: influencing sexual-risk decision-making. *International Quarterly of Community Health Education*, **18**: 139–55.

Nations, M.K. and de Souza, M.A. (1997) Umbanda healers as effective AIDS educators: case-control study in Brazilian urban slums (favelas). *Tropical Doctor*, **27**, Suppl 1: 60–66.

Nations, M.K., de-Sousa, M.A., Correia, L.L. and da-Silva, D.M. (1996) Brazilian popular healers as effective promoters of oral rehydration therapy (ORT) and related child survival strategies. *Bulletin of the Pan American Health Organisation*, 22: 335–54.

Nyandindi, U., Milen, A., Palin-Palokas, T. and Robison, V. (1996) Impact of oral health education on primary school children before and after teachers' training in Tanzania. *Health Promotion International*, 11: 193–201.

Pineda, M.A., Bertrand, J.T., Santiso, R. and Guerra, S. (1983) Increasing the effectiveness of community workers through training of spouses: a family planning experiment in Guatemala. *Public Health Report*, 98: 273–77.

Piotrow, P.T., Rimon, J.G., Winnard, K.D., Lawrence Kinkaid, D., Huntingdon, D. and Convisser, J. (1990) Mass media family planning promotion in three Nigerian Cities. *Studies in Family Planning*, 21: 265–73.

Quigley, P. and Ebrahim, G.J. (1994) Can women's organisations bring about health development? *Journal of Tropical Pediatrics*, 40: 294–98.

Rashid, M., Tayakkanonta, K., Chongsuvivatwong, V., Geater, A. and Bechtel, G.A. (1999) Traditional birth attendants' advice toward breast-feeding, immunisation and oral rehydration among mothers in rural Bangladesh. *Women and Health*, 28: 33–44.

Reeta, M. and Rajeev, M. (1998) Impact of NGO intervention in the knowledge and practices of tribal women of West Bengal. *South Asian Anthropologist*, 19: 87–93.

Reis, R. (1994) Evil in the body, disorder of the brain. Interpretations of epilepsy and the treatment gap in Swaziland. *Tropical Geographical Medicine*, 46: S40–43.

Rogers, E.M. and Shoemaker, F.F. (1971) *Communications of Innovations – A cross-cultural Approach*. New York: Free Press.

Rogers, E.M., Vaughan, P.W., Swalehe, R.M.A., Rao, N., Svenkerud, P. and Sood, S. (1999) Effects of an entertainment-education radio soap opera on family planning behaviour in Tanzania. *Studies in Family Planning*, 30: 193–211.

Röhr-Rouendaal, P. (1997) *Where There is No Artist – Development Drawings and How To Use Them*. London: Intermediate Technology Publications.

Rubabt, M., Chikoko, A., Glik, D., Jere, S., Nwanyanwu, O., Zhang, W., Nknoma, W. and Ziba, C. (1999) Implementing a malaria curtains project in rural Malawi. *Health Policy and Planning*, 14: 313–21.

Rusakaniko, S., Mbizvo, M.T., Kasule, J., Gupta, V., Kinoti, S.N., Mpanju-Shumbushu, W., Sebina-Zziwa, J., Mwateba, R. and Padayachy, J. (1997) Trends in reproductive health knowledge following a health education intervention among adolescents in Zimbabwe. *Central African Journal of Medicine*, 43: 1–6.

Russel-Browne, P., Rice, J.C., Hector, O. and Bertrand, J.T. (1992) The effect of sex education on teenagers in St Kitts and Nevis. *Bulletin of the Pan American Health Organisation*, 26: 67–78.

Schellenberg, J.R., Abdulla, S., Minja, H., Nathan, R., Mukasa, O., Marchant, T., Mponda, H., Kikumbih, N., Lyimo, E., Manchester, T., Tanner, M. and Lengeler, C. (1999) KINET: a social marketing programme of treated nets and net treatment for malaria control in Tanzania, with evaluation of child health and long-term survival. *Transactions of the Royal Society of Tropical Medicine and Hygiene*, 93: 225–31.

Shuey, D.A., Babishangire, B.B., Omiat, S. and Bagarukayo, H. (1999) Increased sexual abstinence among in-school adolescents as a result of school health education in Soroti district, Uganda. *Health Education Research: Theory and Practice*, 14: 411–19.

Simooya, O. and Sanjobon, N. (2001) 'In But Free' – an HIV / AIDS intervention in an African prison. *Culture Health and Sexuality*, 3: 241–51.

Skinner, D., Metcalf, C.A., Seager, J.R., de-Swardt, J.S. and Laubscher, J.A. (1991) An evaluation of an education programme on HIV infection using puppetry and street theatre. Special Section: AIDS–the first ten years. *AIDS Care*, **3**: 317–29.

Speizer, I.S., Tambashe, B.O. and Tegang, S.P. (2001) An evaluation of the 'Entre Nous Jeunes' peer-educator program for adolescents in Cameroon. *Studies in Family Planning*, **32**: 339–51.

Ssembatya, J., Coghlan, A., Lumala, R. and Kituusibwa, D. (1995) Using participatory rural appraisal to assess community HIV risk factors: experiences from rural Uganda. *PLA Notes – International Institute for Environment and Development*: 62–65.

Storey, D., Boulay, M., Karki, Y., Heckert, K. and Karmacharya, D.M. (1999) Impact of the Integrated Radio Communication Project in Nepal, 1994–1997. *Journal of Health Communication*, **4**: 271–94.

Swaddiwudhipong, W., Boonmak,C., Nguntra,P., and Mahasakpan,P. (1998). Effect of motorcycle rider education in changes in risk behaviours and motorcycle-related injuries in rural Thailand. *Tropical Medicine and International Health*, **3**: 767–70.

Swaddiwudhipong, W., Chaovakiratipong, C., Nguntra, P., Khumklam, P. and Silarug, N. (1993) A Thai monk: an agent for smoking reduction in a rural population. *International Journal of Epidemiology*, **22**: 660–65.

Tambashe, B.O., Speizer, I.S., Amouzou, A. and Djangone, A.M. (2003) Evaluation of the PSAMAO 'Roulez Protégé' mass media campaign in Burkina Faso. *AIDS Education and Prevention*, **15**: 33–48.

Terefe, A. and Larson,C.P. (1993) Modern contraception use in Ethiopia: Does involving husbands make a difference? *American Journal of Public Health*, **83**: 1567–71.

Thevos, A.K., Quick, R.E. and Yanduli, V. (2000) Motivational interviewing enhances the adoption of water disinfection practices in Zambia. *Health Promotion International*, **15**: 207–14.

Uchoa, E., Barreto, S.M., Firmo, J.O., Guerra, H.L., Pimenta, F.G. Jr. and Costa, M.F. (2000) The control of schistosomiasis in Brazil: an ethnoepidemiological study of the effectiveness of a community mobilisation program for health education. *Social Science and Medicine*, **51**: 1529–41.

UNICEF (1976) *Communicating with pictures in Nepal – report of a study by NDS and UNICEF*, Kathmandu: UNICEF.

Valente, T.W. and Bharath, U. (1999) An evaluation of the use of drama to communicate HIV/AIDS information. *AIDS Education and Prevention*, **11**: 203–11.

Valente, T.W., Poppe, P.R., Alva, M.E., Vera de Briceño, R. and Cases, D. (1994) Street theatre as a tool to reduce family planning misinformation. *International Quarterly of Community Health Education*, **15**: 279–89.

Vaughan, P.W. and Rogers, E.M. (2000) A staged model of communication effects: evidence from an entertainment-education radio soap opera in Tanzania. *Journal of Health Communication*, **5**: 203–27.

Vaughan, P.W., Regis, A. and St Catherine, E. (2000b) Effects of an entertainment-education radio soap opera on family planning and HIV prevention in St Lucia. *International Family Planning Perspectives*, **26**: 148–57.

Vaughan, P.W., Rogers, E.M., Singhal, A. and Swalehe, R.M. (2000a) Entertainment-education and HIV/AIDS prevention: a field experiment in Tanzania. *Journal of Health Communication*, **5**: 81–100.

Visrutaratna, S., Lindan, C.P., Sirhorachai, A. and Mandel, J.S. (1995) 'Superstar' and 'model brothel': developing and evaluating a condom promotion program for sex establishments in Chiang Mai, Thailand. *AIDS*, **9** Suppl 1: S69–75.

Visser, M. (1996) Evaluation of the First AIDS Kit, the AIDS and lifestyle education programme for teenagers. *South African Journal of Psychology/Suid-Afrikaanse Tydskrif vir Sielkunde*, **26**: 103–13.

Walden, V.M., Mwangulube, K. and Makhumula-Nkhoma, P. (1999) Measuring the impact of a behaviour change intervention for commercial sex workers and their potential clients in Malawi. *Health Education Research: Theory and Practice*, **14**: 545–54.

Westoff, C.F. and Rodriguez, G. (1995). The mass media and family planning in Kenya. *International Family Planning Perspectives*, **21**: 26–31,36.

WHO (1999) *TB advocacy – a practical guide*. Geneva: WHO/TB/98.239 WHO Global Tuberculosis Programme.

Wilson, D., Greenspan, R. and Wilson, C. (1989) Knowledge about AIDS and self-reported behaviour among Zimbabwean secondary school pupils. *Social Science and Medicine*, **28**: 957–61.

Wong, M.L., Chan, K.W. and Koh, D. (1998) A sustainable behavioral intervention to increase condom use and reduce gonorrhea among sex workers in Singapore: 2-year follow-up. *Preventive Medicine*, **27**: 891–900.

Wong, M.L., Chan, R., Lee, J., Koh, D. and Wong, C. (1996) Controlled evaluation of a behavioural intervention programme on condom use and gonorrhoea incidence among sex workers in Singapore. *Health Education Research: Theory and Practice*, **11**: 423–32.

Yoder, P.S., Hornik, R. and Chirwa, B.C. (1996) Evaluating the program effects of a radio drama about AIDS in Zambia. *Studies in Family Planning*, **27**: 188–203.

Young, E. (1998) *Health into science*. London: Child-to-Child Trust.

Yuan, L., Manderson, L., Tempongko, M.S., Wei, W. and Aiguo, P. (2000) The impact of educational videotapes on water contact behaviour of primary school students in the Dongting Lakes region, China. *Tropical Medicine and International Health*, **5**: 538–44.

Zimmerman, M.A., Ramirez-Valles, J., Suarez, E., de la Rosa, G. and Castro, M.A. (1997) An HIV/AIDS prevention project for Mexican homosexual men: an empowerment approach. *Health Education and Behavior*, **24**: 177–90.

CHAPTER 12

Trends and Factors in the Development of Health Promotion in Africa, 1973–2003

DAVID NYAMWAYA

The chapter discusses the major developments in health promotion in sub-Saharan Africa, hereafter referred to as the region, during the last three decades, roughly from 1973 to 2003. It was during this time that health promotion policies, structures and programmes in the region went through fundamental changes. By the end of the period all countries had attained political independence and were thus able to develop health initiatives independent of former colonial rulers. Lastly, over these years the region became fully involved in global events and debates relating to the development and implementation of health promotion.

From the outset mention must be made of the fact that use of the term health promotion in this chapter does not necessarily imply the existence of a unified conceptualisation of health promotion. There are at least two clearly distinguishable conceptualisations of health promotion in the region, one held by its practitioners and the other by academicians and some senior public health professionals. The conceptual differences arise mainly from the contrasting interests of health promotion practitioners and academicians. The practitioners wish to emphasise the specific disciplines and methods in which they are trained or those they use when delivering services to the public. They, therefore, see health promotion primarily as a tool or set of tools for health action, comprising health education, behaviour change communication, social mobilisation and others. On the other hand, academicians and some public health managers are more interested in explaining the general contribution of health promotion to the health and related development processes. At this level, emphasis is placed on strategic health promotion attributes, that is, empowerment of individuals and communities for health action, support for the creation of environments that are supportive of health, and advocacy for health as an investment and not merely as a social service. This issue is discussed further in the last section of the chapter (for other examples of dichotomies around which health promotion is organised, see Part I, Chapter 5).

It is also necessary at this point to state that due to the paucity of published sources, much of the material used in the chapter is drawn from the author's personal and published experiences on the subject, interviews with colleagues and a few published sources.

Progress in health promotion policy development

By the mid 1970s, most countries of the region had attained political independence. During this period, investments in education, health and the economy were regarded as pillars of the development process embarked on by the newly independent countries. The state was the major provider of health services. The prevailing view was that health could be achieved mainly through the provision of biomedical, and in particular curative, services. The focus of health development, therefore, was on health facility construction or expansion besides the training of medical personnel at various levels. The state was primarily responsible for financing the services. Faith-based organisations working in the continent also focused on provision of curative health services. It is, therefore, understandable that most health policies put in place during this period reflected the overriding concern for curative services and, therefore, included little about health promotion per se or its constitutive fields.

The main motivation for systematic incorporation of health promotion in health systems of the region was provided by the declaration of Health for All (HFA) of the World Health Assembly in 1977 followed by the adoption in Alma Ata the following year of the primary healthcare approach (PHC). Health education was listed as one among eight major components of PHC. This explains why many countries of the region started including health education, information, education and communication (IEC) and behaviour change communication (BCC) in national health policy documents from the early 1980s. Few countries, however, developed and elaborated fully fledged national health promotion policies. It is important to indicate that while various health promotion components expanded in the 1980s, they were mostly implemented by health personnel who had had limited or no professional training in health promotion or its constituent components.

In the mid-1980s, countries of the region resolved to involve the general public more actively in health promotion through the Bamako Initiative (Ridde, 2003), which sought to revive PHC and community participation in health development (WHO/AFRO, 2002). This focus on community participation contributed significantly to the subsequent development of health promotion policy in the region as indicated later in the third section of this chapter.

It was only in the 1990s, that the region started to take part effectively in global developments relating to health promotion. For example, while there were no official delegates from the region at the first global conference on health promotion which took place in Ottawa in 1986, there were a number of official delegates at the third one in Sundsvall on supportive environments for health in 1991 and by the time the Mexico ministerial conference on health promotion was held in 2000, about a third of the countries of the region were represented. It was at the Mexico conference that delegates from countries of the region resolved to support and ensure development of national policies and plans for health promotion.

Soon after the Mexico meeting, the adoption of the Health for All policy for the twenty-first century by the regional committee of ministers of health (WHO/AFRO, 2002) provided another significant push for health promotion within the region. In 2000, for the first time ever, 46 health ministers, under the auspices of WHO/AFRO, recognised the importance of developing HFA policies with strong health promotion components and pledged to support them. Adoption of the policy has had and continues to have far-reaching influences on the development of health promotion policies, structures and programmes.

Also in 2000, the committee of ministers of health of the region adopted a resolution calling for urgent action to address the emergent epidemic of noncommunicable diseases (WHO/AFRO, 2000). Among the actions recommended were use of health promotion approaches to respond to closely interrelated risk factors for noncommunicable diseases. This recent recognition (WHO/AFRO, 2000; van der Sande, 2003) of the threat of noncommunicable diseases in the region has provided further impetus for the development of health promotion policies. In countries such as Mauritius and South Africa where noncommunicable diseases have already become a serious threat, recent tobacco legislation and implementation of regulations about salt in processed foods are good examples respectively of appropriate health promotion policies.

Increasingly, health promotion policies and strategies in the region that hitherto have existed in draft form are now being reviewed and rewritten (Lambo and Sambo, 2003). Rewriting of the policies is accelerating partly due to the adoption in 2001 of a regional health promotion strategy by ministers of health of 46 countries of the region. The strategy strongly affirms the importance, indeed the necessity, of health promotion for three reasons. It suggests that there is evidence that it works in terms of empowerment for health action, healthy public policies and increased community involvement. It draws attention to the effectiveness of health promotion to health development by the way it integrates different approaches and methods. It is central to the creation and management of enabling environments for health (WHO/AFRO, 2003).

With the adoption of the regional health promotion strategy, it can be argued that the perception of health promotion as a means for increasing societal responsibility for health and as a combination of diverse approaches now exists in all countries of the region.

Developments in health promotion structures

The majority of countries of the region have established within national or state ministries of health, units, departments or divisions for handling health promotion. South Africa, Uganda, Mauritius and Niger are good examples. In the Anglophone countries, the structures are usually referred to as health education while in the Francophone countries the acronym for information, education and communication (IEC), is most commonly used. Relative to other structures in national health systems in general, the health promotion structures are in most cases very poorly resourced in human, financial and material terms. The majority of health promotion personnel are trained only to certificate or diploma level, with few having university degree qualifications. The reasons for the poor staffing relate to the emphasis on curative services and the consequent low status of health promotion in health systems described in the first section of this chapter.

A typical national health promotion unit or department includes an audio-visual materials production centre, a mass media section, specific projects sections, as well as a public relations component. In most countries, the unit is responsible for writing speeches for the minister and top civil servants in the ministry of health. It also provides the master of ceremony during public functions. The main outputs of these units are audiovisual materials (Nyamwaya and Ndavu, 1997).

While all countries of the region have some official organisation for health promotion at national level, only a few, most notably Botswana, Kenya, Mauritius, Nigeria, Uganda, South Africa and Zimbabwe, have regional or state/district level structures. Some such as Eritrea and Zambia have no structures at local level.

Currently, the development of health promotion structures in the region is accelerating rapidly due to the factors described in the first section of this chapter. In fact, several countries are currently reviewing and in most cases expanding and consolidating existing health promotion structures to cater for the broader health promotion policies being developed. In some, most notably Guinea Conakry, South Africa, Mauritius, Niger and Uganda, fairly comprehensive health promotion entities have been established during the last few years. In these countries, due to the demands generated by the double burden of disease (South Africa and Mauritius) or HIV/AIDS (Uganda), structures have been created which can deliver programmes based on a broad conceptualisation of health promotion. The expanded health promotion organisations deal with areas such as social mobilisation, advocacy, legislative actions and support for health policy development.

A number of private and parastatal corporations have established health promotion structures as part of their staff health service programme. Examples include the Electricity Company of South Africa (Eskom), Telkom Kenya and Ethiopian Airways. These deal mainly with staff education but others provide counselling support as well, especially with regard to HIV/AIDS. They also manage general occupational health matters. The magnitude and coverage of these structures is diverse and there are no standards or guidelines applicable nationwide. No systematic external evaluation of the functioning of the health promotion structures established by parastatal organisations has so far been carried out. Similarly, non-health ministries such as education, agriculture/livestock and related others have established some units that perform health promotion matters. The directorate of health promotion in South Africa is a good example as shown in Part II. The ministry of agriculture in several countries, for example, provides education and support on nutrition matters, focusing on food production, processing and preparation. Health promotion structures have also been established in ministries of education as indicated in the next section.

Developments in health promotion programmes

The socioeconomic conditions of the region have to a very large extent influenced the approaches, issues and actors in health promotion programmes. For example, due to the high incidence and prevalence of communicable diseases and related conditions health promotion interventions are primarily directed towards assisting people to attain better personal hygiene through acquisition of health knowledge and skills. Likewise, low levels of literacy have led to the development and use of innovative indigenous media such as drama and music to communicate health messages (see, for example, Vaughan et al., 2000). In large part, due to general poverty and inadequate understanding of the role of health promotion in development, the main actor in health promotion has been government. The following paragraphs show that several changes are taking place and with radical changes to health promotion programmes for the region in terms of approaches, issues of focus and actors.

It has been shown that in most countries of the region, the most commonly used strategy in health promotion is empowerment for communities and individuals with health knowledge and skills (AMREF, 2000). Health personnel usually seek to impart knowledge to the general public through various episodic interventions, which are not always organised in a programme or even a project format. Key messages are passed on in a prescriptive fashion, in many cases at health service delivery points (Nyamwaya, 2003). The most popular explanation given for this focus on the hierarchical communication of health information is linked to the thinking among health professionals that people engage in unhealthy behaviour mainly because of ignorance resulting from the low levels of formal education in much of the region.

Health promotion programmes in the region usually rely on one or a few specific media. The most commonly used medium continues to be print. Radio (Mohammed, 2001), focus group discussion (Bosompra, 1992), various folk media, interactive theatre, puppetry and television are also used to various degrees in different countries (WHO/AFRO, 2003). Drama and the mass media for example have been used extensively in Tanzania (see, for example, Agha and Rossem, 2002) and Southern Africa in HIV/AIDS prevention programmes (Skinner et al., 1991). Song and dance are being used widely especially in fertility control interventions (for a sustained discussion of mass media techniques of health promotion in low income countries including those of Africa, see Part III, Chapter 11).

Generally, governments have not supported the use of social mobilisation, activism and advocacy interventions funded with public money. This is because such techniques are seen to have the potential of creating awareness about community rights and the responsibility of government to respond, which could lead to political unrest (Nyamwaya, 2003).

During the last two decades, health promotion programmes that seek to combine communication strategies with support for the creation of environments supportive of health have been emerging in several countries. An example of such programmes is the Education for Community Health Action programme (ECHA) the implementation of which started in Kenya during the late 1980s (Okedi, 1993).

The Ministry of Health designed ECHA with technical support from various non governmental organisations (NGOs). Programme activities would start with a consultation, involving a community and personnel from the ministry of health and an NGO. The community would be assisted in identifying health and related needs and the required responses.

The responses planned in ECHA programmes are aimed at addressing the underlying causes of identified problems. Actions to reduce malnutrition, for example, may involve provision of knowledge about its causes, and training in skills on food production, storage and processing. This was done, for example, in Mukurweini, Nyeri district, Kenya in the 1980 and 1990s. Appropriate units of the ministries of health and agriculture handle rehabilitation of severely malnourished children. Community leaders have became actively involved in ECHA and lobbying with political leaders and private enterprises for support to the communities to address major health problems. Rules regulating feeding of children are put in place and families encouraged to adhere to them.

ECHA thus touches on three key strategies of health promotion, the empowerment of individuals and communities, the provision of supportive environments and advocacy for health. Health promotion programmes similar to ECHA have been implemented in other countries including Benin, Botswana, Ethiopia, Ghana, Mali, Tanzania, Uganda and South Africa (Okedi, 1993).

The bulk of health promotion programmes in the region are designed to address one specific health issue, such as personal hygiene, malaria, immunisation, fertility control and recently, HIV/AIDS, depending on prevailing epidemiological patterns. Selection of a single issue for health promotion programmes interventions is usually dictated by the source of funding especially when programmes are externally resourced (AMREF, 2000). Most donors stipulate that their funds must be used solely for the specific health problem in which they are interested.

While this single issue approach may facilitate sharper focus on programme objectives, it has its limitations (Brugha and Walt, 2001). In responding to cholera epidemics, for example, governments have tended to favour knowledge-focused interventions, leading to repeated outbreaks of the same disease, because underlying determinants were not adequately addressed. A case in point is that of Kwazulu Natal Province in South Africa during the last few years. It is not unusual to find interventions for fertility control, HIV/AIDS prevention and unwanted pregnancy prevention programmes being implemented in parallel, with little collaboration among implementers, though the beneficiary may be the same community. Examples are found among current projects in Nyanza Province, Kenya.

In recent years, good progress has been achieved in integrating various issues in health promotion programmes (for one discussion, see Lush et al., 2001). Nine countries are now implementing the adolescent health programme known as the Alliance of Parents Adolescents and Communities (APADOC), which addresses problems such as substance abuse, unsafe sex, HIV/AIDS, mental health and noncommunicable diseases comprehensively. The programme is based on the premise that the risk factors of the various adolescent health problems are closely interrelated. It is known for example, that the behaviours that are responsible for sexually transmitted infections, HIV/AIDS and unwanted pregnancies are more or less similar. Therefore, similar approaches can be used to address all or several of these problems at the same time. Another reason for integration of issues in this programme arises from the realisation that, unlike health workers, the beneficiaries, and especially young people, do not compartmentalise the issues. APADOC is now being implemented in East, Central and South Africa and will soon be introduced in West Africa through support from the Regional Office of the World Health Organisation (Maruping, 2003; http://www.afro.who.int/press/2003/pr20031025.html).

Three kinds of health promotion programmes in the region are normally distinguished according to the primary agency. There are those that are government run, those that are managed by NGOs, and to a small extent, those of the private sector. The latter type tends to be better resourced, has adequate qualified staff and embraces a wider range of strategies than the former. In Zambia for example, there is only one health promotion staff at the Central Board of Health, which serves the whole country, while NGOs dealing with HIV/AIDS and population issues have several well-qualified staff among them who deal with much smaller populations. Increasingly, various NGOs are working with government departments to implement comprehensive health promotion strategies involving multiple actors. Within this context, NGOs and professional pressure groups have actively supported development of health promotion programmes with significant legislative and policy development components. This is becoming more evident in tobacco control and food/nutrition initiatives being carried out in Guinea, Kenya, Mali, Mauritius, Senegal and South Africa, This trend of collaboration between NGOs and government departments in health promotion programmes seems to be increasing especially due to the momentum generated by negotiations leading to the Framework Convention on Tobacco Control agreed to this year (see also Part II, particularly Chapter 8).

School health programmes being implemented in most countries of the region show the ever-increasing involvement of diverse government as well as NGO actors and the increasing efforts by the education sector in particular to facilitate health promotion. With support from WHO, UNESCO, UNICEF and World Bank, many countries in the region have established what is known as the Health Promoting School Initiative (HPSI) (www.afro.who.int/ healthpromotion/project.html). The HPSI programme in Erongo Region of Namibia is an excellent example. HPSI is based on actions called for in both the Ottawa Charter for Health Promotion and Education for All goals and follows the call for mobilisation of new players for health promotion in the Jakarta Declaration. The HPSI is aimed at increasing international, national and local capacity in order to improve the health of students, school personnel, families and community members in the vicinity of the school.

HPSI interventions are aimed at addressing a wide range of health and related issues such as school health policy and/or regulations, the development of a safe, healthy environment in both physical and psychosocial terms and the provision of health and related services such as nutrition, health education and community outreach services. Advocacy, networking and collaboration, resource mobilisation, capacity building and operations research together with process documentation are key components of the Initiative. The multi-issue, multiple strategy nature of HPSI (UNESCO, 2000) facilitates the involvement of diverse actors in health promotion action (for further discussion of the role of advocacy, communication and schools initiatives in low income countries, including those of Africa, see Part III, Chapter 11).

Challenging the public health paradigm

In this section, further examination of some of the matters so far discussed is done with a view to clarifying more the major influences on health promotion and identifying the challenges that need to be addressed to ensure sustainability of the current efforts to expand the field.

It has been indicated in this chapter that print media has been the main channel of communicating health messages in health promotion, in spite of the generally low literacy rates in the region. This situation can be explained through closer examination of the public health paradigm that pervades health systems of the region. The public health model implies approaches in which health, particularly medical, experts identify a problem and recommend, or more accurately prescribe, the solution considered appropriate. According to the model, individuals as well as the public as a whole are expected to accept the solution passively and comply with the stipulated action. This thinking is illustrated by the numerous complaints of health workers (AMREF, 2000) about lack of compliance on the side of users of health systems as the main reason for poor health status of populations in the region.

The conventional public health view can also to some extent explain the inadequate attention health workers pay to the socioeconomic context within which health promotion interventions are implemented. For example, health personnel trained in this model find it difficult to accommodate the views of the public in the implementation of health promotion programmes. In Kenya's Makueni district, the author participated in a community health project in which ordinary people wanted treatment of domestic animals included among priority project interventions while public health officials resisted the inclusion, until a non governmental organisation intervened. In this case, goats are the main source of livelihood and these would ensure human health. With the assumption that health workers alone hold answers to all health problems, few health promotion programmes do audience research to determine people's needs and the appropriate modes of communication that should be used in programmes. Likewise, there is limited operations research carried out to determine which approaches are most relevant in specific programmatic circumstances.

The public health model also accounts for the limited development in the use of indigenous approaches and techniques in health promotion. Since the model raises biomedicine as the pinnacle of modernity, health workers do not encourage use of indigenous resources because they are viewed as connoting backwardness. It is important to note however, that there are now encouraging positive changes taking place in the region with regard to the perception and use of both indigenous concepts and techniques for communicating health messages and motivating health action as indicated in Part II. Examples of such development may be seen in the use of music, drama and poetry to address HIV/AIDS issues in Tanzania by both the Ministry of Health and a non governmental organisation, the African Medical and Research Foundation.

To a large extent the health problems that have so far been the focus of health promotion interventions, reflect closely the prevailing socioeconomic and related epidemiological profiles in the region. Most countries of the region may be considered as low income, with poor housing, low literacy rates and inadequate health systems. Poor governance, human disasters such as civil disturbances, and natural disasters such as floods and droughts compound these conditions. The conditions lead to poor personal hygiene and sanitation. Many communicable diseases such diarrhoea, malaria, vaccine preventable diseases (especially tuberculosis), abound. The last two decades have witnessed the emergence of HIV/AIDS as a major public health problem in the region. It is understandable, therefore, that most health promotion programmes have been directed at communicable disease control.

The rapid increase in noncommunicable diseases in several countries (WHO, 2002) is imposing another obstacle in health promotion programming. It is estimated however that unless urgent preventive and control actions are taken now, the noncommunicable diseases will soon catch up or even overtake communicable diseases as the main causes of morbidity and mortality in the region (WHO/AFRO, 2002). This possible scenario calls for drastic adjustments in health promotion strategies. Positive health promotion responses to the increasing noncommunicable diseases are already being seen in comprehensive health promotion policies in some countries as already indicated in the previous section of this chapter. Ironically, increases in the incidence and prevalence of noncommunicable diseases are leading to more use of advocacy, policy development, and legislation for health promotion far more than was the case when only communicable disease were the focus of programmes. The best illustration of this is the work being done by the Ministry of Health and NGOs of South Africa in diet, nutrition and anti-tobacco campaigns to reduce risks for cancer, heart disease and diabetes.

The global trends towards democratisation and involvement of communities in political action are increasingly leading to the involvement of more actors in health promotion. Indeed, the spectrum of participants in health promotion is widening. NGOs, the private sector and non-health sectors such as education, are becoming more involved. This is a great improvement from the 1970s when the government was the only significant actor in health promotion. While government-led health promotion action emphasises acquisition of knowledge and skills, the partners encourage mobilisation, advocacy, activism and lobbying and policy development as health promotion approaches. There are cases where governments show concern about and sometimes opposition to these latter approaches. This concern by African governments is understandable and exists in other low income regions. It is thought by governments that if communities are mobilised to take part in community action, the consciousness raised can be redirected to political action. Only in countries with well-developed democratic tendencies (especially in high income regions) do we find ministries of health supporting large-scale social mobilisation for health. Professional development of health promotion practitioners in the region has been slow. Only a limited number of health promotion associations exist and most are not active, leading to limited professional debate and interaction. Few universities in the region offer health promotion degrees. Only in South Africa is progress being made in the development of health promotion professional standards. This is an ongoing process but already there is general consensus agreement on the need to have standards and that the standards should cater for the wide range of processes and actors in health promotion.

A number of national associations relating to the constituent components of health promotion and especially health education and IEC exist in several countries. These associations are at the moment grappling with the emergence of health promotion as an area of specialisation. There is serious discussion as to whether health promotion should be regarded as a parallel field or accepted as the broader, integrative process it is. This debate has not been brought into the open and is limited to constructive dialogue in national institutions especially in terms of funding. Expansion of the existing agenda of the associations to accommodate health promotion is a real challenge requiring attention. Collaboration between these associations and the International Union for Health Promotion and Education (IUHPE), which has a regional office in Nairobi, is slowly but steadily emerging.

Due to human and financial resource limitations, research in and evaluation of health promotion in the region is limited and standards of documentation and record keeping is poor. However, the region is getting prepared for involvement in the Global Programme on Health Promotion Effectiveness with support from the IUHPE and the WHO (www.who.int/hpr/ncp/hp.effectiveness.shtml). The region is actively involved in the Global Youth Tobacco Surveys as well as the Global Student Health Studies being supported by WHO and the Centers for Disease Control and prevention.

From the foregoing discussion, it is possible to say that health promotion in the region has been negatively impacted upon by the dominance of curative services health systems in which the public health paradigm predominates. The slow rate of professionalisation made worse by wholesale poverty also hampers more rapid development of health promotion. On the positive side, health promotion has made a strong entry into health systems of the region as evidenced by ongoing review of policies, the initiation of integrated interventions and more involvement of non-health agencies. Finally, since some of the problems affecting the development of health promotion in the region are global in nature, there is need for global collaboration to ensure faster development of health promotion.

References

African Medical and Research Foundation, AMREF. (2000) *Health Promotion and Health Education in the Anglophone African sub-Region.* Nairobi: AMREF.

Agha, S. and Rossem, R.V. (2002) Impact of mass media campaigns on intentions to use the female condom in Tanzania. *International Family Planning Perspectives*, **28**: 151–57.

Bosompra, K. (1992) The potential of drama and songs as channels for AIDS education in Africa: a report on focus group findings from Ghana. *International Quarterly of Community Health Education*, **12**: 317–42.

Brugha, R. and Walt, G. (2001) A global health fund: a leap of faith? *British Medical Journal*, **323** (7305): 152–54.

Lambo, E. and Sambo, L.G. (2003) Health sector reform in sub-Saharan Africa: a synthesis of country experiences. *East African Medical Journal*, **80** (Suppl 6): S1–20.

Lush, L., Walt, G., Cleland, J. and Mayhew, S. (2001) The role of MCH and family planning services in HIV/STD control: is integration the answer? *African Journal of Reproductive Health*, **5** (3): 29–46.

Maruping, A. (2003) Regional Adviser for Child and Adolescent Health, WHO/AFRO: Personal communication based on unpublished material.

Mohammed, S. (2001) Personal communication networks and the effects of an entertainment-education radio soap opera in Tanzania. *Journal of Health Communication*, 6: 137–54.

Nyamwaya, D.O. and Ndavu, E. (eds) (1997) *Health Promotion and Health Education in English speaking Africa*. Nairobi: AMREF.

Nyamwaya, D.O. (2003) Health promotion in Africa: Strategies, players, challenges and prospects. *Health Promotion International*, 18 (2) (editorial).

Okedi, W.N. (1993) Community involvement in health promotion and development: A case study of the Gitie community-based health promotion project in Kenya. Masters Dissertation. Scotland: University of Glasgow.

Ridde V. (2003) Fees-for-services, cost recovery, and equity in a district of Burkina Faso operating the Bamako Initiative. *Bulletin of the World Health Organisation*, 81(7): 532–38.

Skinner, D., Metcalf, C.A., Seager, J.R., de-Swardt, J.S. and Laubscher, J.A. (1991) An evaluation of an education programme on HIV infection using puppetry and street theatre. Special Section: AIDS – the first ten years. *AIDS Care*, 3: 317–29.

UNESCO (2000) *School Health and Nutrition*. Paris:UNESCO.

van der Sande, M.A. (2003) Cardiovascular disease in sub-Saharan Africa: a disaster waiting to happen. *Netherlands Journal of Medicine*, 61 (2): 32–36.

Vaughan, P.W. and Rogers, E.M. (2000) A staged model of communication effects: evidence from an entertainment-education radio soap opera in Tanzania. *Journal of Health Communication*, 5: 203–27.

WHO Regional Office for Africa (2000) *Noncommunicable Diseases: A Strategy for the African Region*. Harare: WHO/AFRO.

WHO Regional Office for Africa (2002) *Health-for-all Policy for the 21st Century in the African Region: Agenda 2020*. AFR/RC50/8Rev.1. Brazzaville: WHO/AFRO.

WHO Regional Office for Africa (2003) *Health Promotion: A strategy for the African Region*. Brazzaville: WHO/AFRO: 18–19.

World Health Organisation (2002) *The World Health Report: Reducing Risks, Promoting Healthy Life*. Geneva: WHO.

CHAPTER 13

Health Promotion in Latin America

HIRAM ARROYO

From an institutional perspective, health promotion emerged as a movement and a global strategy at the first international conference on health promotion held in Ottawa, Canada in 1986. Latin America was one of the world regions that incorporated, more through discourse than practice, the values of health promotion in a relatively short period of time. In 1987, for example, the Pan American Health Organisation (PAHO), suggested that health promotion was both the main objective for the development and the major reason of any social policy (PAHO, 2002). In 1992, in the City of Santa Fé de Bogotá, Colombia, the international conference of health promotion was held, sponsored by the Department of Health of Colombia and PAHO (see Chapter 1 for further discussion of the significance of the Ottawa Charter for global health promotion).

Consequently, the first declaration to conceptualise health promotion in Latin America emanated from here and, in essence, tied it to a political and economic role. The Santa Fé de Bogotá declaration, *Health Promotion and Equity*, not only linked health promotion in Latin America with the need to create the conditions to guarantee the general wellbeing of the population, which it saw as the fundamental purpose of development, it also suggested that such a strategy presupposes the interrelationship of health and development (PAHO, 1996: 374). The strategy was to involve the tackling of exclusionary policies by reconciling economic interests with the need for wellbeing, solidarity and social equity (PAHO, 1996: 374).

In 1993, the Caribbean countries accepted the relevance of health promotion in the *Caribbean Statement for Health Promotion*. The declaration was approved at the first conference of health promotion of the Caribbean, held between 1 and 4 June 1993, at Puerto España, Trinidad and Tobago. At this time, the values of health promotion were distinguished as strengthening the capabilities of the individual and the community, taking preventive actions, disease control and health and wellbeing, inter-sectoral collaboration, developing creativity and productivity, and establishing good interpersonal relationships and peace (PAHO, 1996).

Other historical instances of critical reflection on health promotion in Latin America have been promoted by WHO, PAHO, the International Union for

Health Promotion and Education (IUHPE), and other public and private entities in the region. Among those worth mentioning are the XVI World Conference on Health Promotion and Health Education, sponsored by IUHPE, which was held from 21 to 26 June 1998 in San Juan, Puerto Rico and, in 2000, the organising of the Fifth Global Conference on Health Promotion, in Mexico City, sponsored by WHO and PAHO, under the motto *Health Promotion: Bridging the Equity Gap*. The conference promoted a declaration, the *Mexico Ministerial Statement for the Promotion of Health*, which committed the states' members to strengthen the planning of health promotion activities in their political agendas and in local, regional, national, and international programmes (Cerqueira, 2000).

Conceptualisation of health promotion in Latin America

In Latin America, the coexistence of diverse concepts of health promotion impedes a homogeneous frame of reference. It adversely affects and contra indicates the discourse and the policies of health and health promotion of the countries in this region. The conceptual and interpretative differences towards health promotion and its applications are motivated by experiences, problems, and the historical context of each country in Latin America (Westphal, 2000).

The relative consensus is that it would not be ethical to develop a single concept and methodology for health promotion in the context of Latin America because increasing differences in politics, economy and culture entitle countries to claim the development and contextualisation of their own national models for health promotion. However, there is interest in exploring mechanisms to evaluate and identify proof of effectiveness of health promotion. For this a clear concept of health promotion is important (Castro-Albarrán, 2003) because, with different paradigmatic referents, intervention models of health promotion cannot be subject to a uniform mechanism of validation. Castro-Albarrán (2003) identifies the paradigms of health promotion that coexist in Latin America. The paradigm categories of preventive medicine, individual behaviour, and socio-political context are shown in Table 13.1 (for further discussion of the importance of proof for health promotion, see Part III, particularly Chapters 11, 14 and 19).

It is sometimes suggested that health promotion in Latin America has not generated real cultural changes and that health promotion has exclusively functioned as a new rhetoric formula (Cardaci, 1999), with determinants of health being shaped by socio-political events. There are several political and social structural circumstances that characterise the reality of Latin America (Cardaci, 1999). As well as being perhaps the most inequitable global region in economics, welfare and health (Alleyne, 2001; Almeida-Filho et al., 2003) it is marked by epidemiological complexity due to the coexistence of degenerative chronic illnesses, preventable illnesses, poverty-related illnesses, and diverse manifestations

Table 13.1   Health promotion paradigms (Castro-Albarrán, 2003)

Paradigms	Applications of health promotion
Medical prevention	– Health promotion focuses on the traditional interventions of disease prevention. It consists of a basic clean environment, health education, risk control, favouring individual hygiene practices, and organising medical care into levels of prevention. – The proof of effectiveness of the actions is assessed with indicators of incidence/prevalence of disease, of relationship, and of epidemiological impact.
Individual behaviour	– Prioritises on individual behavioural change by means of interventions directed to the individual without ignoring the emphasis on disease. – Incorporates healthy lifestyles and proper health practices.
Socio-political	– It is based on the values of equity, social transformation and human rights. Fosters collective action, advocacy, empowerment, sustainable human development, establishing social alliances, among others.

of violence (Cardaci, 1999). Yet it is making encouraging progress with the epidemiological transition with age-adjusted mortality rates from communicable diseases showing dramatic falls by around 50 per cent over the 15 years to the year 2000, with the greatest progress where rates were previously highest. Despite fears about malaria, prospects continue to look good (Alleyne, 2001). In contrast, increases of noncommunicable disease reach near-epidemic proportions with cardiovascular diseases already making up one third of the risk of death for both sexes. Obesity with its associated diseases shows rapid rates of increase (Uauy et al., 2001) and with the number of cases of diabetes expected to more than double by the year 2025 (Aschner, 2002) a reorientation of health promotion strategies towards those focused on behaviour changes is called for (for further discussion of changes in health promotion strategies in the context of the epidemiological transition, see Chapters 5, 6 and 15).

The consolidation of an economic model based on cuts in social expenses, on the progressive privatisation of the health sector, and on the redistribution of responsibilities between the state and the individual has led to concerns about equity and the potentially damaging health consequences (Cardaci, 1999; Armada et al., 2001). The growing significance of supranational financing agencies on the definition of social policies (Armada et al., 2001; Iriart et al., 2001), the lack of assurance in compliance with environmental protection policies of free commerce treaties and the inefficacy of updating and training programmes pertaining to health promotion (Cardaci, 1999) is changing, in part, the role of health ministries from delivering services to the monitoring of the quality and equity of provision (Alleyne, 2001).

Indeed, there is a need for the civil society, also, to continue increasing its participation in the formulation of solutions for institutional policy in order to counteract excessive centralisation (Westphal, 2000) and for health promotion to build partnerships with a strengthened civil society. Other challenges of health promotion in Latin America include facing resistance and criticism to the health promotion model, encouraging equity movements, solving distortions and disparities at the different health levels of the population groups, and finding ways for achieving democratic political decisions (Westphal, 2000).

Possibly, the Declaration of Sao Paulo is the most recent expression evoking the ideals and values of health promotion in Latin America. The declaration was developed at the Third Regional Latin American Conference on *Health Promotion and Health Education*. The event was organised by IUHPE with the Regional Office for Latin America (ORLA) and took place in Sao Paulo, Brazil on 10–13 November 2002. The document outlines the following challenges of health promotion:

1. Promote an integrated social agenda that looks for alternatives to development which are focused on the human being. This implies exalting the values of equity, respect for disparities, building solidarity and peace.
2. Adopt democratic processes for true and effective social participation in the promotion of health and quality of life policies.
3. Recognise the diversity of knowledge and culture, and the need to decentralise power.
4. Work towards overcoming fragmentation of healthcare and attention. Promote communication between the state, the civil society and the communities.
5. Develop public health systems committed to collective health actions and to assuring quality attention of the needs of the population (Carta de Sao Paulo, 2002).

These challenges suggest specific courses of action for health promotion: to defend public and universal health systems of the countries; to develop integrated health agendas responsive to human development and to principles of equity; to assure greater investments in the development and training of professionals who attend to the perspectives of health promotion; to foster the creation of social networks and the social participation in support of the actions of health promotion and of an integrated attention to health; and to develop a culture of dialogue between the state, the civil society and the communities with the purpose of promoting policies which favour health and quality of life (Carta de Sao Paulo, 2002).

Health promotion and health education in Latin America

In Latin America, the concepts of health promotion and health education are difficult to separate due to the interdependent relationship that exists between them. Participation in health education and community action has followed a long path that cannot be ignored. These actions have been prototypes of models and conceptual and methodological approaches that have been practiced globally. A great part of the conceptual, strategic and methodological richness that today is associated with the health promotion movement worldwide has been historically present in the discourse and practice of health education in Latin America (Arroyo, 2002). The shifts in emphasis of the paradigms and the policies promoted by WHO, PAHO and IUHPE on health education versus health promotion have adversely affected Latin America. They contribute to the confusion and the overlapping of concepts and methods between the two approaches, an underestimation of the advancements achieved in health education in the region, the elimination of health educational structures in the health sector, and the lack of an aggressive plan for training of personnel (Arroyo, 2002). Latin America is in a process of conceptual and strategic transition regarding health promotion. Whilst health education has a long history, both in the health sector and the educational sector in all Latin American countries, so that it is deep rooted and linked to many programmes and substantial areas; it is also a field of knowledge in transition (Cerqueira, 1997: 38; Arroyo, 2001).

The purpose of health education consists of providing the population with the necessary knowledge, capabilities and skills for promoting and protecting individual, family and community health (Cerqueira, 1997). It is suggested that this can be achieved by developing personal capabilities and skills for active participation in defining the needs, and negotiating and implementing their own proposals for achieving health goals. Certain strategies for a new health education in Latin America have been recommended (Arroyo, 1997; Cerqueira, 1997). These include strengthening policies and actions at the community and school level and expanding the bonds with non governmental organisations; fostering the consolidation of social pacts, conventions, and agreements with diverse social sectors; supporting the expansion of research activities in health education; establishing working alliances with the mass media and maintaining ideas and approaches for a critical reflexive analysis and popular education. Guaranteeing the continuity and permanence of programmes and services in health education as well as investment in actions for developing and training human resources, is also seen to be important.

Health promotion structures

During the last few years, Latin American countries have promoted structural reforms in the area of health promotion. These reforms have varied presentations in content and in the way of focusing principles, postulates and health promotion policies. A representation of the changes in the health promotion strategies in a sample of Latin American countries is shown in Table 13.2. Of concern is that at a time when these countries, motivated by the policies

Table 13.2   Relationship of changes in the institutional structures of health promotion in various Latin American countries

Country	Period of change	Structural changes
Argentina	1999–2001	– Creation of a Division of Promotion and Prevention within the Department of Health. – Creation of the Office of Operations Coordination of Healthy Municipalities – Creation of a Coordinating Unit for the Network of Healthy Municipalities.
Brazil	1998–2002	– Creation of the National Program for Health Promotion under the Secretary of Health Policies of the Department of Health.
Chile	1998	– Creation of the National Council for Health Promotion VIDA CHILE. – Development of the National Plan for Health Promotion following a decentralised and inter-sectoral model.
Colombia	1995–1999	– Promotion of a strategy for Healthy Municipalities for Peace by the Department of Health.
Cuba	1994	– Creation of the National Center for Health Promotion and Education (CNPES, Spanish acronym).
Ecuador	2002	– Development of a National Committee of Health Promotion by the National Council of Health with inter-sectoral representation for advocacy of health actions.
Mexico	1995	– Substitution of the Health Education General Office for the Health Promotion General Office.
Panama	1994	– Creation of the Health Promotion Office and definition of health policies, objectives, and strategies for the years 1994–99.
Peru	2002–03	– Creation of the Health Promotion General Office. – Development of the Strategic Plan for Health Promotion. – Health Promotion becomes a principal objective in the National Health Plan for the period of 2001–06.
Puerto Rico	2001–03	– Creation of the Auxiliary Office for Health Promotion within the Department of Health. – Creation of the Initiative for Special Communities of Puerto Rico fostering social participation and creation of inter-sectoral alliances.
Dominican Republic	2002	– Creation of the General Department of Health Promotion and Education.
Uruguay	1995–2003	– Creation of the Office of Health Promotion within the Department of Health. – Initiation of the Healthy Uruguay 2010 Programme in 2001. – Refocus of the national network of health services towards Primary Care in Health in 2003.

established by PAHO, have made advancements in their health promotion structures, PAHO headquarters in Washington, DC has incorporated changes to their internal structures in 2003. These changes seem questionable and contradictory, and generate confusion and destabilise advances to health promotion in the region. Dissatisfaction has grown because changes have taken place without accompanying evidence of their effectiveness even though they may serve as precursors for further change. This situation of political and administrative instability of the organisational structures of health promotion at both international and national level is one of the principal barriers of the health promotion movement in the region.

Based on a recent analysis of the status of health promotion in some Latin American countries, different common barriers to the advancement of health promotion have been identified (Arroyo, 2004) including a lack of a general understanding of the scope and benefits of health promotion, the exaggerated importance to the curing model as well as administrative weaknesses such as financing requirements, extensive bureaucracy, a lack of training and development of human resources and the need for decentralised actions. There is also political instability, which generates a precipitated turnover of health officials and changes to policies and programmes. Finally there is a need to identify proof of effectiveness of the actions taken.

The effectiveness of health promotion

At the global and regional level there is interest in strengthening research evaluation activities to determine the effectiveness of health promotion interventions (for further discussion of the global strengthening of research evaluation see Chapter 11). This has been possible through the development of projects sponsored by leading international health promotion organisations. An example is the regional project for proof of effectiveness in health promotion in Latin America. This project became official on November 2002, at Sao Paulo, Brazil. The initiative was promoted by the IUHPE, the PAHO, and the Centers for Disease Control and Prevention (CDC), at Atlanta, Georgia. The regional project seeks to develop evaluations of effectiveness that allow the building of proof in health promotion in Latin America, as well as the strengthening of the capabilities, the knowledge, the methodologies, the infrastructure and the investment in the different countries. The main office of the project is at the Universidad Del Valle in Cali, Colombia (Salazar, 2003).

The objectives of the project are to contribute to the construction of proof of effectiveness in the Latin American region; to identify and develop methodologies, instruments and indicators for proof of effectiveness in health promotion in Latin America; to elaborate a document that synthesises and systematises the experiences in health promotion and in evaluation of effectiveness that have taken place in the region; to strengthen the local and regional capability to evaluate effectiveness in health promotion; to develop courses for training the trainers on the evaluation of methods in health promotion; and to disseminate information of proof of effectiveness.

Programmatic priorities of the Pan American Health Organisation

The Pan American Health Organisation (PAHO) has been one of the leading institutions to establish policies and strategic orientations on health promotion in Latin America. Following the Ottawa Declaration of 1986, PAHO sponsored the Bogotá Declaration of 1992, the Caribbean Conference on Health Promotion of 1993, and the Fifth Global Conference on Health Promotion of 2000 in Mexico. PAHO has promoted various events in the Latin American countries or at the sub-regional level (Arvizu and Buelow, 1999). The executive director of PAHO has acknowledged that several countries have incorporated health promotion strategies into their national health plans. In this effort, the contributions and advancements made by Chile, Colombia, Cuba, El Salvador, Guatemala, Mexico and Nicaragua have been particularly recognised (PAHO, 2000).

The health promotion proposals elaborated by PAHO have been presented in different technical documents. For example, the 1994–98 regional plan of action highlights the importance of healthy settings or spaces and the development of alliances with diverse bodies, including institutions for developing human resources. It also emphasises the importance of technical programmes for the following areas: adolescent health, health education, social communication, tobacco control, community mental health and violence. With the aim of improving lifestyles and reducing risky health behaviours PAHO gives support to the education for health and social communication focus on the health behaviour of the population. Priority is given to sexual and reproductive health, tobacco use reduction adequate nutrition for mother and child, child abuse and negligence and other manifestations of violence against children and adolescents (PAHO/WHO, 2001). The 1999–2002 PAHO document outlining strategic and programmatic orientations for health promotion reiterates the relevance of previous programmatic emphasis on healthy settings or spaces, fostering healthy public policies, mental health, tobacco control, prevention of substance abuse, food and nutrition, family health throughout the life cycle and sexual and reproductive health (PAHO/WHO, 2001).

The focus on healthy settings or spaces intends to foster the creation and maintenance of the physical and psychosocial means for people to live healthy lives. This approach is put into action in the projects of healthy cities, healthy municipalities or communities, healthy workplace, and schools as promoters of health (PAHO, 2000; PAHO/WHO, 2001). The initiative for healthy municipalities and communities facilitates and promotes community participation and strengthens community action for improving the conditions and the quality of life (Cerqueira, 1997). The initiative is institutionalised in the Latin American region by the regional network for healthy municipalities and communities established in Campinas, Brazil in 1966. By 1999, PAHO had introduced this concept into the plans of action and policies of the departments of health in the Latin American and Caribbean countries. In the 2001 annual report, the executive director of PAHO highlights the actions taken towards facilitating the establishment of this initiative in the following 13 countries: Bolivia, Brazil, Colombia, Chile, Cuba, Ecuador, El Salvador, Guatemala, Honduras, Mexico, Peru, Dominican Republic and Venezuela (PAHO, 2001).

The initiative of health promoting schools was strengthened by the creation of the Latin American network of health promoting schools in 1996. By 1998, the network reached a membership of 20 countries. Establishing a health promoting school is seen to be a process of social development and as response to the biological, psychological and social needs of children (PAHO, 2001). The emphasis of the programme for the health promoting schools initiative for the years 2000, 2001 and 2002 is shown in Table 13.3. The technical collaboration of PAHO with the Latin American countries in the area of school health focuses on the following aims: revising and updating school health policies, establishing and strengthening the inter-sectoral coordination between health and education, incorporating health promotion contents to school study plans and training of teachers (Cerqueira, 2000; PAHO2001).

Table 13.3   Programmatic priorities of the schools promoters of health initiative in Latin America for the years 2000, 2001 and 2002

2000[a]	2001[b]	2002[c]
– Aptitudes for life. – Improvement of infrastructure for watersupply and sewerage. – Solution of conflicts. – Violence prevention. – Adaptation of instruments for the surveillance of youth risk behaviour. –Needs assessment and diagnosis of health status.	–The right of children and adolescents to health and education. –The right to sexual and reproductive health. – Aptitudes for life. – Education for family life. – Communication among family members. – Exercise and healthy life style.	– Integral development of citizens. – Care for individual and family health. – Teaching aptitudes for life. – Protection of the environment. – Healthy habits. – Promote self esteem. – Foster environmental health. – Strengthening of the inter-sectoral working relationship between Health and Education. – Parent integration and participation in school activities.

Sources: [a] Pan American Health Organization (2000)
[b] Pan American Health Organization (2001)
[c] Pan American Health Organization (2002)

Development of human resources in health promotion

Consensus exists as to the importance of the development and training of human resources in health promotion in Latin America, a consensus that has been helped forward by the health promotion global movement. During the 1990s and early 2000s, important academic developments have taken place. The relation between education and initiatives for training and development of human resources for health promotion in selected Latin American countries is shown in Table 13.4.

As has already been pointed out, the health promotion movement in Latin America is difficult to describe without considering the context of health education as an antecedent. Human resource data demonstrate that, currently, in Latin America, most established academic programmes offer health education and that there are a limited number of academic degrees focused on health promotion. Nevertheless, in the last few years, health education programmes have incorporated into their curricula the basic theory and strategies associated with health promotion. Nevertheless, academic institutions are evaluating their projections for the development of programmes that offer a degree in health promotion (Arroyo, 2000–01; Arroyo, 2002). Moreover, Latin American schools of public health have come to analyse the practice and applications of health promotion as an integral part of public health, particularly the view that health promotion plays a linking role between the functions of the state and that of other social components contributing to a collective community effort (Kickbusch, 2001).

In 1996, the Interamerican Consortium of Universities and Training Centers of Health Education and Health Promotion Personnel (CIUEPS) was instituted. This initiative was sponsored by the former division of social participation and health education of the Pan American Health Organisation and the department of social sciences of the graduate school of public health of the University of Puerto Rico. CIUEPS was constituted as a network of institutions with a mission to strengthen the bonds, cooperation, solidarity and collaborative relationships and academic exchange between members for the development of human resources in health education and health promotion. It is an active discussion forum of current study plans for developing staff in health education and health promotion and a promoter of joint actions directed to fostering and improving the development of theory, methodology, practice of teaching and research in this field in the American regions (CIUEPS, 1996). General assemblies have been held in Puerto Rico, Mexico city and Sao Paulo. CIUEPS is constituted of more than 30 university institutions from the Americas, the Caribbean and Spain. The work of CIUEPS is based on the development of collaborative projects between its members, which include designing curricular alternatives, offering international courses, developing publications and exchanging information by electronic, research and academic means(CIUEPS, 1998, 2000, 2003).

Table 13.4 Initiatives and challenges in the development of human resources for health promotion and health education in Latin America

Country	Initiatives for development	Challenges
Argentina	1. Health Education Programme at the University of Santiago del Estero. 2. In 2003, a Health Promotion and Education degree will be implemented at the Universidad Nacional de Cuyo. 3. In 1987, the Interdisciplinary Health Education Residence is created. It responds to the Office of Training and Development of the Department of Health of the Autonomous Government of the City of Buenos Aires.	1. Inclusion of Health Promotion and Health Education as a requirement of the pre- and post-degree for health professionals. 2. The possibility of having an integral point of view in the academic environment, beyond a fragmented view of the object of study (Ruiz and Dakessian, 2004).
Brazil	1. Public Health Schools offer fellowships and post-degree courses in Health Promotion and Health Education. 2. The Brazilian Association of Post Degree in Collective Health has two working groups: one in Popular Education in Health and another in Health Promotion.	1. The commitment of the Universities is required (by way of the Schools of Public Health, Departments of Preventive Medicine and Collective Health Groups) for creating new programmes for professional development.
Chile	1. An agreement was established between Canada and Chile for the transferring of technology with the University of Toronto and MINSAL in 1999–2001. 2. Implementation of the Network of Academic Centers for Health Promotion of Chile. 3. Since 2000, a Masters degree in Public Health is offered with a Distinction in Health Promotion at the School of Public Health of the University of Chile.	2. The following strategies were prioritised to strengthen the development and training activities: theory and practice of training, clerkship exchange programmes, development of innovating teaching materials, use of interactive technology and creation of working networks (Salinas and Escribano, 2004).

Table 13.4 Continued

Country	Initiatives for development	Challenges
	4. Since 2002, a degree in Health Promotion was offered by INTA at the University of Chile. 5. In 2003, a degree in Good Practices in Health Education and Communication was implemented at the School of Public Health. Other universities have incorporated courses in Health Promotion or Health Education, among them: Pontificia Universidad Católica, Universidad Católica del Maule, Universidad Adventista, Universidad del Bio-Bio y Universidad de Los Lagos.	
Colombia	1. Existence of a Masters Degree in Public Health and Community Health at the University of Antioquía. The Masters Degree Programmes integrate modules in health promotion and health education (Martínez, 2004)	1. The Masters Degree in Collective Health at the School of Nursing of the University of Antioquia has established the need for research in health promotion (Escobar and Torres, 2004).
Cuba	1. In 2001, a Masters Degree in Health Promotion and Education initiated at the National School of Public Health. 2. A degree in Health Promotion and Education is expected to be initiated by 2004. 3. The existence of a degree in Social Communication.	1. The activities directed to the development of human resources are decentralised and offered at the provinces. 2. Continue to offer courses for the advancement and updating of the CNPES programme and the Health Promotion Programme (Sanabria, 2004).
Ecuador	1. The State University of Cuenca has developed a post-degree in Public Health with emphasis in Health Promotion. 2. The Polytechnic School of Chimborazo has developed a post-degree in Health Promotion and Education. 3. The University of San Francisco de Quito has developed a Masters degree in Public Health in which	1. The universities of Ecuador should promote training activities that focus on the health status of the country, work with other professionals in a coordinated fashion, and foster the participation of the population (Puertas et al. 2004).

Table 13.4 Continued

Country	Initiatives for development	Challenges
	Health Promotion is its focal point. 4. The Technical University of Portoviejo has developed a post-degree in Health Promotion. 5. The Simón Bolívar Andean University has developed a School Health Programme.	
Mexico	1. Development of a degree in Health Promotion at the University of Mexico City. 2. The Interamerican Center for the Study of Social Security offers a course in Health Promotion, Communication and Marketing since 1992.	1. It is suggested that the development of human resources in health promotion and health education respond to global strategic planning and not to isolated initiatives (Cardaci, et al. 2004).
Panama	1. Since 1996, the University of Panama offers a Masters Degree in Public Health with emphasis in Health Promotion. 2. Existence of a post-degree in Health Promotion at the Latin University. 3. A degree in Health Promotion and Health Education is in the process of development.	1. Continue revising the study plan for the Masters degree in Public Health with emphasis in Health Promotion at the University of Panama (Muñoz, 2004).
Peru	1. The General Office of Health Promotion of the Department of Health offers training activities. 2. The Cayetano Heredia University is developing a Masters degree in Health Promotion.	1. The need to increase the number of accredited human resources in health promotion is presented (Peñaherrera, 2004).
Puerto Rico	1. The Masters degree Programme in Health Education of the Graduate School of Public Health of the University of Puerto Rico integrates into its curriculum the concepts, approaches and strategies on Health Promotion (Arroyo and Rivera, 2004).	1. Achieve a greater academic-curricular integration between the Bachelor and Masters degrees in Public Health Education.

Table 13.4   Continued

Country	Initiatives for development	Challenges
	2. In 2004, the University of Puerto Rico will establish the Graduate Certificate Programme in School Health Promotion. 3. The country has two Bachelor degree programmes in Health Education. 4. The Graduate School of Public Health of the University of Puerto Rico maintains the main office of the Interamerican Consortium of Universities (CIUEPS).	
Dominican Republic	1. The General Office for Health Promotion and Education, along with the Autonomous University of Santo Domingo, is offering a diploma in Health Promotion.	1. Continue offering training activities originated by the General Office of Health Promotion and Education.
Uruguay	1. Currently, there are no academic programmes offering a degree in Health Promotion at the universities of the country (González, 2004). 2. Various institutions offer specialised courses in health promotion and health education.	1. Continue exploring the possibilities for developing academic programmes in health promotion in the country. 2. Develop training activities at all levels of the system (Gonzáles, 2004).

Faced by the challenges of a globalising world with the concomitant changes in health challenges such as the epidemiological transition, the need to focus on lifestyle changes and a shifting balance between private and public provision, Latin American health promotion is in a period of rapid transition. Although the imprecisions and limitations of the establishment of health promotion in Latin America are well recognised, it has emerged as a body of knowledge, a study discipline and a health intervention strategy of vast possibilities. The permanence of its values, concepts, methodologies and operations will depend on complex factors of a social, ethical, political and institutional nature. Likewise, the enthusiasm generated for qualifying and quantifying the consistency and proof of effectiveness of its actions must be closely observed. It is important that a respect for evidence as the basis for practice is shared among the public, private, community and professional sectors since the permanence of existing practice or its substitution for new health promotion policies in Latin America is the sole responsibility of these sectors.

References

Alleyne, G.A.O. (2001) Latin America and the Caribbean. In Everett Koop, C., Pearson, C.E., Schwarz, M.R. (eds) *Critical Issues in Global health*. San Francisco, CA: Jossey-Bass.

Almeida-Filho, N., Kawachi, I., Filho, A.P. and Dachs, J.N. (2003) Research on health inequalities in Latin America and the Caribbean: biometric analysis (1971–2000) and descriptive content analysis (1971–95). Review. *American Journal of Public Health*, **93** (12): 2037–43.

Armada, F., Muntaner, C. and Navarro, V. (2001) Health and social security reforms in Latin America: the convergence of the World Health Organisation, the World Bank, and transnational corporations. Review. *International Journal of Health Services*. **31** (4): 729–68.

Arroyo, H.V. (2000/01) Training in health promotion and health education in Latin America. *Promotion and Education*, **7** (1): 19–22.

Arroyo, H.V. (2002) Reorientación Conceptual y Estratégica de la Educación para la Salud según referencial de la Promoción de la Salud. Ponencia presentada en la III Conferencia Regional Latinoamericana de Promoción de la Salud y Educación para la Salud. Sao Paulo, Brasil, del 10 al 13 de Noviembre de 2002.

Arroyo, H.V. (ed.) (2001) *Formación de Recursos Humanos en Educación para la Salud y Promoción de la Salud: Modelos y Prácticas en las Américas*. Puerto Rico: Editorial de la Universidad de Puerto Rico.

Arroyo, H.V. (ed.) (2004) *La Promoción de la Salud y la Educación para la Salud en América Latina: Modelos, Estructuras y Visión Crítica*. Puerto Rico: Editorial de la Universidad de Puerto Rico.

Arroyo, H.V. and Cerqueira, M.T. (eds) (1997) *La Promoción de la Salud y la Educación para la Salud en América Latina. Un Análisis Sectorial*. Puerto Rico: Editorial de la Universidad de Puerto Rico.

Arroyo, H.V. and Rivera, W. (2004) La Promoción de la Salud y Educación para la Salud en Puerto Rico. En Arroyo, H.V. (ed.) *La Promoción de la Salud y Educación para la Salud en América Latina. Modelos, Estructuras y Visión Crítica*. Puerto Rico: Editorial de la Universidad de Puerto Rico.

Arvizu, A. and Buelow, J. (1999) Health and health promotion in Latin America. A social change perspective. In Bracht, N. (eds) *Health Promotion at the Community Level 2*. New Advances. Thousand Oaks, CA: Sage Publications.

Aschner, P. (2002) Diabetes trends in Latin America. *Diabetes/Metabolism Research Reviews*, **18** (Suppl 3): S27–31.

Cardaci, D. (1999) Promoción de la Salud: ¿cambio cultural o nueva retórica?. En Bronfman, M. y Castro, R. (eds) *Salud, Cambio Social y Política. Perspectivas des de América Latina*. EDAMEX, S.A. de C.V. e Instituto Nacional de Salud Pública. México.

Cardaci, D., Cavazos, M.A. and Díaz, B. (2004) ¿En un mar de ambigüedades? Políticas, Programas y Estrategias de Formación en Promoción y Educación para la Salud en México. En Arroyo, H.V. (ed.) *La Promoción de la Salud y Educación para la Salud en América Latina. Modelos, Estructuras y Visión Crítica.* Puerto Rico: Editorial de la Universidad de Puerto Rico.

Carta de Sao Paulo (2002) *Documento declaratorio de la III Conferencia Regional Latino americana de Promoción de la Salud y Educación para la Salud.* Sao Paulo, Brasil, 10–13 de Noviembre de 2002.

Castro-Albarrán, J.M. (2003) *Reflexiones Conceptuales sobre la Promoción de la Salud.* Unpublished monograph.

Cerqueira, M.T. (1997) Promoción de la Salud y Educación para la Salud: retos y perspectivas. En Arroyo, H.V. and Cerqueira, M.T. (eds) (1997) *La Promoción de la Salud y la Educación para la Salud en América latina. Un Análisis Sectorial.* Puerto Rico: Editorial de la Universidad de Puerto Rico.

Cerqueira, M.T. (2000) Health Promotion in the Americas: toward bridging the equity gap. *Promotion and Education, 7* (4): 4–7.

CIUEPS (1996) *Memorias de la Asamblea Constitutiva del Consorcio Interamericano de Universidades y Centros de Formación de Personal en Educación para la Salud y Promoción de la Salud.* San Juan, Puerto Rico.

CIUEPS (1998) *Memorias de la II Asamblea General del Consorcio Interamericano de Universidades y Centros de Formación de Personal en Educación para la Salud y Promoción de la Salud.* San Juan, Puerto Rico.

CIUEPS (2000) *Memorias de la III Asamblea General del Consorcio Interamericano de Universidades y Centros de Formación de Personal en Educación para la Salud y Promoción de la Salud.* México, D.F.

CIUEPS (2003) *Memorias de la IV Asamblea General del Consorcio Interamericano de Universidades y Centros de Formación de Personal en Educación para la Salud y Promoción de la Salud.* Sao Paulo, Brasil.

Escobar, M.L. and Torres, B.P. (2004) El Estado de la Discusión y de la Práctica en Promoción de la Salud en Colombia 1991–99 (Resumen) En Arroyo, H.V. (ed.) *La Promoción de la Salud y Educación para la Salud en América Latina. Modelos, Estructuras y Visión Crítica.* Puerto Rico: Editorial de la Universidad de Puerto Rico.

González, M. (2004) La Promoción de la Salud y Educación para la Salud en Uruguay. En Arroyo, H.V. (ed.) *La Promoción de la Salud y Educación para la Salud en América Latina. Modelos, Estructuras y Visión Crítica.* Puerto Rico: Editorial de la Universidad de Puerto Rico.

Iriart, C., Merhy, E.E. and Waitzkin, H. (2001) Managed care in Latin America: the new common sense in health policy reform. *Social Science and Medicine, 52* (8): 1243–53.

Kickbusch, I. (2001) Reflexiones sobre la Salud Pública en las Américas. *En Educación en Salud Pública. Nuevas Perspectivas para las Américas.* Organización Panamericana de la Salud y Asociación Latinoamericana y del Caribe de Educación en Salud Pública. Washington, DC.

Martínez, A. (2004) La Promoción de la Salud y Educación para la Salud en Antioquía, Colombia. En Arroyo, H.V. (ed.) *La Promoción de la Salud y Educación para la Salud en América Latina. Modelos, Estructuras y Visión Crítica.* Puerto Rico: Editorial de la Universidad de Puerto Rico.

Muñoz, H.I. (2004) Evolución de la Promoción de la Salud y Educación para la Salud en Panamá. En Arroyo, H.V. (ed.) *La Promoción de la Salud y Educación para la Salud en América Latina. Modelos, Estructuras y Visión Crítica.* Puerto Rico: Editorial de la Universidad de Puerto Rico.

Pan American Health Organization (PAHO) (1996) *Promoción de la Salud: una antología.* Publicación Científica No. 557. Washington, DC.

Pan American Health Organization (PAHO) (2000) *El Progreso en la Salud de la Población. Informe Anual del Director– 2000.* Documento Oficial de la OPS #298. Washington, DC.

Pan American Health Organization (PAHO) (2001) *Promoción de la Salud en las Américas. Informe Anual del Director– 2001.* Documento Oficial de la OPS #302. Washington, DC.

Pan American Health Organization (PAHO) (2002) *Nuevos Rumbos para la Salud en las Américas. Informe Cuadrenial del Director*, Edición 2002. Washington, DC.

Pan American Health Organization PAHO/WHO (2001) *Strengthening Health Promotion Planning for Action in the Americas. A Document Prepared for the Subcommittee on Planning and Programming.* Washington, DC.

Peñaherrera, E. (2004) La Promoción de la Salud en el Perú. En Arroyo, H.V. (ed.) *La Promoción de la Salud y Educación para la Salud en América Latina. Modelos, Estructuras y Visión Crítica.* Puerto Rico:Editorial de la Universidad de Puerto Rico.

Puertas, B., Herrera, M., and Aguinaga, G. (2004) La Promoción de la Salud y Educación para la Salud en Ecuador. En Arroyo, H.V. (ed.) *La Promoción de la Salud y Educación para la Salud en América Latina. Modelos, Estructuras y Visión Crítica.* Puerto Rico: Editorial de la Universidad de Puerto Rico.

Ruiz, G. and Dakessian, M.A. (2004) Situación de la Promoción de la Salud y Educación para la Salud en la Argentina. En Arroyo, H.V. (ed) *La Promoción de la Salud y Educación para la Salud en América Latina. Modelos, Estructuras y Visión Crítica.* Puerto Rico: Editorial de la Universidad de Puerto Rico.

Salazar, L. (2003) *Informe de Progreso del Proyecto Regional de Evidencias de Efectividad en Promoción de la Salud en América Latina. Noviembre 2002–Agosto 2003. Lecciones aprendidas para construir el futuro.* Santiago de Cali, Colombia.

Salinas, J. and Escribano, I. (2004) Promoción de la Salud y Educación para la Salud en Chile. En Arroyo, H.V. (ed.) *La Promoción de la Salud y Educación para la Salud en América Latina. Modelos, Estructuras y Visión Crítica.* Puerto Rico: Editorial de la Universidad de Puerto Rico.

Sanabria, G. (2004) Promoción y Educación para la Salud en Cuba: Apuntes sobre su Desarrollo. En Arroyo, H.V. (ed.) *La Promoción de la Salud y Educación para la Salud en América Latina. Modelos, Estructuras y Visión Crítica.* Puerto Rico: Editorial de la Universidad de Puerto Rico.

Uauy, R., Albala, C. and Kain, J. (2001) Obesity trends in Latin America: transiting from under- to over-weight. *Journal of Nutrition*, **131** (3): 893S–899S.

Westphal, M.F. (2000) Mobilisation of Latin America to promote health. *Promotion and Education*, 7 (4): 2–3.

CHAPTER 14

A Public Health and System Approach to Health Protection and Health Promotion in Hong Kong

SOPHIA CHAN AND GABRIEL LEUNG

The fundamental premise of successful and effective health protection and promotion is the adoption of the public health approach. Keys (1970) and Pickering (1968) first exposed this way of thinking about whole populations and a continuous distribution of risk. Rose developed it further with his prevention paradox, the suggestion that a preventive measure with large community benefits will offer little to each participating individual (Rose, 1981). The corollary is that a large number of individuals exposed to low risk may generate more cases of disease than a small number exposed to high risk. This population perspective depends on recognition that nature is a process or continuum as distinct from a dichotomy and that risk typically varies across the spectrum of a risk factor (Rose, 1992).

The customary categorisation of risk in healthcare does not follow its natural order but rather represents an operational convenience. The deviant minority or high-risk group, such as hypertensives with a systolic pressure over 140 mmHg or a diastolic above 90 mmHg, is part of the risk continuum and not a distinct population. Rose pointed out that any health promotion or disease prevention strategy focusing on the high risk group will deal only with the margin of the problem and will not have any significant impact on the much larger proportion of disease occurring in the majority of individuals who are at mild to moderate risk (Rose, 1992). For instance, people with mild to moderate hypertension account for the largest share of heart disease and stroke in the population whereas those with severe, uncontrolled high blood pressure are only responsible for a small minority of the population's cardiovascular disease burden. In contrast, and herein lies the prevention paradox, reducing blood pressure through medications and regular aerobic exercise will bring much greater personal benefit to high-risk individuals compared to those with more modest risk profiles.

As a cardiovascular epidemiologist, Rose cited most of his examples from that literature, but his concepts are equally applicable in other fields.

The present preoccupation with genetics and the molecular basis of disease within medicine brings into sharp relief the critical need to understand the prevention paradox. Germ line mutations in the *BrCA1, BrCA2, p53* and *AT* genes (the latter two are tumour suppressor genes) confer a very high risk of breast cancer, among other malignancies, in those exhibiting the mutant genotype. However, they account for no more than 5 to 10 per cent of all breast cancer cases in the population. Put in another way, at least 90 per cent of the population's incident breast cancer burden does not arise from a monogenic aberration. In addition, there are as yet no preventive interventions that can alter the risk associated with such genetic predisposition (Nass et al., 2001).

To take this line of reasoning further, with the many recent technical advances that facilitate the identification of defective genes and polymorphisms have come increased efforts in the promotion of screening and surveillance (Khoury et al., 2003). Wilson and Jungner's (1968) first principle mandates that only important health problems in terms of both disease severity and frequency on the public health level should be screened. However, most monogenetic disorders and diseases associated with polymorphisms do not qualify on the latter axis. Lay fear of disease, a defensive medico legal culture and a weakly regulated marketplace mean that purveyors of at-risk testing will proliferate resulting in unforeseen social and psychological harms. As the breast cancer example demonstrates, once genetic variants are identified, what then? In the dawn of genomic medicine, it must be acknowledged that genetic screening identifies many conditions for which no treatment, clear understanding of appropriate management or preventive strategies exist. While some have justified such screening on the basis that it can help avoid 'diagnostic odysseys' if low probability health problems emerge (Khoury et al., 2003), they fail to mention that mass genetic screens almost guarantee an epidemic of therapeutic odysseys as anxious patients seek multiple treatments for diseases that may never manifest. While identification of people at risk from important diseases like diabetes mellitus would be helpful, health workers are poor at effecting and maintaining preventive behaviour change in such individuals. Much greater value for money can be achieved by addressing those problems which are already known to be important influences on health: tobacco and alcohol consumption, weight reduction, cholesterol-lowering through exercise and dietary improvements (WHO, 2002), than are likely to be gained by screening of genetic profiles (Fielding et al., 2003).

In the past decade or so, there have been major efforts directed at educating the public about various risks to health and the message that one can prevent a particular disease by altering certain behaviours or exposures has been widely conveyed, where such dissemination activities have formed the main platform of some health promotion agencies. In parallel, chronic disease epidemiologists have produced a torrent of relative risks, odds ratios and hazard ratios associated with different conditions. However, it remains unclear whether knowledge of such probabilistic associations can bring about substantive health improvements on the personal level. While comparative risk estimates often appear impressive, risk factors per se are poor predictive tools at the individual level. This is a fact of statistical reality where most risk-factor disease associations in chronic disease epidemiology are modest and most epidemiologic risk models have correspondingly suboptimal discriminatory or concordance accuracy for individuals (Rockhill, 2001). It is suggested that the ability to predict individual futures will always be uncertain despite advances in knowledge of factors, including that of genes, which may elevate risk (Rockhill, 2001). There are further potential pitfalls about designating the individual as the main locus of risk. One danger is the exacerbation of social inequalities in health because individuals from lower socioeconomic strata will invariably have less capacity to understand and deal with such information about personal health risks. Moreover, the overt individualisation of risk may project the impression that patients are to be blamed regarding their illness (Berkman and Kawachi, 2000; Rockhill, 2001) which in turn fosters an indifference to the wider social, economic and political determinants of health (for a comparable discussion of the individualisation of risk, see Part II, Chapter 11).

A system approach to health promotion

Having recognised and accepted that health promotion should be viewed from the public health perspective, it follows that a system approach be adopted to formulate, develop, implement and evaluate interventions and programmes designed to protect and promote the public's health. But why do health systems matter? Since the late 1970s there has been accumulating evidence showing that the financing, organisation and delivery of care and services make a substantial impact on health outcomes (Morris, 1980) even without further advances in fundamental science (WHO, 2000). The Evidence and Information in Policy team at WHO calculated that between 1960 and 1990, almost 50 per cent of the reduction in mortality in 115 low to middle income countries could be attributed to the generation and utilisation of knowledge as developed and applied by the health system (WHO, 2000). Nevertheless, health systems worldwide can and should accomplish much more with the available scientific understanding of how to improve and promote health. The failings, which limit greater health improvements, stem from the misapplication of best current evidence rather than a lack of understanding about appropriate interventions; it arises from systemic rather than technical or scientific failures.

James Reason (2000) advocated the system approach to averting medical errors. He pointed out that the person or individualist approach focuses on the errors of individuals, blaming them for forgetfulness, inattention or moral weakness whereas the system approach concentrates on the conditions under which individuals work and tries to build defences to avoid errors or mitigate their effects. Highly reliable and successful organisations, such as the military, airlines and nuclear power plants, which have less than their fair share of accidents, recognise that human variability is a root cause of errors and work hard to reduce that variability (Kohn et al., 1999). Shewhart (1931) and Deming (1990), the fathers of quality control, devised early methods to quantify variability in manufacturing processes which directly led to the unprecedented post-war productivity gains in Japan, then in North America and Europe. More recently, Mohammed and colleagues (2001) demonstrated, using six case studies including the Bristol, UK paediatric cardiac surgery debacle and the UK Harold Shipman murders, a central role for Shewhart's control charts in operationalising clinical governance using a system approach to protecting and improving health. This is analogous to the myriad health promotion programmes and activities currently in place and those being planned, where significant health gains can be and have been realised from careful systemic implementation and evaluation. The following section details a comprehensive system framework for health protection and promotion.

A framework for health protection and promotion

Population distributions of the determinants of health

Figure 14.1 shows a schematic of key inputs and outcomes in health protection and promotion. In the planning stages of any health promotion programme or intervention, such as annual reviews or strategic development exercises, the first task is to define the scope of the programme being considered, which in turn depends on the purpose or aim of the particular programme. Part of this task involves measuring the baseline or pre-intervention health (or disease) burden within the context of that particular health promotion programme in the community being targeted. In measuring the population health burden, there must be explicit acknowledgement and full accounting of the multiple, wider determinants of health. Numerous models of population health have been developed over recent decades. Perhaps the most representative and comprehensive conceptual framework is that of Evans and Stoddart (1990). Current thinking in population health recognises that individuals are endowed with a unique set of genetic characteristics from the time of conception that has deterministic (mostly monogenetic disorders) as well as potentially modifiable (polymorphisms) influences on future health throughout the life course. By way of mechanisms that are not yet understood, genetic factors, manifested through biological processes of the host, interact with the epidemiologic triangle of external environmental factors, psycho-behavioural traits, and socioeconomic as well as geopolitical factors to determine human health, illness and disease. Two issues bear special attention. The cumulative effects of risks throughout the life course and those at critical junctures both play an important role in pathogenesis (Barker, 1998; Davey Smith et al., 1998). In addition, echoing Rose's emphasis on the continuum

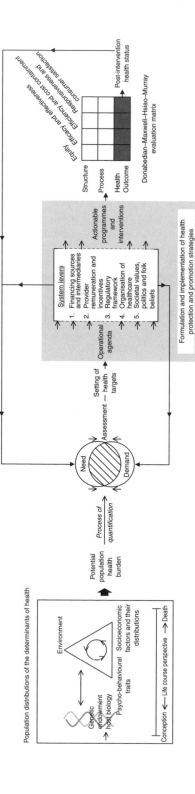

Figure 14.1   Key system inputs and outcomes in health protection and promotion

of risk, it is crucial for programme planners to comprehend that how a certain health risk is distributed across the community matters as much as, if not more so in some cases, than the absolute level of that risk.

Need and demand assessment

Since a landmark global burden of disease study (Murray and Lopez, 1996), a number of methodologies have been devised and refined to quantify the attributable, and therefore avoidable, burden of morbidity and mortality on the population level (Peto et al., 1992; Mathers et al., 1999). Common among them are several key components espoused by the WHO including standardised comparisons and common outcome measures; comprehensive assessment of protective and hazardous factors, as well as the joint effects of competing risks; inclusion of both proximal and distal causes; consideration of the distribution of risk in the population in addition to the identification of high-risk individuals; an evidence-based approach to estimating and projecting certain and probable risks to health; and computation of attributable and avoidable health burden using appropriate counterfactual risk levels and distributions as reference (WHO, 2002).

The systematic measurement of the population health burden and its attendant risks establishes a normative level of need, which may be and frequently is different to what individuals or special interest groups demand. There is no single correct definition of need but so long as the measurement yardstick remains constant pre and post intervention for a particular health promotion activity, relative changes can be objectively quantified and easily assessed. Communities must be brought together, through an open and transparent political process, to agree on a common set of measurement techniques that can accommodate normative needs as perceived by public health and health promotion professionals as well as felt or expressed demand that reflect consumers' beliefs and broader societal values. The goal is to achieve as much overlap as possible between the two subsets of need and demand in the Venn diagram (Figure 14.1).

Formulation and implementation of health protection and promotion strategies

Need assessment then leads to the setting of health targets. The concept of targeting for health began with the WHO in 1977 when it issued *Health for all by year 2000*. From this campaign grew a revolutionary approach to policy making which redefined the responsibilities of government in this field. Health targets are specific and measurable goals for improving the health of individuals and populations. Documents such as *Saving lives: our healthier nation* in the UK (UK Department of Health, 1999) and *Healthy people 2010* in the US (US Department of Health and Human Services, 2000) set out the overarching national vision in health whereas plans like the condition-specific national service frameworks in the UK National Health Service serve as concrete objectives. Hong Kong has yet to issue similar population health targets.

Once an agreed set of health promotion objectives has been processed through the target setting exercise, it enters the operational agenda of health agencies where implementation plans should be formulated and developed, and the output consists of specific actionable programmes and interventions. Need will almost always exceed the available supply of resources for health and healthcare. In low income countries, such as those in sub-Saharan Africa, the problem is mainly due to the lack of financial resources, often accompanied by geopolitical instability, and the continuing scourge of infectious diseases such as tuberculosis, malaria, and HIV/AIDS. In Europe, Australia and North America, high income, developed economies have been struggling with the demographic, epidemiologic, technologic and economic transitions and the associated pandemic of chronic diseases since the Second World War (Leung, 2002). Middle or low income countries, including China and India, suffer from the double burden of the old diseases of the poor while simultaneously having to deal with the rapid growth of noncommunicable conditions. Therefore, a system of prioritisation follows to determine which programmes or interventions should proceed (for more on the epidemiological transition in different regions, see Chapters 6, 12, 13 and 15).

In considering and filtering out competing programmes for health protection and promotion, it is important to keep in mind the underlying forces which shape health policy in general. William Hsiao (1999) proposed five key system levers or control knobs. First, an understanding of the financial dimensions of healthcare systems is increasingly recognised as an important contribution to health policy development. In the industrialised countries, especially those belonging to the Organisation of Economic Cooperation and Development (OECD), systematic accounting of national health expenditures, in the form of National Health Accounts (NHA), has been carried out for several decades. The creation of standardised definitions and accounting methods across countries and the routine collection of data have provided the means for informative and productive inquiry into the financial and health implications of different national patterns of healthcare financing. NHA are a set of descriptive accounts that describes systematically and accurately the totality of healthcare expenditure flows in both the government and non-government sectors. NHA achieve this by identifying the sources of all funds utilised in the sector, ascertaining the uses of these funds and demonstrating how they are spent. Overall, NHA provide essential data for health sector planning and management, in the same way that national income accounts and vital statistics information provide essential data for macroeconomic planning, and population and service planning respectively (OECD, 2000).

As with any initiative, promoting health requires resources. A close examination of Hong Kong's Domestic Health Accounts reveals that only 2.3 per cent of total health expenditure is currently targeted at health promotional activities (Hsiao and Yip, 1999). Figure 14.2 illustrates the health financing paradox, a phenomenon that is not unique to Hong Kong. Since Last (1963) and White et al. (1961) first described the iceberg concept of disease and the medical ecology of care respectively, studies have confirmed that the majority of the population, some apparently healthy and some unwell, do not present to the formal care system at any particular point in time and therefore form the eligible group for health promotion activities. However, only a tiny fraction of the total resources in the system is targeted at this large group to enhance their social and personal resources for everyday living (WHO, 1986).

The extent to which the entire reimbursement structure in the healthcare sector is tied to patterns of disease diagnosis and treatment, rather than to health promotion and disease prevention, deserves special attention and reconsideration. This illustrates the importance of a related but separate system lever, that of provider remuneration and incentives. To achieve better health for more people, a fair and adequate remuneration system is required for doctors, and in particular other healthcare professionals, to provide health education advice and disease prevention counselling. For instance, extending health insurance coverage to smoking cessation interventions (Schauffler and Parkinson, 1993), or providing payment for diabetic education sessions can facilitate the promotion of health (Schwartz et al., 1985). Providing that impact and outcomes, the government should encourage all third party payers, public and private, to reimburse for health promotional activities. They should no longer be an afterthought.

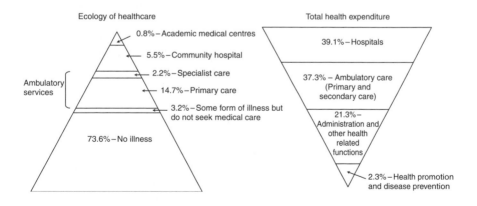

Figure 14.2   The health financing paradox

Source: Government of Hong Kong SAR, (2002); Government of Hong Kong SAR, (1997)

The third policy lever concerns the regulatory or governance framework of the system. Professional licensing regulations, principles of medical jurisprudence, pharmaceutical and food product evaluation and labelling, stewardship of healthcare organisations all contribute to the effectiveness and impact of this system lever on health protection and promotion interventions. For example, Hong Kong recently negotiated a free trade agreement (Closer Economic Partnership Agreement or CEPA) with mainland China in which provisions have been made to allow for reciprocal recognition of medical qualifications between certain Chinese medical schools and their Hong Kong counterparts. Before all the details of CEPA are finalised, an interim arrangement permits Hong Kong registered doctors to obtain a temporary mainland license for three years. This has enormous implications for cross-border workforce planning, especially in the Pearl River Delta of which Hong Kong is a part with a population in excess of 50 million, equivalent to the whole of the United Kingdom or one-fifth of that of the United States. Secondary effects of this closer economic integration with this hinterland specific to health promotion and protection would influence the way such activities as social marketing campaigns, health education classes, and the planning of mass vaccination and screening services are conducted.

Fourth, the way services and facilities are organised have important consequences for how health promotion should be structured, and ultimately the health status of whole populations. Figure 14.3 gives an overview of Hong Kong's health system. Barbara Starfield's landmark ecological study in the OECD countries, where she found that those countries with weak primary care infrastructures had higher costs and poorer health outcomes, provided the first evidence that an intact primary care network should underpin all health systems (Starfield, 1994). Within country studies (Farmer et al., 1991; Shi, 1992 and 1994) and numerous individual level research reports (Starfield, 1985; Shea et al., 1992; Franks and Fiscella, 1998) have confirmed these correlational findings. *World Health Report 2003* reaffirms the recognition that progress in health is dependent of improved health systems vitally based on primary healthcare (WHO, 2003). In Hong Kong, a functional primary care network does not yet exist. Most ambulatory practice is still based on the solo practitioner model. The first cohort of trained family physicians are only beginning to graduate from residency programmes, let alone realising a multidisciplinary primary care team of nurse practitioners, physician assistants and social workers. The lack of such a core infrastructure hampers the delivery of health education, counselling, primary and secondary screening interventions and perhaps accounts for part of the reason why Hong Kong is a relative latecomer to participating in the full range of health promotional activities, especially outside the government sector (Figure 14.3).

Finally, all the system levers detailed previously are ultimately underpinned by prevailing attitudes, folk beliefs and societal values. A liberal democratic political system, like that found in most high income countries, would facilitate the translation of the people's values in a shorter time frame compared to

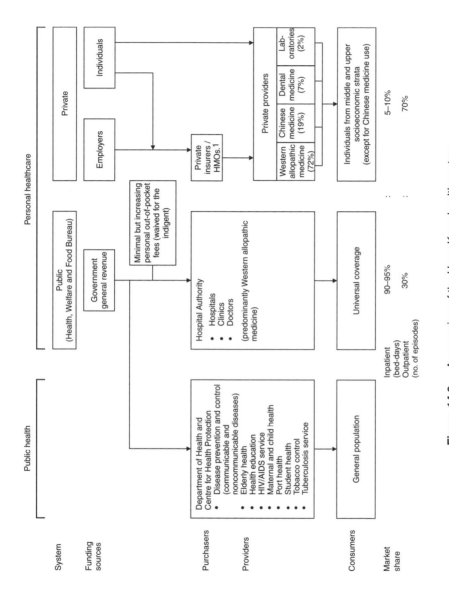

Figure 14.3 An overview of the Hong Kong health system

Note: 1. Health maintenance organisation

less open, more opaque systems, which tend to delay such a process. Of course, among the myriad other issues competing for the political stage at any one point in time it should be borne in mind that health, while a top fixture issue in US and UK elections in recent memory, generally occupies a much less important position on the political agenda in other less progressive economies, including Hong Kong (for a discussion on the part played by political factors in health promotion in the USA, see Chapter 19).

The Donabedian–Maxwell–Hsiao–Murray evaluation matrix

The central importance of an evaluative culture within health protection and promotion, indeed all of healthcare, needs no justification here. Muir Gray (2001) summarised well the essence of evaluating the quality of health interventions: does the programme do the *right* thing *right*, to the *right* people at the *right* time. In the following paragraphs a possible, systematic way to think about auditing programmes and interventions that have passed through the filter of system levers in the formulation and implementation process will be outlined. Figure 14.1 shows a prototype evaluation matrix. The rows represent the three core Donabedian axes of structure, process and outcome, or resource, action, and result (Donabedian, 1980).

Maxwell suggested the six intersecting dimensions of effectiveness, efficiency, acceptability, access, equity, relevance, which form the basis of quality of care and service (Maxwell, 1984 and 1992). Hsiao (1995), from the health system perspective, defined the goals of healthcare as equity, efficiency, effectiveness, cost containment, and quality of care. Although not without controversy and criticism, Murray and colleagues (WHO, 2000) argued that good health, responsiveness to the expectations of the population, and fairness of financial contribution as measured by seven indices should be used to assess health systems and their component parts. These are disability-adjusted life expectancy, health equality in terms of child survival, responsiveness level, responsiveness distribution, fairness of financial contribution, performance on level of health, and overall health system performance. These variants of quality indices are combined into a single matrix whereby trade-offs between dimensions of quality can be made explicit between different programmes and over time, acknowledging that no single activity or intervention can achieve a satisfactory standard on all the different domains at the same time. For instance, with the dramatic improvements in living conditions and the concomitant reduction in infectious diseases fuelled by an economic transition from an undeveloped British trading outpost to an Asian financial hub since the 1900s, Hong Kong has traditionally traded off efficacy and effectiveness in terms of isolation beds for infection control in the nosocomial setting in favour of cost containment and efficiency of hospital services, while being able to maintain some of the best health indicators in the world. During the severe acute respiratory syndrome (SARS) outbreak in 2003, Hong Kong was caught off guard and isolation facilities were found to be inadequate in number and quality. Painful lessons from SARS tipped the priority balance back towards health protection from communicable diseases and six months since the end of the epidemic, there are now 1400 state-of-the-art isolation beds in negative pressure rooms that stand ready for another similar infectious disease outbreak.

Output from the evaluation matrix should enter a feedback loop to programme planners and practitioners in order to improve future performance and quality. In particular, findings on the health outcome axis indicate the post intervention health status and thus can inform the next iteration of need and demand assessment. This last step closes the continuous quality improvement cycle (Deming, 1990; Muir Gray, 2001).

Two case examples

Two case examples from some of our work in Hong Kong complete this chapter. The first involves the secondary preventive strategy of population screening for breast cancer among Chinese and East Asian women, and the second case outlines a successful local experience with tobacco control, specifically smoking cessation, where tobacco consumption is the single most preventable health risk estimated to be responsible for 8.8 per cent of all deaths and 4.1 per cent of disability adjusted life years (DALYs) worldwide (WHO, 2002; see also Part II, Chapters 6 and 8 for further discussions of cancers and tobacco consumption).

Breast cancer screening by mammography in East Asia

Breast cancer is the commonest female malignancy and the third leading cause of cancer-related mortality among women in Hong Kong. It was previously found that the average annual per cent change of the age-standardised incidence was 1.2 per cent from 1973 to 1999. The increase was mostly concentrated in the younger age groups and appeared to be accelerating (Leung et al., 2002a). These grim facts, coupled with the desperate desire to find something, anything, that might help in this terrible disease, have led many to believe that one of the best hopes for improving health outcomes must lie with earlier diagnosis, and in particular, through mass screening. Screening by regular testing has been billed as a 'motherhood and apple pie' issue. Since it is intuitively attractive and apparently free of downside risks it *must* be the right to thing to do. Whereas screening by mammography for the early diagnosis of breast cancer has become routine practice in many western countries, the benefits, as well as inherent risks and costs, of mass population mammography screening, have yet to be rigorously considered in Chinese women, a group that comprises one fifth of the world's female population.

This is particularly important because the epidemiology and clinical patterns of breast cancer differ markedly between Chinese and Western women, which may have serious implications for many healthcare interventions including mammography screening. Despite this lack of evidence, there have been wide-spread suggestions and unqualified recommendations for whole population screening, and the aggressive promotion of mammographic examination in Chinese women.

Having determined the population burden of disease and quantified the rate of change in breast cancer incidence (Leung et al., 2002a), the research team proceeded to a formal need assessment exercise by systematically reviewing the evidence base for population-based screening in early breast cancer detection through an updated meta analysis of the literature, and examined the applica-bility of these results to Chinese women by epidemiologic projections using the relevant outcome measures of breast cancer-related mortality, the number needed to screen (NNS) and positive predictive value (PPV) statistics. It was concluded that there was insufficient evidence to support mammography screening in Hong Kong, and indeed all East Asian, women. The underlying reason was a relatively much lower disease rate in this population compared to Western Europeans and North Americans, from whom all of the research evidence supporting screening has been derived. More specifically, Figure 14.4 gives the estimated age-specific incidences of breast cancer for the age group 50 to 69 years, comparing the rates in East Asian regions with those of populations from Canada, Scotland, Sweden and the US where the primary studies were performed. There is at least a one- to two-fold difference in breast cancer risk between the two groups. These differences imply that the PPV of any test, which depends on prevalent disease rates in the screened population, will be

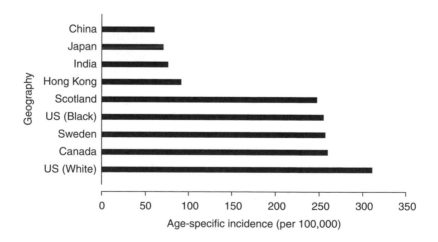

Figure 14.4   Estimated age-specific rates of breast cancer incidence for women aged 50–69 years (adapted from Leung et al., 2002b)

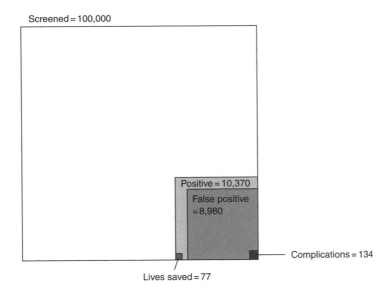

Screened = 100,000

Positive = 10,370

False positive = 8,980

Complications = 134

Lives saved = 77

Figure 14.5 Net balance of benefit and harm per 100,000 women aged 50–69 years over 10 years (adapted from Leung et al., 2002b)

much lower in East Asia than in the West. The NNS will be correspondingly higher and hence less favourable and the absolute number of false positive tests unacceptably high in relation to a relatively modest number of lives saved from mass screening as illustrated by Figure 14.5 (Leung et al., 2002b).

The public health perspective and system approach to assessing need for this potential preventive intervention allowed us to objectively, dispassionately and comprehensively compare and adjudicate, from a professional normative standpoint, the relative merits and demerits of the proposed health promotion programme. An additional lesson to be drawn from this experience is the potential danger of accepting epidemiologic findings wholesale from a different population without careful reappraisal, taking into account geoethnic characteristics (Lam and Leung, 2003).

Broadening the service delivery network for smoking cessation in Hong Kong

The treatment of tobacco dependency has been traditionally identified as the exclusive responsibility of healthcare professionals. However, it is well recognised that only a fraction of those who are ill seek medical attention, and even fewer in the well population attend regular preventive visits. In fact, smokers tend to underutilise healthcare services, given the same state of health, compared to never smokers (Lam et al., 2001). This is particularly true for the elderly who often face compounded difficulties in accessing the healthcare system. Social workers, on the other hand, are trained to identify and counsel socially disadvantaged and marginalised groups in the community, who are at risk for smoking and are either reluctant or have problems accessing smoking cessation services. A population-based health promotion programme was designed to address this service gap (Figure 14.6). A need and demand assessment was undertaken of all social workers in Hong Kong who were working with the elderly via a knowledge, attitudes, practice (KAP) survey (Phase I). Through this questionnaire a susceptible target group was identified

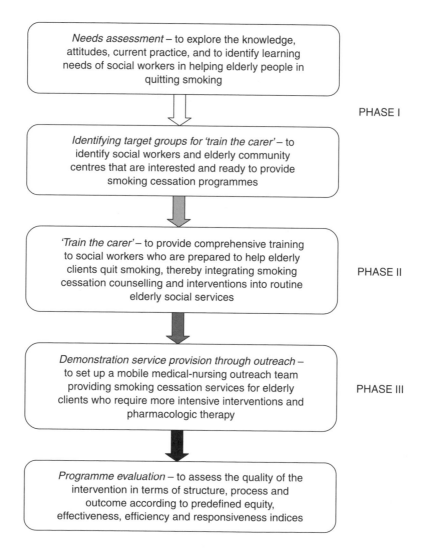

Figure 14.6   Smoking cessation programme for social workers

that was interested in further training and was ready to provide smoking cessation interventions, thereby integrating such a programme into routine elderly social services. Phase II adopted a 'train the carer' approach and involved a short course specifically tailored to social workers' expressed learning needs regarding smoking cessation education and counselling. The last component of this programme involved demonstration service provision through outreach by setting up a mobile joint medical nursing outreach team providing smoking cessation services for elderly clients who require more intensive interventions and pharmacologic therapy. This aimed to support the application of social work where clients with more complex morbidity conditions, identified and initially cared for by social workers, were referred to the mobile clinic (Phase III). In addition, previous studies showed that smoking cessation interventions offered by a team approach including different types of healthcare professionals are most effective (Fiore et al., 2000). Lastly to close the quality improvement feedback loop, this ongoing project will be evaluated using the Donabedian–Maxwell–Hsiao–Murray matrix (see Figure 14.1.).

Preliminary findings from Phase I showed that among 1696/2522 (response rate = 67.3 per cent) social workers surveyed in Hong Kong, most had reasonable knowledge about basic health facts of smoking, recognised the importance of and showed positive attitudes towards tobacco control. However, only 0.4 per cent had received any formal or informal training in providing smoking cessation counselling and 96.3 per cent believed they were unprepared or very unprepared for helping their clients deal with tobacco dependency (Chan et al., 2003a). Three three-hour workshops in Phase II were conducted for 193 respondents where they learned smoking cessation strategies and brief intervention techniques targeted at elderly clients. The course was rated as 'good' and 'excellent' by 79.0 per cent and 10 per cent of the participants respectively (Chan et al., 2003b). The last phase was a multidisciplinary demonstration project where a mobile team of smoking cessation counsellors provided more intensive counselling interventions and nicotine replacement therapy to 500 clients referred by the social worker course participants.

Broadening the service base of tobacco dependency treatment programmes is feasible and social workers were generally enthusiastic about and supportive of the added role of smoking cessation counselling to their service offerings. Future work should focus on confirming the generalisability of these findings and the systematic redesign and implementation of social workers' services to include tobacco dependency management.

References

Barker, D.J.P. (1998) *Mothers, Babies and Health in Later Life*. London: Churchill Livingstone.

Berkman, L.F. and Kawachi, I. (eds) (2000) *Social Epidemiology*. New York, NY: Oxford University Press.

Chan, S.S.C., Lam, T.H., Leung, G.M., Abdullah, A.S.M., Chan, S.K.K., Chi I. and Ng, C. (2003a) Optimising the treatment of tobacco dependency in the elderly: social workers as change agents. *Abstracts of the 12th World Conference on Tobacco or Health*: 3–4.

Chan, S.S.C., Lam, T.H., Leung, G.M., Abdullah, A.S.M., Chan, S.K.K., Chi I. and Ng, C. (2003b) Expanding the role of social workers in the treatment of tobacco-dependency in elderly: a demonstration project. *Abstracts of the 4th International Symposium on Chinese Elderly*: 3–4.

Davey Smith, G., Hart, C., Blane, D. and Hole, D. (1998) Adverse socioeconomic conditions in childhood and cause specific adult mortality: prospective observational study. *British Medical Journal*, **316**: 1631–35.

Deming, W.E. (1990) *Sample Design in Business Research*. New York, NY:Wiley Classics Library Edition.

Donabedian, A. (1980) *Explorations in Quality Assessment and Monitoring*, vol. 1. *The Definition and Quality and Approaches to its Assessment*. Ann Arbor, MI: Health Administration Press.

Evans, R.G. and Stoddart, G.L. (1990) Producing health, consuming health care. *Social Science and Medicine*, **31**: 1347–63.

Farmer, F.L., Stokes, C.S. and Fisher, R.H. (1991) Poverty, primary care and age-specific mortality. *Journal of Rural Health*, 7: 153–69.

Fielding, R., Lam, W. and Leung, G.M. (2003) Population screening. *New England Journal of Medicine*, **348**: 1604–05.

Fiore, M.C., Bailey, W.C. and Cohen, S.J. (2000) *Treating Tobacco Use and Dependence: A Clinical Practice Guideline*. Rockville MD: US Department of Health and Human Services, Public Health Services.

Franks, P. and Fiscella, K. (1998) Primary care physicians and specialists as personal physicians: health care expenditures and mortality experience. *Journal of Family Practice*, **47**: 105–09.

Government of Hong Kong SAR (1997) Estimates of Domestic Health Expenditure, 1986/97. Hong Kong SAR, People's Republic of China.

Government of Hong Kong SAR (2002) Thematic Household Survey Report, No. 12 Census and Statistical Department, Hong Kong SAR, People's Republic of China.

Hsiao, W.C. (1995) Abnormal economics in the health sector. *Health policy*, **32**: 125–39.

Hsiao, W. and Yip, W. for The Harvard Team (1999) *Improving Hong Kong's Health Care System: Why and for Whom?* Hong Kong: Government Printers.

Keys, A. (ed.) (1970) *Coronary Heart Disease in Seven Countries. American Heart Association Monograph 29*. New York, NY: American Heart Association.

Khoury, M.J., McCabe, L.L. and McCab, E.R.B. (2003) Population screening in the age of genomic medicine. *New England Journal of Medicine*, **348**: 50–58.

Kohn, L., Corrigan, J. and Donaldson, M. (eds) (1999) *To Err is Human: Building a Safer Health System*. Washington, DC: Institute of Medicine, National Academy of Sciences.

Lam, T.H., Leung, G.M. and Ho, L.M. (2001) The effects of environmental tobacco smoke on health services utilisation in the first 18 months of life. *Pediatrics*, **107**: e91.

Lam, T.H. and Leung, G.M. (2003) Geoethnic-sensitive and cross-culture collaborative epidemiological studies. *International Journal of Epidemiology*, **32**: 178–80.

Last, J.M. (1963) The iceberg. *Lancet*, **2**: 28–31.

Leung, G.M. (2002) The challenge of chronic conditions in Hong Kong. *Hong Kong Medical Journal*, **8**: 376–78.

Leung, G.M., Thach, T.Q., Lam, T.H., Hedley, A.J., Foo, W., Fielding, R., Yip, P.S.F. Lau, E.M.C. and Wong, C.M. (2002a) Trends in breast cancer incidence in Hong Kong between 1973 and 1999: an age-period-cohort analysis. *British Journal of Cancer*, **87**: 982–88.

Leung, G.M., Lam, T.H., Thach, T.Q. and Hedley, A.J. (2002b) Will screening mammography in the East do more harm than good? *American Journal of Public Health*, **92**: 1841–46.

Mathers, C., Vos, T. and Stevenson, C. (1999) *The Burden of Disease and Injury in Australia*. Canberra: Australian Institute of Health and Welfare.

Maxwell, R.J. (1984) Quality assessment in health. *British Medical Journal*, **288**: 1470–72.

Maxwell,R.J. (1992) Dimensions of quality revisited: from thought to action. *Quality in Health Care*, **1**: 171–77.

Mohammed, M.A., Cheng, K.K., Rouse, A. and Marshall, T. (2001) Bristol, Shipman, and clinical governance: Shewhart's forgotten lessons. *Lancet*, **357**: 463–67.

Morris, J.N. (1980) Are health services important to the people's health? *British Medical Journal*, i: 167–68.

Muir Gray, J.A. (2001) *Evidence-Based Healthcare: How to Make Health Policy and Management Decisions (2nd ed.)*. Edinburgh: Churchill Livingstone.

Murray, C.J.L. and Lopez, A.D. (eds) (1996) *The Global Burden of Disease: A Comprehensive Assessment of Mortality and Disability from Diseases, Injuries, and Risk Factors in 1990 and Projected to 2020*. Cambridge, MA: Harvard University Press.

Nass, S.J., Henderson, I.C. and Lashof, J.C. (eds) for the Committee on Technologies for the Early Detection of Breast Cancer, National Cancer Policy Board (2001). *Mammography and Beyond: Developing Technologies for the Early Detection of Breast Cancer*. Washington, DC:National Academy Press.

Organisation for Economic Cooperation and Development (OECD) (2000) *A System of Health Accounts, vol.10*. Paris: OECD.

Peto, R., Lopez, A.D., Boreham, J., Thun, M. and Heath, C.W. (1992) Mortality from tobacco in developed countries: indirect estimates from national vital statistics. *Lancet*, **339**: 1268–78.

Pickering, G.W. (1968) *High Blood Pressure. 2nd ed.* London: Churchill.

Reason, J. (2000) Human error: models and management. *British Medical Journal*, **320**: 768–70.

Rockhill, B. (2001) The privatisation of risk. *American Journal of Public Health*, 91: 365–68.

Rose, G. (1981) Strategy of prevention: lessons from cardiovascular disease. *British Medical Journal*, **282**: 1847–51.

Rose, G. (1992) *The Strategy of Preventive Medicine*. Oxford: Oxford University Press.

Schauffler, H.H. and Parkinson, M.D. (1993) Health insurance coverage for smoking cessation services. *Health Education Quarterley*, **20**: 185–206.

Schwartz, R., Zaremba, M. and Ra, K. (1985) Third party coverage for diabetes education. *Quality Review Bulletin*, **11**: 213–17.

Shewhart, W.A. (1931) *Economic Control of Quality of Manufactured Product*. New York, NY: D Van Nostrand Company. (Reprinted by ASQC Quality Press, 1980).

Shea, S., Misra, D., Ehrlich, M.H., Field, L. and Francis, C.K. (1992) Predisposing factors for severe, uncontrolled hypertension in an inner-city minority population. *New England Journal of Medicine*, **327**: 776–81.

Shi, L. (1992) The relation between primary care and life chances. *Journal of Health Care for the Poor and Underserved*, **3**: 321–35.

Shi, L. (1994) Primary care, specialty care and life chances. *International Journal of Health Services*, **24**: 431–58.

Starfield, B. (1985) *Effectiveness of Medical Care: Validating Clinical Wisdom*. Baltimore: The Johns Hopkins University Press.

Starfield, B. (1994) Primary care: is it essential? *Lancet*, **344**: 1129–33.

United Kingdom Department of Health, 1999 *Saving Lives Our Healthier Nation: Cm. 4386*. London: HMSO.

United States Department of Health and Human Services (2000) *Healthy People 2010*, 2nd ed. Washington DC: US Government Printing Office.

White, K.L., Williams, T.F. and Greenberg, B.G. (1961) The ecology of medical care. *New England Journal of Medicine*, **265**: 885–92.

Wilson, J.M.G. and Jungner, G. (1968) Principles and practice of screening for disease. *Public Health Papers*, **34**: 11–163.

World Health Organisation (1986) *Ottawa Charter for Health Promotion*. Copenhagen, Denmark: World Health Organisation, European Regional Office.

World Health Organisation (2000) *World Health Report 2000. Health Systems: Improving Performance*. Geneva: World Health Organisation.

World Health Organisation (2002) *World Health Report 2002. Reducing Risks, Promoting Healthy Life*. Geneva: World Health Organisation.

World Health Organisation (2003) *World Health Report 2003. Shaping the Future*. Geneva: World Health Organisation.

CHAPTER 15

Public Health in the Former Soviet Union

JOANA GODINHO

More than a decade after the breakdown of the Soviet Union, the 15 newly independent states still have significant human development problems, due to increasing poverty and inequalities. A recent review considered that some of these countries face major challenges to reach the Millennium Development Goals (MDGs) related to poverty reduction, malnutrition, child and maternal mortality and HIV/AIDS unless major efforts are carried out (World Bank, 2003).

In the 1990s, gross national product (GNP) quickly declined by 50–80 per cent in most countries of the Former Soviet Union (FSU), plunging one-third to half of the population of some countries into poverty. By the mid-1990s, the Ginni coefficient, an indicator of inequality that varies between zero (perfect equality) and 100 (perfect inequality), had raised to 35 in the Baltic countries, 40 in Central Asia and 50 in Russia and Ukraine. Recently, positive growth and reduced poverty have been observed in some FSU countries, such as the Russian Federation and Kyrgyz Republic, but it is not clear whether these have translated into increased likelihood of achieving the MDGs.

As a consequence of increasing poverty and rising inequalities in the ten years since the break up of the Former Soviet Union, public health deteriorated significantly. Life expectancy decreased by two to five years, mostly due to premature adult mortality, as infant mortality decreased in most regional countries, although much less than officially reported in some cases. The most important causes of premature death are cardiovascular diseases (CVDs), cancer and injuries. Smoking, excessive consumption of alcohol and a fatty diet, coupled with lack of physical exercise, play a role in the high premature mortality by CVDs. Traffic accidents are the most important cause of injuries, but domestic and work-related accidents, suicide, violence and war also play a role in the high burden of disease by injuries. Depression may also play a role in the excessive consumption of alcohol, being therefore interlinked with the CVDs and injuries (for further discussion of the impact of inequalities on health in the FSU, see Part I, particularly Chapter 5).

In addition, there is still an unfinished reproductive health agenda in the FSU. While fertility and birth rates drastically decreased throughout the region by between 20 and 50 per cent, maternal mortality either increased or remained high, especially in Latvia, Russia, Belarus, Azerbaijan, Georgia and Central Asian countries; and infant mortality may still be high and has not decreased as much as officially reported in the Caucasus and in Central Asia. Diarrhoeal diseases and acute respiratory infections are still responsible for considerable burden of disease, especially among children in Central Asia. Finally, epidemics of TB, HIV/AIDS and sexually transmitted infections (STIs) have been spreading throughout the region, initially in Russia, Belarus, Ukraine, Moldova and the Baltic states, but more recently also in the Caucasus and Central Asia (see also Part II, Chapter 9 on HIV/AIDS).

The regional governments have continued previous public health best practices, such as maintaining high rates of immunisation, and have adopted some health policies to counteract the effects of lifestyle trends, such as anti-smoking laws. However, most have not yet fully adopted health promotion approaches, neither have they modernised their insolvent public health services.

Deteriorating health status

During the Soviet era, health indicators in the Former Soviet Union (FSU) compared favourably with those of other countries with similar income. However, health status has significantly deteriorated in the FSU more than a decade after the political, economic and social transition began, despite the investments that have been made on health, education and social protection by national and international organisations. Poor health status in the FSU reflects increasing poverty and inequalities, coupled with the population's lack of knowledge, decision making power and options to lead healthier lives, weak

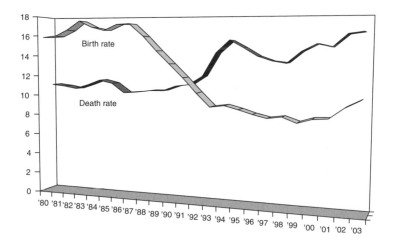

Figure 15.1   The Russian Cross: birth and death rates per 1000, 1980–2003
Source: Russian State Committee for Statistics (2001, 2003 and 2004)

leadership and institutional capacity, and the evident deterioration of health services.

The Russian Federation, for example, is losing almost one million of its population a year due to the combined effect of decreased fertility, increased premature mortality and migration (see Figure 15.1).

Men in the FSU live 10 years less, on average, than men in Western Europe and other developed regions, with premature mortality by CVDs, cancer and injuries accounting for most of the difference. Suicide, homicide and alcohol-related causes are the most important cause of injuries. Noncommunicable diseases (CVDs, cancer, injuries) are the most important causes of burden of disease (BOD) in the FSU, although communicable diseases also have an important and increasing weight in the region's mortality and morbidity.

Noncommunicable diseases

The most important causes of premature death in the Former Soviet Union are CVDs, cancer and injuries. Alcohol may be the main culprit that brings CVDs and injuries to the top of the burden of disease charts. Smoking and a fatty diet, coupled with lack of physical exercise, also play a role in the high premature mortality by CVDs and smoking is the main risk factor for chronic lung disease. As in other low and middle income countries, where 65 per cent of CVDs occur, CVDs in FSU countries may affect younger groups than in high income countries and poorer groups may have similar or higher rates than wealthier groups.

In 1990, smoking was responsible for 12.5 per cent of the total disability adjusted life years (DALYs) in Europe and Central Asia (ECA), while alcohol accounted for 8.3 per cent. Hypertension was identified as the third main risk factor, accounting for about 6 per cent of total DALYs. Diet and physical inactivity (2.8 per cent) are other lifestyle factors that explain the regional health status (Murray and Lopez, 1997). While the estimated proportion of deaths due to alcohol is relatively small (1.4 per cent), the contribution of excessive alcohol consumption to DALYs is large (8.3 per cent), due to the young ages of death and large number of years of life lost attributable to this risk factor. One of the most obvious indicators of alcohol-related harm is mortality by chronic liver disease and cirrhosis, which in Moldova reached 87 per 100,000 in 1998.

Surprisingly, 1998 data show that per capita consumption of alcohol was lower in ten of the ECA countries than in Western Europe as a whole: 6.65 and 9.24 litres of pure alcohol (LPA) respectively. However, estimates show that unrecorded alcohol consumption is a significant problem in the FSU, possibly raising consumption to over 20 LPA at the upper end. Furthermore, while total consumption decreased 6.6 per cent in the EU in the 1990s, it grew 11.6 per cent in ECA. While the EU consumes mostly wine and beer, the FSU consumes hard liquor: wine accounted for 40 per cent of the consumption of pure alcohol in the EU, whereas hard liquor accounted for 70 per cent of the

Table 15.1   Life expectancy (LE) in Russia

	1990	*1991*	*1992*	*1993*	*1994*	*1995*	*1996*	*1997*	*1998*
LE at birth									
All	69.28	69.02	67.90	65.14	64.00	64.67	65.92	66.80	67.24
Female	74.43	74.31	73.77	71.88	71.18	71.71	72.52	72.91	73.26
Male	63.79	63.44	62.02	58.91	57.62	58.30	59.77	60.96	61.46
Difference in LE between female and male	10.64	10.87	11.75	12.97	13.56	13.41	12.75	11.95	11.63

Source: WHO Europe Health for All Database 2000; and estimates from Vinokur et al., 2001

consumption in Russia, Ukraine, Belarus, Moldova, Latvia and Estonia. As a result, per capita consumption of pure alcohol from hard liquor is over twice as high in countries of the FSU (3.3 LPA) than in Western Europe (1.6 LPA) (Vinokur, 2000).

Since 1988, the Russian Federation has had the steepest growth in recorded alcohol consumption in ECA, with vodka accounting for 82 per cent of about 5 litres per capita of official sales of alcohol. Following the Gorbachov anti-alcohol campaign, consumption decreased, but the trend reverted in the late 1980s, with particular high growth rate in 1992–95. After a short drop in 1996–97, it took off again in 1998 (Vinokur, 2000). Signs of recovery in life expectancy were observed in 1994–98, which was attributed to the reduction in the rate of deaths from a group of causes associated with alcohol consumption (Shkolnikov et al., 2001), but in 1999 mortality started increasing again, possibly as a consequence of the financial crisis and decreasing alcohol prices (see Table 15.1).

About 700,000 deaths per year are estimated to be due to smoking in ECA. Death rates are expected to further rise in ECA, including in Central Asia and among women in most countries, as 44 per cent of the adult population are smokers. A detailed analysis and comparison of smoking prevalence in the FSU and high income European countries shows significant differences between and within the two regions. FSU countries have, in general, a smoking prevalence amongst males around or higher than 40 per cent, and increasing, while high income European countries have a prevalence of less than 40 per cent and decreasing.

However, FSU countries have in general a prevalence amongst females under 25 per cent, though it is rising, while high income countries have a prevalence above 25 per cent, and in some cases still rising (WHO, 1997; Corrao et al., 2000).

The price of cigarettes, including retail base prices and taxes, has a significant influence over consumption. In general Eastern European countries, including those of the FSU, sell cigarettes at a low price. Russia has one of the lowest cigarette prices and tax rates in the region and, indeed, the world. This has clearly an impact on the high prevalence of smoking and per capita consumption, which combines prevalence and intensity of smoking (see Figure15.2 and also Part II, Chapter 6 for a discussion of noncommunicable diseases).

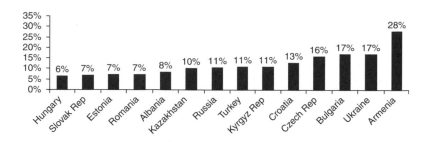

Figure 15.2 A smoker's cigarette expenditure as percentage of monthly average wage in Europe and Central Asia, 1999–2000

Communicable diseases

Acute respiratory infections (ARI) and diarrhoeal diseases are the main causes of death and disease for children. Communicable diseases such as TB and HIV/AIDS are increasingly contributing to the avoidable death and disease toll among, respectively, the population of productive age and young people. Unsafe sex (2.2 per cent), consumption of illicit drugs (1.3 per cent), and poor hygiene are some of the lifestyle factors that explain the regional health status (Murray and Lopez, 1997).

HIV/AIDS infection is still very low and confined to specific groups of the population, such as drug users and commercial sex workers, but some countries in the region, especially the Russian Federation, Belarus, Ukraine, Moldova and the Baltic countries, have the highest growth in the world of new cases of HIV infection. Central Asia has been found at high risk as well, not the least because heroine comes to the FSU and Western Europe through this region.

The rapid increase in HIV/AIDS infection rate is due to the use of intravenous illegal drugs with shared syringes. Infected people have unsafe sex, which then contributes to spread the infection to other groups of the population. The parallel epidemics of HIV, injecting drug use and STIs are associated with the social context of economic crisis, rapid social change, increased poverty and unemployment, growing prostitution, and changes in social norms (UNAIDS, 2000).

The number of reported infections by HIV in ECA has gone from 170,000 in 1997 to over one million in 2003. Ukraine, the hardest hit country in the region, has a reported infection rate around one per cent. Russia, where the infection has the steepest growth, has a reported infection rate of only 0.2 per cent but health authorities estimate that more than one million people are already infected, which brings the percentage of the infected adult population to 1 per cent, and may soon hit the rate of 3 per cent unless the government acts quickly and decisively. In Ukraine, where the number of infected people was of 240,000 by the end of 1999, it is estimated that in a low-case scenario, 600,000 cases will exist in 2006, and in a high-case scenario, 1.4 million cases will exist by the end of the decade.

Tuberculosis is the most common opportunistic infection of AIDS. The prevalent epidemic of TB may become uncontrollable in the presence of even a moderate HIV/AIDS epidemic, as shown in projections carried out in the Russian Federation (Vinokur et al., 2000). Therefore, the potential for further spread and exponential growth of the TB, HIV/AIDS and STIs epidemics is clearly present in the FSU, with possible catastrophic consequences for the lives of young people, and for the shattered economies of those countries (see Part II, Chapter 9 for further discussion of HIV/AIDS).

Reproductive health

In addition to communicable and noncommunicable diseases, there's still an unfinished reproductive health agenda in the FSU, especially in Latvia, Russia, Belarus, Azerbaijan, Georgia and Central Asian countries. While fertility and birth rates drastically decreased throughout the region (20–50 per cent), maternal mortality either increased or was kept at high levels in the countries mentioned above, and infant mortality may still be high and has not decreased as much as officially reported in the Caucasus and in Central Asia. Abortion ratios decreased in most countries in the region, while contraceptive prevalence increased from very low levels to 50–80 per cent. This may have accounted for some decreases in maternal and infant mortality. However, much remains to be done in terms of improvements in prenatal care and obstetric care to ensure that the MDGs for child and maternal mortality are reached. A recent review considered that Armenia is unlikely to reach the MDG for child mortality, and Georgia is unlikely to reach the MDG for maternal mortality, while the Russian Federation, Kazakhstan, Kyrgyz Republic and Tajikistan are unlikely to reach both (World Bank 2003 see Figure 15.3).

Goal 4. Reduce child mortality
Target 5. Reduce by two thirds, between 1990 and 2015, the under-five mortality rate

Goal 5. Improve maternal health
Target 6. Reduce by three quarters, between 1990 and 2015, the maternal mortality ratio

Figure 15.3   Two selected Millennium Development Goals

The root causes: poverty and inequality

A striking fall in income per capita in the FSU may partly explain the premature excessive burden of disease. In the ten years after the break up of the FSU, GNP decreased by 50–80 per cent in most countries, with the exception of the Baltic countries and Belarus (Table 15.1). Nine out of fifteen former middle income countries became low income countries. In the Russian Federation, the 1990s life expectancy decline was specifically blamed on the government 'shock therapy', which abolished price controls in a highly monopolised economy, resulting in soaring consumer prices, rapid decrease in real wages and pensions, and nearly complete loss of personal savings and tremendous increase in the poverty rate (Gravilova et al., 2000; see also Table 15.2).

Starting with FSU countries of Europe and Asia, which previously had been some of the most equal societies in the world, inequalities grew throughout the FSU during the last decade, sometimes dramatically. For example, Armenia, the Kyrgyz Republic, Moldova and Russia are now among the most unequal world societies, with Ginni coefficients nearly twice their pre-transition levels, as is shown by a World Bank study (Selowsky and Mitra, 2002).

The study verified, however, that the more advanced reformers in the ECA region show much more equal outcomes. The study adds that the causes of the huge rise in inequality in some FSU countries lie in the prevalence of widespread corruption and rent seeking; the capture of the state by narrow vested interests, which have modified policy to their advantage, often at a high social cost; and the resulting collapse of formal wages and income opportunities.

Table 15.2 GNP per capita and per cent change 1991–2000

GNP/capita	1991	2000	Change
	US $	US $	%
Tajikistan	1,050	170	−84
Turkmenistan	1,700	840	−51
Uzbekistan	1,350	610	−55
Kyrgyz Republic	1,550	270	−83
Moldova	2,170	400	−82
Armenia	2,150	520	−76
Kazakhstan	2,470	1,190	−52
Azerbaijan	1,670	610	−63
Ukraine	2,340	700	−70
Russian Federation	3,220	1,660	−48
Georgia	1,640	590	−64
Lithuania	2,710	2,900	7
Estonia	3,830	3,410	−11
Latvia	3,410	2,860	−16
Belarus	3,110	2,990	−4

Source: World Development Indicators Database: Adapted from Arnstein, 1969

Rising inequalities have a clear negative impact on health. In Western countries, the burden of disease amongst the poorest groups is several times higher than amongst the richest. The same is true in the FSU, as shown by the limited regional evidence available (Gwatkin, 2001): poorer groups have the worst health status and less access to healthcare (on the relationship between inequality and health, see Part I, particularly Chapters 3 and 5).

Obsolete public health services

About one quarter of the difference in male life expectancy and 40 per cent of that in female life expectancy between countries of the FSU and EU countries have been attributed to differences in health system performance and the unavailability of modern healthcare (European Health Forum, 2000). The health system of the FSU has several weaknesses. These include the use of clinical and public health practices not based on evidence. These countries also maintain outdated public health services unable to deal with the epidemiological transition, including noncommunicable diseases and new and resurgent communicable diseases, and use available resources inefficiently.

The governments of the newly independent countries have continued previous public health best practices, such as maintaining high rates of immunisation, and have adopted some health policies to counteract the effects of lifestyle trends, such as anti-smoking laws. However, most have not yet fully adopted health promotion approaches, nor have they modernised their insolvent public health services.

Action to decrease the main causes of burden of disease and control the epidemics of HIV/AIDS and STIs has been taken. Significant examples are the Gorbachov 1985–87 campaign to reduce the availability of alcohol and the approved or proposed legislation to ban smoking in some public places and ban or restrict advertising of cigarettes in Estonia, Latvia, Russian Federation, Belarus, Moldova, Romania, Georgia and Kazakhstan. However, pressed by more urgent issues or interests, constrained by traditional practices, and forced by lack of, or misuse of resources, the governments of the FSU have shown reluctance to change and have been slow to adopt the most cost-effective interventions.

To a large extent, the public health sector continues to use outdated, costly and ineffective strategies for the prevention, diagnosis and treatment of the main diseases. FSU countries lack health policy development capacity, and health promotion has never been developed properly in many countries, with the two remarkable exceptions of Estonia and Kyrgyz Republic. The completeness, timeliness and quality of existing disease surveillance data vary from country to country, and were qualified as poor in many countries by a recent review (Miller and Ryskulova, 2004).

Health services have deteriorated significantly, and despite the development of general practice or family medicine throughout the region, the system is still mostly hospital-centred. While health budgets have decreased, few countries have moved decisively to get rid of excess capacity that consumes most resources. Public health and medical training has yet to be evidence-based, and training in health financing and management is in its infancy.

In what concerns alcohol policy, available data on trends in real prices of alcohol during the 1990s shows that the situation was not conducive to lowering consumption in the most affected countries, such as Latvia, Estonia, Russia, Ukraine, Georgia and Moldova. On the contrary, in Ukraine and Latvia real prices were falling for all sorts of alcohol; in Russia and Georgia, real prices were falling for hard liquor; and in Moldova and Estonia, while real prices of beer and wine were rising, real prices of hard liquor were stable (Vinokur, 2000).

In the 1990s, FSU countries started adopting smoking control measures that have been successfully launched in the European high income countries since the late 1970s. These measures aim at encouraging non-smokers to continue a smoke free lifestyle; protecting non-smokers from involuntary exposure to environmental tobacco smoke; and discouraging smokers from smoking. Anti-smoking laws have been approved in the 1990s in some FSU countries, such as Estonia, Latvia, Lithuania and the Russian Federation; and drafted in some other countries, such as Albania, Georgia and Turkmenistan. Excise taxes on tobacco in ECA normally range from 40 per cent in Estonia to 70 per cent in Albania. However, even where taxes are a reasonably high percentage of the retail price, retail prices are generally very low and it is the final price to the consumer that influences consumption. Some ECA countries, such as Slovakia, have been following the Finnish example of allocating excise taxes on tobacco and alcohol to health promotion and anti-smoking activities. Estonia has allocated a small percentage of the medical insurance proceeds to financing health promotion. However, public services are still mainly in charge of financing health promotion and anti-smoking activities from meagre state budgets and providing those services directly (for tobacco strategies and taxation see also Chapters 6 and 8 in Part II).

National and international NGOs and bilateral organisations have developed many pilot projects throughout the FSU to initiate HIV/AIDS and STIs prevention, mainly through harm reduction. These organisations have had a crucial role in stimulating regional governments to take action to improve the health of the population, especially of the poorest and most discriminated groups. The Soros Foundation/Open Society Institute and Medecins Sans Frontieres have provided some remarkable examples, amongst others, in the regional fight against TB, HIV/AIDS and STIs. Attitudes of FSU governments regarding these initiatives have varied from open hostility, passing by and non-interference, to supporting pilot projects. However, some FSU governments have requested grants and loans from the World Bank, and grants from the Global Fund to Fight AIDS, TB and Malaria (GFATM) exclusively to finance the control of TB, HIV/AIDS and STIs and, in some cases, follow up on the innovative pilot work.

The economic costs of disease

Disease and death further contribute to increasing poverty and disparities. The potential economic impact of disease and premature death caused by, among other risk factors, excessive alcohol consumption, smoking and use of illegal drugs in the FSU is severe. The estimates of total costs of alcohol use and abuse include household costs, direct healthcare expenditures, premature death, impaired productivity, motor vehicle accidents, crime and social welfare. Data indicate that family members in particular pay a part of the price for the excessive alcohol consumption by one or more members of the household.

A study of the potential economic effects of an unchecked HIV/AIDS epidemic in the Russian Federation suggests that GDP could be 4.15 per cent lower in 2010. Without intervention the loss would rise to 10.5 per cent by 2020. The uninhibited spread of HIV would diminish the economy's long-term growth rate, reducing growth by half a percentage point annually by 2010, and a full percentage point annually by 2020. Investment would decline by more than production. In the pessimistic scenario, investment would decline by 5.5 per cent in 2010 and 14.5 per cent in 2020, indicating a growing impediment to growth (Rühl et al., 2002).

Recent modelling carried out in Central Asia indicates that, even in an optimistic scenario, mortality rates would increase nearly tenfold from 2005 to 2020, accounting for about a hundred deaths a month, and the cumulative number of HIV-infected individuals would rise to tens of hundreds by 2020. In the pessimistic scenario, in all three countries studied (Kazakhstan, Kyrgyz Republic and Uzbekistan), GDP in 2010 would be about 5 per cent lower, and without any intervention the loss would rise to roughly 10 per cent by 2020. As in the Russian Federation, the uninhibited spread of HIV/AIDS would significantly diminish the economy's long-term growth rate (Vinogradov, 2004). Clearly, the time to address this problem is now if the region is to prevent a potential catastrophic impact on the wellbeing of the population, health services expenditures and the economy.

Managing health risks

The balance between the costs of doing nothing to deal with the main threats to the health and lives of people in the FSU, and the costs of adopting evidence-based and cost-effective approaches, is certainly in favour of the latter. By comparison with the potential economic impact of disease and premature death, costs of intervention are relatively small. However, they are well above what regional governments can afford. The amount of money necessary to curb the epidemics of noncommunicable and communicable diseases is staggering. The identification of sustainable sources of funding to prevent and reduce harm caused by legal and illegal recreational drugs in the FSU, and other risk factors, is required. For example, in countries that have from

US $20 to US $200 per capita to spend on health, the estimated US $30 per drug user that harm reduction costs and the over US $1,000 per year per patient that anti-retroviral treatment costs are simply unaffordable. Therefore, investing in the poor to increase their socioeconomic and health status raises two difficult problems, which have not been solved satisfactorily so far: finding sustainable sources of significant funding and reaching the poor.

National and international organisations, including NGOs and bilateral and multilateral agencies, have had a crucial role in stimulating governments in the FSU to take action to improve the health of the population, especially of the poorest and most discriminated groups. However, efforts so far have failed to reverse the tide of avoidable death and disease by CVDs, cancer, injuries and communicable diseases. In addition, these countries will have to deal with an ageing population and growing numbers of chronically ill in the near future.

FSU countries present a challenging environment for managing public health problems. These range from cultural norms that may lead people to find practices such as excessive alcohol consumption and smoking socially acceptable, to structural problems that may prevent implementation of cost-effective programs, such as rising poverty and inequalities. Evidence-based and cost-effective approaches to address the main risk factors have to be implemented if governments want to decrease the main causes of burden of disease. These approaches can be summarised under the four headings of facilitation, incentives, regulation and restructuring.

Facilitation and educational activities include for example, advocacy, increasing health literacy, harm reduction, establishing help lines, and providing social support. These might be supported by incentives such as increases in prices and taxes on alcohol, cigarettes and illegal drugs (if the supply becomes scarce, prices go up). Incentives are unlikely to be effective without regulation such as, for example, bans or restrictions on advertising cigarettes and alcoholic drinks, a ban on smoking in public buildings and laws on drunk driving.

Further laws might be designed to protect drug users and commercial sex workers from discrimination and authorise harm reduction activities, including decriminalisation of drug use, commercial sex work and homosexuality. However, incentives and legal changes are unlikely to be effective without a restructuring of organisation. These could include shifts from central to regional or local control and from vertical to horizontal structures. With less hierarchical control a movement from sectoral to inter-sectoral structures might be encouraged. In health administration a shift from tertiary care to public health and primary healthcare is to be encouraged with a concomitant decrease in excess capacity.

The final priority is that of restructuring health services. It is important to establish health policy development capacity at the highest government levels, for the development of regulation, health promotion, disease prevention and treatment.

Developing, preferably integrated, modern health promotion and environmental health services should reform public health services.

Other restructuring would include the development of evidence-based pre- and post-graduate public health and medical training and training in health financing and management. In terms of care it is important to develop primary healthcare focused on immunisation, maternal and child health, diagnosis and treatment of highly prevalent conditions such as sexually trans- mitted infections, hypertension, diabetes and depression. It is also important to develop emergency services focused on prevention of death and disability by CVDs and injury and to improve surgery services.

Health promotion and stakeholder participation

An assessment of health promotion development in European and Central Asian countries (Godinho, 1998) made the following recommendations regarding the development of health promotion programmes in the countries of the FSU. They should develop health promotion activities in the context of a health strategy with defined and achievable targets. They should establish specific, measurable and modest health promotion objectives. These might be sustained by setting clear and working financing mechanisms and by allocating more modest budgets to health promotion activities (in one specific project, of the US $14 million allocated to health promotion, only 30 per cent were committed in four years).

Strategies would include both top-down approaches, such as policy and legislative initiatives, and bottom-up approaches, such as community-based activities and demand-driven initiatives. Again, modesty is recommended in the design and operational implementation arrangements. It is recommended that innovative mechanisms, such as inter-sectoral or expert committees should be backed up by a reliable administrative structure that will ensure that the mechanism works.

Finally, it is perhaps worth saying a word about processes and instruments for investments in health promotion and public health. Stakeholders belong to interest groups that not only have different perceptions, attitudes and practices in relation to different issues, which should all be taken into account in analyses and interventions, but also have different or even conflicting interests. On many occasions, the diversity of stakeholder interests is not sufficiently taken into account, though stakeholders try to call the attention of external and inter- nal partners to their different concerns and interests. Issues should be discussed with as many stakeholders as possible and not only with a small fraction of them. One of the most common mistakes in externally assisted interventions is to deal with a reduced number of stakeholders, and to rely heavily on external technical assistance. Good technical level may be achieved, but not ownership.

Instruments that increase impact on human development (HD) should be used, and processes that increase participation and ownership should be followed. Investments on inter-sectoral HD programmes could increase the impact on HD outcomes. Inter-sectoral action involving sectors such as health, education, social protection, infrastructure and environment should be revived, for example, to decrease injuries (transport operations), or to prevent HIV/AIDS and STIs. Social funds are the best example of human development operations, and the approach deserves to be extended to other areas. The Africa region has moved to sector-wide approaches to increase sector sustainability and coordinate donor investments, and this could also prove relevant in the FSU.

More than a decade after the breakdown of the Soviet Union, FSU countries still have significant human development problems, due to increasing poverty and inequalities. The potential impact on the economy of the main threats to the health and lives of people in the FSU suggest that these countries would greatly benefit from adopting evidence-based and cost-effective approaches to deal with the main risk factors. Funding available is far from enough and it is not properly organised to achieve the best results. Approaches for reaching vulnerable groups have been piloted, but they need to be evaluated and scaled up. The international community has been and can continue to be of assistance to the FSU in raising the funding, organising its use, piloting and evaluating cost-effective approaches to reach the poor, and advocating the scaling up of interventions that give the best results in terms of lives saved and wealth created.

References

The American European Health Forum (2000) *Creating a Better Future for Health in Europe* September. Gastein: Information and Communication in Health.

Arnstein, S. (1969) A ladder of citizen participation. *Journal of the American Planning Association*, **35** (4): 216–24.

Corrao, M.A., Guindon, G.E., Sharma, N. and Shokoohi, D.F. (2000) *Tobacco Control Country Profiles*. The 11th World Conference on Tobacco or Health. Atlanta.

Godinho, J. (1998) *Health Promotion in Bank-Financed Projects in Europe and Central Asia. ECSHD*. Washington DC: The World Bank.

Gravilova, N.S., Semyonova, V.G., Evdokushkina, G.N. and Gavrilov, L.A. (2000) Health responses to economic change in Russia. The Reves International Network on Health Expectancy and the Disability Process. Presentation. University of South California.

Gwatkin, D.R. (2001). Inequalities in access to health care in developing countries: what should be done? Washington DC: The World Bank

Miller, D. and Ryskulova, A. (2004) *Surveillance Systems in Eastern Europe and Central Asia*. Washington DC: The World Bank.

Murray, C. and Lopez, A. (1997) Global mortality, disability, and the contribution of risk factors: Global Burden of Disease Study. *The Lancet*, **349**: 1436–42.

Rühl, C., Pokrovsky, V. and Vinogradov, V. (2002) *The Economic Consequences of HIV in Russia*. Moscow: The World Bank.

The Russian State Committee for Statistics (2001) *Russian Statistical Yearbook 2001*. Moscow: The Russian State Committee for Statistics.

The Russian State Committee for Statistics (2003) *Russian Statistical Yearbook 2003*. Moscow: The Russian State Committee for Statistics.

The Russian State Committee for Statistics (2004) Natural Dynamics of the Population in the Russian Federation in 2003. *Statistical Bulletin.* Moscow: The Russian State Committee for Statistics.

Selowsky, M. and Mitra, P. (2002) *Transition: The First Ten Years.* Washington DC: The World Bank.

Shkolnikov, V., Mckee, M. and Leon, D.A. (2001) Changes in life expectancy in Russia in the mid-1990s. *Lancet,* **357**: 9260, 917–21.

UNAIDS (2000) Fact Sheet. *HIV/AIDS in the Newly Independent States.* Geneva: UNAIDS.

Vinogradov, V. (2004) *Economic Consequences of HIV in Central Asia*: Simulation Model Approach, in Reversing the Tide: Priorities for HIV/AIDS Prevention in Central Asia Washington DC: The World Bank.

Vinokur, A. (2000) *Trends in Alcohol Consumption and Alcohol-related Harm in Europe and Central Asian Region 1980–98.* Washington DC: The World Bank.

Vinokur, A., Godinho, J., Dye, C., and Nagelkerke, N. (2001) The TB and HIV/AIDS epidemics in the Russian Federation. Washington DC: The World Bank.

WHO (1997) Tobacco or health: A global status report. Geneva: WHO.

World Bank (2003) *The Millennium Development Goals in Europe and Central Asia.* Washington DC: The World Bank.

CHAPTER 16

Health Promotion Development in Europe: Barriers and New Opportunities

ERIO ZIGLIO, SPENCER HAGARD AND CHRIS BROWN

In 1984, a set of possible concepts and principles for health promotion was put forward for discussion by the WHO Regional Office for Europe WHO (WHO, 1984). Those concepts and principles informed and underpinned the Ottawa Charter two years later (WHO, 1986). They have provided the basis for the many health promotion innovations and developments which have emerged from Europe ever since. These have included a range of pan-European projects, and national projects and programmes, including the settings approach, for example, Healthy Cities, Health Promoting Schools, Health Promoting Hospitals, and numerous initiatives on health topics and specific risk factors. In the late 1990s, the Investment for Health approach to implementing health promotion also had its origins in the European region (Ziglio et al., 2000).

Although innovations related to health promotion often found their origins in the European region (Ashton, 1992; WHO-EC-CE, 1992; WHO, 1992, 1994, 1998b; Grossman and Scala, 1993; Pelikan et al., 1998), nevertheless, the health promotion concepts and principles of the mid-1980s have not become mainstream in most European countries. The explanation for this is probably complex, including both the existence of a policy climate hostile to the underlying concepts and principles of the Ottawa Charter in many western European countries in the mid to late1980s and also the sudden and dramatic political changes which took place in the central and eastern countries of the region from 1989–91. Other factors include the enormity of changes in the subsequent course of political, economic, social and health status and development in those countries as well as the constant emergence of new challenges across Europe over the past 15 years (Ziglio, 1993, 1998).

This chapter takes a developmental approach to European innovations in health promotion, in the context of the remarkable changes which have been transforming European society. Partly based on the analysis of Ziglio et al.,

(2000), the chapter considers the kind of health promotion strategy likely to be most effective in Europe in the future and concludes that it is vital to reassert the centrality of health to human and social development. For the purposes of this chapter, Europe is defined as lying within the boundaries of the European region of the World Health Organisation (WHO), and European countries are defined as the member states of WHO that are located within its European region.

Evidence requiring action

Since the appalling downturns in health status and life expectancy in most countries of central and Eastern Europe in the early 1990s, there has been some degree of recovery in many countries (Figure 16.1).

Despite this improvement overall, across Europe there are continuing huge inequalities in levels of health and illness, both between countries and between population groups within the same country. For example, a baby born in Tajikistan is five times more likely to die in infancy than a baby born in Finland. Likewise children born in the UK to the least affluent families are 2.5 times more likely to fail to thrive during the first year of life than children born into the most affluent families. In some Eastern European countries adult male mortality remains below the retirement age, while in some cities of Western Europe men in more affluent areas live on average ten years longer than those in the least affluent areas of the same city. Figure 16.2 illustrates that even across the European Union, an estimated 60 million citizens, accounting for

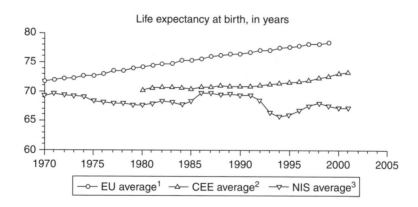

Figure 16.1   Years of life expectancy at birth, Europe, 1970–2001

Notes

1 Europe Union average
2 Central and Eastern Europe average
3 New Independent States average

Source: WHO, 2002a

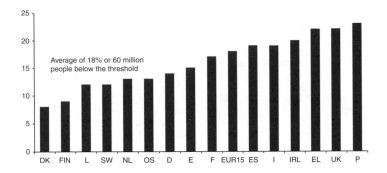

Figure 16.2   Percentage of people at risk of poverty and social exclusion,
European Union, 1997

Source: European Commission (1997)

18 per cent of the total EU population, were living at or below the poverty threshold in 1997 (for further discussion of inequalities, see Chapters 3 and 5 in Part I).

There are many reasons for these profound differences, but adverse economic, social and psychosocial circumstances are now considered to be paramount. The scientific evidence shows that large differences in health status can only be partially explained by the differences in available healthcare, and that in the fast changing European context, social and economic factors, in addition to environmental factors, have a stronger impact upon determining population health outcomes than do healthcare services (Evans et al., 1994; Wilkinson, 1996).

In comparison with most of the rest of the world, Europe is economically well off. The region is therefore not the main focus of the global debate about development in general and about the Millennium Development Goals (MDG), despite the fact that a significant number of countries in Eastern Europe and in the central Asian part of the region now display per capita incomes broadly comparable with the low income countries of Africa and southeast Asia. In 2000, eight European countries were classified as low income countries (annual gross national income (GNI) per capita below 745 United States dollars (US $)), and ten were in the lower middle income category (GNI per capita from US $745 to 2975) (World Bank, 2002) as can be seen in Table 16.1, which relates income levels in European countries in 2000 to three key mortality indicators in that year (for a sustained analysis of the health consequences of falling incomes in Russia, parts of East Europe, and Central Asia, see Part III, Chapter 15).

Much of current low income levels in these 18 countries is the result of the substantial fall in output, which took place during the decade of transition from planned to market economies, and from which the output in many countries has not yet fully recovered. This has had a huge impact on poverty: of all regions in the world, Eastern Europe has experienced the largest relative

Table 16.1 The European region by income and WHO mortality stratum
(Classified by GNI per capita in US $ in the year 2000)

High income (> US $9,265)		Higher middle income (US $2,996–9,265)		Lower middle income (US $756 – 2,995)		Low income (< US $756)	
Andorra	A	Croatia	A	Albania	B	Armenia	B
Austria	A	Czech Republic	A	Belarus	C	Azerbaijan	B
Belgium	A	Estonia	C	Bosnia and Herzegovina	B	Georgia	B
Denmark	A	Hungary	C	Bulgaria	B	Kyrgyzstan	B
Finland	A	Poland	B	Kazakhstan	C	Moldova	C
France	A	Slovakia	B	Latvia	C	Tajikistan	B
Germany	A	Turkey	B	Lithuania	C	Ukraine	C
Greece	A			Romania	B	Uzbekistan	B
Iceland	A			Russia	C		
Ireland	A			FYR Macedonia	B		
Israel	A			Turkmenistan	B		
Italy	A			Yugoslavia	B		
Luxembourg	A						
Malta	A						
Monaco	A						
Netherlands	A						
Norway	A						
Portugal	A						
San Marino	A						
Slovenia	A						
Spain	A						
Sweden	A						
Switzerland	A						
UK	A						

Notes: Mortality strata: A = 'very low child-, very low adult mortality', B = 'low child-, low adult mortality', C = 'low child, high adult mortality'

Source: World Bank (2002), World Development Indicators 2002

setback in achieving the principal MDG on poverty reduction, as illustrated in Figure 16.3.

Moreover, many of the transition countries became unable to afford the huge social infrastructures they inherited, resulting in the reversal of many social indicators. Most countries in the poorest part of the region have now begun to restore positive economic growth, and this is starting to lead to poverty reduction, for example in Russia. However, it remains to be seen if this will translate into comparable progress toward meeting the education, health, and environmental MDGs, which will require significant resource reallocations and major public sector and institutional reforms (www.developmentgoals.org, 2004). Strong national and international commitment will be required to reach these goals by 2015.

Meanwhile, two European countries classified as lower middle income in 2000, together with five classified as higher middle income, and two in the high income category, are due to join the existing high income 15 countries of the European Union on 1 May 2004.

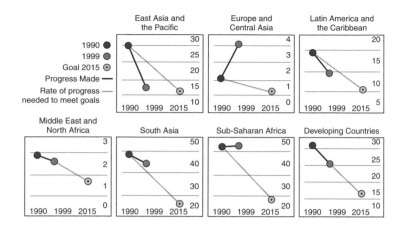

Figure 16.3 Progress towards the poverty goal (percentage of people living below US $1 or US $2 per day)

Source: www.developmentgoals.org, 2004

Health promotion in practice

Since the Ottawa Charter, much health promotion activity has taken place in Europe and the practice of health promotion within a number of countries has developed considerably. The implementation of a wide range of health promotion initiatives in Europe has generated much collective experience and added considerably to both knowledge and progressive change (for more on the influence of the Ottawa Charter on global health promotion, see Chapter 1).

Specific segments of the population, for example older people, young people, women, migrants, disabled and chronically ill people, have been involved in a variety of activities aimed at improving or gaining more control over their health (WHO, 1998b). Programmes and projects have been conducted in a variety of regional and social settings including those of cities, schools, workplaces and healthcare organisations.

At the same time, the European Union, comprising 15 member states with a combined population of around 300 million, has developed a role in public health through the Treaties of Maastricht and Amsterdam (but the promotion of population health has been outside the scope of the negotiations for the accession of new EU members). Some international projects, for example the WHO/Council of Europe/European Commission Health Promoting Schools project, have provided for health promotion development in a particular setting to be systematically planned, implemented, monitored, evaluated and developed, step by step on a multi-country basis, with strong international sharing of experience. In their turn, such projects have helped to stimulate moves in some countries towards a more strategic approach to programme development and towards a more ecological approach to health through inter-sectoral action and community development at the local level (WHO-EC-CE, 1992, 1997, 1998).

Moreover, with their focus on equity and healthy public policy, the health promotion concepts and principles set down in the mid-1980s appeared to be well matched to the challenges of the 1990s and the new century, as set out above under *Evidence requiring action*. However, in practice, they have generally not been equal to the challenge.

Despite the indisputable growth in health promotion activities, the continent is as divided in health promotion as in most aspects of economic, social and health development. In the east there has been a dearth of modern concepts of health promotion, as well as negligible resources, little public policy development and numerous one-off, discontinuous project activities, while in the west, despite substantially greater funding and an apparently greater continuity of development, there are not only widespread discontinuities of both policy development and interventions in health promotion but also a continuing reliance in many countries on approaches that have little obvious relationship to the accepted concepts and principles of health promotion (for more on the discontinuous and fragmented health promotion development in parts of Eastern Europe, see Chapter 15). Moreover there is a continuing preoccupation with individual risk behaviours and the promotion of healthy lifestyles, limited development of the investment for health approach within countries, and little evidence of the creation of the institutions and systems necessary to sustain the development of effective population health promotion (WHO, 2002b; EC/IUHPE, 1999; www.HP-source.net; 2004).

Investment for health

The international literature demonstrates that investing to address social and economic determinants of health is essential to improve the impact and sustainability of lifestyle interventions. Additionally, the evidence shows that when addressing the health needs of vulnerable groups and people living in poverty, isolated lifestyle and behaviour change programmes have limited impact. Incorporating actions to address the social and economic determinants of health into population health promotion can however improve the overall effectiveness, efficiency and sustainability of a country's approach to health promotion (Levin and Ziglio, 1997; WHO, 2002a).

Correspondingly, there is growing evidence and recognition of the value of good health as a reliable indicator of future economic development (UNICEF 1997). Hence, interventions that bring about the social conditions that create good health contribute in addition the added value of helping to build a strong and stable civil society. This in turn is an asset for economic development. Thus health, in addition to being a fundamental human right, is also an asset for broader regional or national development and stability (for more on

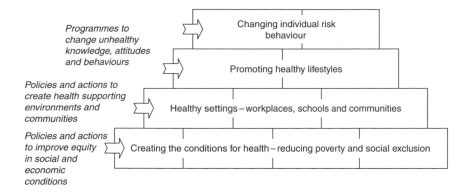

Figure 16.4   The building blocks to sustainable population health promotion

the relationship between health, inequality and welfare, see Part I, particularly Chapters 3 and 5).

Figure 16.4 illustrates how a robust and coherent approach to promoting population health requires a solid foundation, built through investing in policy actions that create the conditions for good health, and complemented by programmes to create healthy settings and promote healthy lifestyles (Ziglio and Brown, 2003).

A key priority for development is therefore to ensure the establishment of a sustainable infrastructure and systems to promote population health, which are competent to address not only individual risk behaviours, but also health related policies, and the social and economic conditions for good health. Recent evidence indicates that even in European countries with long traditions in the development of health promotion, both infrastructure and systems for these purposes remain seriously incomplete (WHO, 2001, 2002b; www.HP-Source.net, 2004).

Sustaining the vision but revisiting the means

The principles underlying the Ottawa Charter still stand. However, this review points to the need to revisit the means by which its vision of health promotion can be realised, especially in view of the many changes which have occurred in Europe in the last decade (Ziglio et al., 2000).

This implies a new dialogue with those who govern expenditure and policy throughout Europe, to engage their interest in the consequences of their actions for health and the corresponding implications for long-term social and economic development. With well-planned, concerted and sustained action in many societies over many years, the principles and values that underpin health promotion might be progressively brought to the forefront of public policy. By this means, the determinants of health might be influenced in the long term, which could have a significant impact on the quality of life of European people and their ability to realise their full potential. That is a long-term social investment issue not a series of short-term financial tactics (Ziglio et al., 2000).

European countries continue to experience major challenges to delivering robust and coherent population health promotion strategies in a systematic manner and concerns about performance and effectiveness are high priorities. The key areas where countries are requesting particular support from WHO include guidance about how to develop an effective health promotion infrastructure fitting countries' specific needs, and policy-making structures, both national and sub-national; advice about how to establish funding arrangements to ensure sustainable investment in an area which has been characterised by chronic underinvestment, fragmented mechanisms and short-term approaches; and help with the utilisation of appropriate methods for the evaluation of health promotion policies, programmes and initiatives. They also ask for guidance about how to plan, sustain and/or modernise human resource skills to enable robust health promotion development in European countries; how to ensure evidence-based best practice in health promotion and how to provide prompt information, with specific examples, on health promotion activities in other countries especially on any of the above issues (for a discussion of comparative research and evidence-based practice in global health promotion, see Part III, Chapter 11).

In these domains there is an urgent need to support countries to strengthen policy action, to increase capacity and to develop the skills, tools and technologies, working arrangements as well as the systems for translating scientific evidence into effective and sustainable practice across Europe. The Venice Office of WHO has been established to respond to this need. It has been given the mandate to perform the focal point function on these policy and capacity development issues.

Lessons learnt and priorities for action in Europe

The outstanding observation from the past two decades is that nowhere in Europe is population health promotion firmly established. This determines that the overriding priority for action is advocacy for the potential of population health promotion to enhance and support the rest of the social and economic development agenda in European societies.

For this to happen, better networks will be needed across Europe to evaluate and share knowledge of good practices in health promotion systems development, policy making and implementation. Three important elements of this will be benchmarking health promotion policies, strategies, institutions and infrastructures in different European countries; assessing on a pan-European basis the skills needed for the broad field of population health promotion, and designing appropriate education and training programmes;

and identifying and sharing practical solutions to the chronic shortage of resources which has hindered development from the outset.

References

Ashton, J. (1992) *Healthy Cities.* Buckingham: Open University Press.

European Commission (1997) *Public Health in the European Community. Health Promotion Programme (1996–2000).* Luxemburg: European Commission, D.G.V.

European Commission and International Union for Health Promotion and Education (1999) *The Evidence of Health Promotion Effectiveness.* Paris: International Union of Health Promotion and Education.

Evans, R.G., Barcer, M.L. and Marmot, T.R. (eds) (1994) *Why are Some People Healthy and Others Not?* New York: Aldine De Gruyter.

Grossman, R. and Scala, K. (1993) *Health Promotion and Organisational Development. European Health Promotion Series, No. 2.* Copenhagen: World Health Organisation, Regional Office for Europe.

Levin, L. and Ziglio, E. (1997) Health promotion as an investment strategy: a perspective for the 21st century. In Sidell, M., Johns, L., Katz, J. and Peberdy, A. (eds) *Debates and Dilemmas in Promoting Health.* London: MacMillan Press.

Pelikan, J. M., Garcia-Barbero, M., Lobnig, H. and Krajic, K. (eds) (1998) *Pathways to a Health Promoting Hospital.* Gamburg, Germany: G. Conrad, Health Promotion Publications.

UNICEF (1997) Children at Risk in Central and Eastern Europe: Peril and Promises. *Economies in Transition Studies, Regional Monitoring Report, No. 4.* Florence: Unicef, International Child Development Centre.

Wilkinson, R.G. (1996) *Unhealthy Societies.* London; Routledge.

World Bank (2002) *World Development Indicators, 2002.* Washington; The World Bank.

World Health Organisation (WHO) (1984) *Health Promotion: A Discussion Document on the Concept and Principles.* Copenhagen: World Health Organisation, Regional Office for Europe.

WHO (1986) *Ottawa Charter for Health Promotion.* World Health Organisation, Health and Welfare Canada, Canadian Public Health Association. Ottawa Charter for Health Promotion, Ottawa, Ontario, Canada. 21 November l986. (Available through Copenhagen: World Health Organisation, Regional Office for Europe.)

WHO (1991) *The Budapest Declaration of Health Promoting Hospital.* Copenhagen: World Health Organisation, Regional Office for Europe.

WHO (1992) *Twenty Steps for Developing a Healthy Cities Project.* Copenhagen: World Health Organisation, Regional Office for Europe.

WHO (1994) *National Healthy Cities Networks in Europe.* Copenhagen: World Health Organisation, Regional Office for Europe.

WHO (1998a) *The World Health Report.* Geneva: World Health Organisation.

WHO (1998b) *Health 21 – Leadership Guide to the Policy for Health for All in the European Region.* Copenhagen: World Health Organisation.

WHO (2001) *Investment for Health Appraisal in Malta.* Copenhagen: World Health Organisation.

WHO (2002a) *The European Health Report 2002.* Copenhagen: World Health Organisation.

WHO (2002b). *Review of National Finnish Health Promotion Policies and Recommendations for the Future.* Copenhagen: World Health Organisation.

WHO (2002c). *Investment for Health: A Discussion of the Role of Economic and Social Determinants.* Copenhagen: World Health Organisation.

WHO-European Commission-Council of Europe (1992) *The European Network of Health Promoting Schools.* Copenhagen: World Health Organisation, Regional Office for Europe.

WHO-European Commission-Council of Europe (1997) *The European Network of Health Promoting Schools. (Updated Version).* Copenhagen: World Health Organisation, Regional Office for Europe.

WHO-European Commission-Council of Europe (1998) *The Health Promoting School – An Investment in Education, Health and Democracy.* Conference Report. (First Conference of the European Network of Health Promoting Schools, Thessaloniki–Halkidiki, Greece, 1–5 May 1997.) Copenhagen: World Health Organisation, Regional Office for Europe.

www.developmentgoals.org (2004) Progress towards the poverty goal.

www.HP-Source.net (2004), accessed 5 February 2004.

Ziglio, E. (1993) *European Macro Trends Affecting Health Promotion Strategies.* WHO/EURO Working Paper. Copenhagen: World Health Organisation, Regional Office for Europe, Health Promotion and Investment Programme.

Ziglio, E. (1998) Key issues for the new millennium. *Promoting Health: The Journal of Health Promotion for Northern Ireland,* **2**: 34–37.

Ziglio, E., Hagard, S. and Griffith, J. (2000) Health promotion development in Europe: achievements and challenges. *Health Promotion International.* **15**(2): 143–54.

Ziglio, E. and Brown, C. (2003) *Strengthening Health Promotion in the European Region of WHO.* Venice: WHO European Office for Investment for Health and Development.

CHAPTER 17

Health Promotion in Australia and New Zealand: The Struggle for Equity

SHANE HEARN, HINE MARTIN, LOUISE SIGNAL
AND MARILYN WISE

Over the last twenty years health promotion has developed in Australia and New Zealand into an accepted discipline for solving public health problems. These countries have much in common, and are often compared, although, from the size and composition of their populations and economies to their history or geography, there are significant differences. This chapter outlines the health status of their peoples and describes the development of health promotion in both countries. It highlights successes, notably the successful delivery of programmes and infrastructures for health promotion. The chapter also draws attention to challenges that remain, particularly that of unacceptable inequalities in health.

The populations of New Zealand and Australia have life expectancies that are among the best in the world (World Health Organisation, 2000) although, in common with other economically developed nations, the socioeconomic gradient applies and mortality rates and years of life lost have been shown to increase with increasing socioeconomic disadvantage (Mathers et al., 1999; Howden-Chapman and Tobias, 2000). Of further concern in both countries is the fact that the greatest and most persistent inequalities in health status are those experienced by our indigenous populations. Indigenous life expectancy is poorer, and mortality rates higher, than those of non-indigenous New Zealanders of similar socioeconomic status (Howden-Chapman and Tobias, 2000; Reid et al., 2000).

For this reason a common theme for both post-colonial countries has been the struggle for equity in health since the colonisation had direct and serious impact on the health of indigenous communities, which persists to this day (Durie, 1998; Trewin and Madden, 2003). The different colonial experiences have, however, resulted in differences in the way health promotion has been undertaken. Critical to Māori, the indigenous people of New Zealand, is te Tiriti o Waitangi, a contract between Māori and the British Crown. Signed in 1840 the agreement, in which Māori exchanged sovereignty for protection

239

of their interests and the same citizenship rights as other British subjects, was largely ignored until 1975. Since then, however, it has provided an avenue for the settlement of Māori grievances with, in some cases, the return of control of lands, fisheries and forests or monetary compensation where this has been impossible. Further, the relevance of Te Tiriti has been acknowledged in social policy areas, including those of health.

In Australia, the consequences of having been colonised under the legal framework of terra nullius have been profound, excluding Aboriginal peoples and Torres Strait Islanders from citizenship in their own country for almost 200 years. Until 1967 they were left without a legal framework within which to claim rights to political and social self-determination, and to their land.

Health status

The patterns of life expectancy in the populations of New Zealand and Australia tell two seemingly incompatible tales. On the one hand there is the improving health of a majority, on the other, a failure to reduce the equity gap between the indigenous and non-indigenous people. Life expectancy in Australia and New Zealand has increased steadily over the last 40 years and is now, on average, 76 and 74 respectively for males and 83 and 79 years for females (Australian Institute of Health and Welfare, 2002). However, in 1999, Māori life expectancy at birth was approximately ten years less than for non-Māori. This was a significant increase in the gap in survival chances between Māori and non-Māori from 1980 (Ajwani and Blakely, 2003). Moreover the average life expectancy of indigenous Australian males born in 1998–2000 is expected to be 56 years for males and 62 years for females (Australian Institute of Health and Welfare, 2002). The differential between indigenous and non-indigenous Australians has remained unchanged for decades.

Clearly, neither all successes nor all failures to improve the health of populations can be attributed to health promotion. Nevertheless through encouraging strategic interventions and through advocacy, health promotion has a vital role to play. The chapter explores key aspects of health promotion strategy in both countries.

Underpinning values and ideas of health promotion

In contrast to Australia, where Ottawa Charter principles seem generally to have gained acceptance, there is a developing debate among New Zealand health promoters about health promotion values. Themes include the critical importance of indigenous rights, equity of health outcomes and capacity building (Health Promotion Forum, 2000). The Ottawa Charter has been significant in framing health promotion in New Zealand. In part, this is because it was promoted by leading players and organisations but also because the ideas resonated with concepts of health and health development. Māori New Zealanders, in particular, have begun to formulate their own health promotion philosophy, theory and practice (Waa et al., 1998; Durie, 1999; Ratima, 2001).

A key development has been TUHA-NS, a tool to assist in the application of Te Tiriti o Waitangi in health promotion practice (Martin, 2000). Indigenous Australians, also, have developed their own definition of health (National Aboriginal Health Strategy Working Party, 1989), and there is a growing body of evidence of effective indigenous health promotion interventions (National Health and Medical Research Council, 1997a; Northern Territory Health, 2001). There has been a gradual shift in indigenous health promotion in Australia toward the adoption of more policy- and systems-driven approaches, highlighting not only the need for community control of individual projects, but for active engagement of indigenous people in the decision making processes.

Rhetorically, social justice and equity remain at the core of health promotion in both countries, although it has proven to be a continuing challenge to align investment, practice and research with these values (for further discussion of the significance of the Ottawa Charter for health promotion, see Chapter 1).

Infrastructures and strategies for health promotion

Australia is a federation. All three tiers of government have some responsibility for funding and providing components of the nation's public health services. The states and territories have principal responsibility for public health policy, health promotion policy, funding, and programme design and delivery, although the Commonwealth health authority and local government also undertake significant health promotion.

Within each state and territory, the responsibility and accountability for the design and delivery of local and regional health promotion programmes has been organised differently. But in each jurisdiction programmes are delivered by specialist health promotion services, community health and primary healthcare services, hospitals, and general practice. In addition, NGOs and community organisations and components of the private sector also fund and deliver health promotion. Aboriginal medical services, controlled and staffed, principally, by Aboriginal and Torres Strait Islander health professionals, provide a range of primary healthcare services and health promotion to more than 50 communities. Other government sectors develop policies and programmes that contribute to health including occupational health and safety legislation, urban planning or waste management regulations and programmes.

The plethora of funders and providers of health promotion has resulted in some confusion about roles and responsibilities, and about leadership. A National Public Health Partnership has been established to develop a more consistent, comprehensive approach to identifying and solving public health problems (National Public Health Partnership, 1999; National Aboriginal and Torres Strait Islander Nutrition Working Party, 2000).

A major issue for the future is to make more efficient, effective use of the considerable infrastructure available for health promotion in Australia. The compelling need is for a client-defined infrastructure for health promotion to take forward actions to promote the health of indigenous Australians (National Health and Medical Research Council, 1997a).

New Zealand is a unitary state where central government, augmented by local government, funds much of health promotion. Public health organisation in New Zealand has undergone frequent, costly and disruptive change since the late 1980s with varying degrees of devolution and market orientation (Ashton 1999; Devlin et al., 2001). Currently, the Ministry of Health's Public Health Group advises on health promotion policy and legislation. Contracts for public health services having moved away from a quasi market approach to one based on local governance, cooperation and population health. This change was made by a centre left government in the face of a perception (Devlin et al., 2001) that market approaches had neither increased efficiency, nor sufficiently attended to quality nor focused on health outcomes (for a discussion of a comparable dilemma about health promotion strategy in Canada, see Part III, Chapter 18).

Contracted providers, including NGOs, public health services and community groups, deliver health promotion services. Indeed, a wide range of organisations is now engaged in providing health promotion services, as indicated by the size of the Health Promotion Forum, which now has more than 200 member organisations amongst its constituents. The number of Māori health providers, often involving health promotion activities, has also increased significantly in the last decade to 240. There has been a smaller, but measurable, increase in Pacific providers. Other sectors of government, such as the Land Transport Safety Authority and the Accident Compensation Corporation, also develop policies and programmes that explicitly promote health.

Although the personal health sector has not had a strong role in health promotion in New Zealand, primary care is currently undergoing change. New entities called Primary Health Organisations (PHOs), which are required to increase community participation including that of Māori, are being introduced with responsibility for population health gain and reduction in health inequalities. Supported by some new funding, their role in health promotion is likely to strengthen.

Public health legislation defines responsibilities and sets standards in a range of areas including water quality, environmental health, food safety and communicable disease control. In New Zealand new public health legislation is urgently needed as key statutes, particular the Health Act 1956, are outdated. Both countries have succeeded in implementing legislation and policy as components of comprehensive health promotion interventions to address major public health problems. Examples include legislation governing blood alcohol levels in drivers, bans on tobacco advertising and sales to minors, and school policies to reduce children's sun exposure.

Strategic approach

Both countries developed health goals frameworks in the late 1980s (Health Targets and Implementation Committee, 1988; Minister of Health, 1989) and revised them as new governments chose to revisit them (Nutbeam et al., 1993; Commonwealth Department of Human Services and Health, 1994; Ministry of Health, 1997; Minister of Health, 2000). The National Aboriginal Health Strategy (NAHS), released in 1989, was a landmark document that set the agenda for Aboriginal and Torres Strait Islander health (National Aboriginal Health Strategy Working Party, 1989). Although never fully implemented, the NAHS remains the key document to guide policy makers and planners. In 2003 a complementary framework was released (National Aboriginal and Torres Strait Islander Health Council, 2003). The NAHS established health goals and targets but the action to achieve these was never fully implemented. The 2003 framework identifies the infrastructure development that is needed to make progress. Ratification by the federal government and all the state and territory governments, itself, represents considerable progress.

New Zealand's current goals framework is broad, including goals for both healthy social and physical environments (Minister of Health, 2000). The 13 national priorities focus on individual risk factors and disease outcomes such as reducing smoking, improving obesity, and reducing the incidence and impact of cancer and cardiovascular disease. A parallel Māori health strategy has also been developed (Ministry of Health, 2002b). Australia's health priority areas now include seven major causes of disease, namely cardiovascular diseases, cancers, injuries, mental health problems, diabetes mellitus, asthma, arthritis and musculoskeletal conditions (Australian Institute of Health and Welfare, 2002). A range of national public health strategies is linked with the achievement of these goals. At both state and local levels the mix of specific programmes being implemented in relation to each of the priorities is dependent upon matching local, regional and state needs, with priorities and resources.

This strategic approach has provided a valuable framework for health promotion in both countries, assisting in determining priorities for public health investment, coordinating action to implement these priorities and focusing on health outcomes to measure effectiveness. However, the opportunity has been missed to prioritise broader determinants of health and their unequal distribution and therefore focus the sector's efforts in these critical areas.

Priority health promotion programmes

Over the last two decades comprehensive health promotion interventions have been implemented to address priority health issues. In New Zealand these include tobacco control, mental health promotion, road safety and reducing inequalities for all, including those of Māori and Pacific peoples (Minister of Health, 2000). Health promotion has yet to demonstrate more than limited progress in this last area although appropriate steps are being taken in some quarters (Signal et al., 2003). In terms of Māori health, for example, mainstream providers are required to prioritise health needs and provide services that are effective for Māori (Ministry of Health 2002c). Increasingly, Māori are developing and providing services to meet the needs of their own communities (Ministry of Health, 1998; Ratima, 2000). Likewise, the increasing numbers of Pacific providers are implementing 'by Pacific for Pacific' programmes (Ministry of Health, 2003b).

Even with respect to the national priority issues, Australia's national health promotion interventions have not always been nationally planned nor implemented systematically across the nation. Nonetheless, where there has been sufficient political commitment and leadership, sustained investment in intervention, and a comprehensive range of strategies, there have been some notable successes (National Health and Medical Research Council, 1997c; NSW Public Health Bulletin, 2003). There are also many examples of aboriginal communities having succeeded in implementing effective health promotion programmes to address priority issues they have identified (Health Promotion Journal of Australia, 1998).

The National Public Health Partnership has been developing national, coordinated strategies to address priority public health issues, and to contribute to strengthening infrastructures for public health and health promotion but there has been slow progress toward the routine consideration of equity within national issue-specific strategies and policies (National Public Health Partnership, 2003). Recently there has been greater emphasis on using advocacy, policy and partnerships to change the environments and structures that influence or determine the health choices of communities. In addition, both countries have been effective in using community development, the mass media and community education to inform, educate and mobilise communities to take or support action to promote health. There has been some progress in working in settings, the most successful of which has been health promoting schools (James, 2001) that have developed into a strong movement in Australia and has been growing in strength in New Zealand (for a further discussion of the possibilities of advocacy, the mass media and schools, see Chapters 4 and 11).

Overall, then, there is an increasing body of evidence that health promotion interventions have brought about positive changes. Although it is difficult to attribute the subsequent reductions in the prevalence of risk behaviours and in premature mortality to health promotion interventions, only, there is growing acknowledgement that such interventions can assist in bringing about sustained changes in the health of the population. Further, there is some evidence of the economic benefits that have resulted from these improvements (Applied Economics, 2001).

Capacity building for health promotion

Australia and New Zealand have worked to build skilled health promotion workforces. Both countries have identified health promotion workforce competencies (Health Promotion Forum of New Zealand, 2000; Shilton et al., 2001) but there is debate about whether introducing a system of professional accreditation would help to strengthen the quality of health promotion research and practice.

In Australia, specialised tertiary education programmes in health promotion, environmental health, mental health and health economics have been developed. Moreover the range of tertiary education in public health, including that for indigenous public health and health promotion professionals, has broadened (Standing Committee on Aboriginal and Torres Strait Islander Health, 2002; Commonwealth Department of Health and Ageing, 2003). A need remains for programmes to enable aboriginal health workers to add knowledge and skills in health promotion to their clinical, community and cultural skills and experience.

In New Zealand training options are more limited, especially for those outside the main centres. Many workers come into health promotion without formal training, although often they bring skills from other professions or from work with their own communities. Larger trained Māori and Pacific workforces are urgently needed, as are more Pakeha (non-Māori) workers who are skilled at working across cultures.

As yet many health professionals within the personal health sector of both countries have no access to adequate education in health promotion in general, and in indigenous health promotion in particular.

Research and development

In Australia there has been an ongoing effort to expand the funding of policy-driven, intervention research that will contribute to the evidence base for health promotion. The National Health and Medical Research Council, a strategic body responsible for public health research and policy advice, with some of the state health departments, has invested in research capacity building. There have also been encouraging steps to build indigenous research capacity (National Health and Medical Research Council, 2003) and the Cochrane Collaboration on Health Promotion is also contributing to the development of the evidence base (for evidence-based comparative research, see Part III, Chapter 11).

In New Zealand, the Health Research Council is the major government-funded agency responsible for health research. Its current priority areas include health and independence of population groups, the determinants of health, and Māori health. In both countries, the focus on evidence-based practice has pointed to the need for increased investment in intervention research, evaluation research and dissemination research including active programmes to encourage the early inclusion of research results in policy and programmes (Ministry of Health, 1997; National Health and Medical Research Council, 2003)

Little research has been commissioned to identify effective interventions to improve health equity, particularly interventions that address the social, economic and environmental determinants of health. There has been surprisingly limited engagement by the health sector in the development of wider aspects of public policy that influence the conditions in which individuals and communities make health choices. An evidence base for this will be required to enable the health sector to participate actively in policy debate and development with other sectors in the future (for comparable dilemmas, see the discussion of Canada in Part III, Chapter 18).

Evaluation and monitoring

Both countries report regularly on progress of their health strategies, (Australian Institute of Health and Welfare, 2002; Ministry of Health, 2002c) and are continually improving the information systems required for this. A coordinated national population survey programme has been proposed in New Zealand, but has yet to be implemented (Ministry of Health, 2002e). This has the potential to significantly strengthen monitoring relevant to health promotion.

Australia has continued to invest in developing effective national health monitoring and surveillance systems including routine monitoring of progress toward improved population health status and disparities in health status among different population groups. Gradually, the monitoring and surveillance systems have expanded to include social, economic and environmental determinants of health (Australian Institute of Health and Welfare, 1999; Australian Health Ministers' Conference, 2001). There are biennial reports on progress in improving Australia's health and welfare (Australian Institute of Health and Welfare, 2002, 2003). There has also been progress in developing comprehensive information and reporting on the health and welfare of Aboriginal and Torres Strait Islander peoples (Trewin and Madden, 2003).

As yet, there is no systematic measurement of the inputs to, or quality of health promotion in either country. These are future challenges. There is also the need to develop better methods and measures and to assess the effectiveness of comprehensive health promotion programmes in improving health and reducing inequalities (Speller et al., 1997; McQueen, 2001).

Investments for health development and health promotion

Governments provided more than two thirds of funding for health expenditure in Australia in 2001–02 (Australian Institute of Health and Welfare, 2003).

A 1.5 per cent levy on taxable income provides all citizens with free access to medical and hospital services. Estimated public expenditure on dedicated health promotion infrastructure and programmes, included in public health expenditures, represented approximately 1.9 per cent of all government health expenditures in 1995/96 (Deeble, 1999). Less than 2 per cent of New Zealand's tax-based health budget is allocated specifically for public health (Ministry of Health, 2002a). However, in both countries, these figures significantly underestimate total government expenditure on health promotion, particularly when the contributions of sectors other than health are included.

There is no reliable data on funding health promotion for indigenous peoples in Australia. However, it is possible to say that, despite the significantly poorer health status, the proportion of the population who live in remote areas where the costs of delivering health services are higher, and the evidence of high levels of social and economic disadvantage, the average expenditure per person on health services for Aboriginal and Torres Strait Islander peoples was similar to that for the rest of the population (Commonwealth Department of Health and Ageing, 2000; Trewin and Madden, 2003).

Both countries have relied, largely, on government investment to fund health promotion infrastructure and programmes. However, three state governments in Australia have imposed special taxes on tobacco products, a proportion of which are used to establish health promotion foundations. The funding available through the foundations is approximately equal to the amount of state or territory government funding for health promotion in each of their respective states, representing a considerable additional investment. A similar New Zealand organisation is the Health Sponsorship Council. The foundations have replaced tobacco sponsorship with health sponsorship, developed a range of innovative community and settings-based programmes and contributed to intervention research and capacity building (Healthway, 2002; VicHealth, 2002).

NGOs are becoming increasingly important in the overall national investment in health promotion and they can play a particularly valuable role as health advocates, especially in relation to health equity (Nathan et al., 2002). Neither country has a strong record of investment in health development and health promotion by the private sector, although interest is increasing. There is concern that the role of some parts of the private sector in promoting health raises ethical conflict.

Collaboration and partnerships for health

Public engagement is a feature of much health promotion endeavour. Community needs assessments that are based on some level of community participation are common features of many local programmes. Public consultation is routine in the development of national health promotion policy in New Zealand, where consultation is a statutory obligation of the Public

Health Group of the Ministry of Health. A key development in New Zealand, in line with te Tiriti, has been the increasingly active participation by Māori in defining and addressing their own public health needs (Wehipeihana and Burr, 2001; Ministry of Health, 2003a).

In Australia there has been considerable rhetoric about the need for greater community participation in health sector decision making, but there are few examples of this having developed into sustained, empowering processes that engage communities. This has been the case for indigenous communities, in particular, but non-indigenous rural and remote communities and outer urban communities, too, have recently succeeded in drawing attention to their needs (Premier's Department, NSW, 2000).

Examples of collaboration that have been effective in addressing specific public health problems include, the Coalition for Gun Control in Australia and the Aparangi Tautoko Auahi Kore (the Māori Smokefree Coalition) of New Zealand. The Australian Indigenous Health Promotion Network, the Health Promotion Forum of New Zealand, the Australian Association of Health Promotion Professionals, and the Public Health Associations of Australia and New Zealand are examples of networks of individuals and organisations that support health promotion practice.

Collaboration between health promotion agencies and healthcare services is not as strong, although often the principal delivery mechanisms for health promotion at the local level are primary healthcare agencies. Collaboration with other sectors has contributed, for example, to reductions in transport-related deaths and injuries, and to reductions in the prevalence of smoking. There are many other examples of successful collaboration, such as the Families First programme in New South Wales (NSW Cabinet Office, 2003) and the New Zealand Ministerial Committee on Drugs (Signal, 1997). There is a growing understanding of the factors that enhance collaboration between sectors (Harris et al., 1995; Fear and Barnett, 2003). Experience in New Zealand and Australia has shown that although it is possible to work with other sectors, it is not simple, particularly when the area of overlapping interests between organisations is small. To meet the complex challenges to the health of populations the health sectors in both countries must build their capacity to collaborate with other sectors. The use of Health Impact Assessment as a tool to highlight the role of all sectors in health development is being explored in both countries (Mahoney et al., 2002; Public Health Advisory Committee, 2003).

Health promotion challenges

This brief overview indicates that health promotion has developed into an accepted public health discipline in Australia and New Zealand and the Ottawa Charter has gained wide acceptance as the framework for health promotion, to which each country has added its own perspectives and ways of working. Both nations have established a health promotion infrastructure to identify priority issues, to allocate and distribute resources and to design and deliver national and local intervention strategies, including policies and legislation. Each has networks of health promotion providers. Both have demonstrated that comprehensive, sustained interventions can succeed in improving the health status of the population (Hawe et al., 2001; Ministry of Health, 2002c). The health sector's organisational capacity for health promotion includes systems for monitoring and surveillance, workforce development, research and development, and programme evaluation. Government, which has invested the greatest volume of resources in health promotion, has contributed policy leadership. Nevertheless tax-funded foundations, NGOs and community-based organisations are also important contributors. Collaboration and partnership have been strong features of health promotion in both countries.

However, there are weaknesses in health promotion in both Australia and New Zealand. Constant restructuring of the sector has made sustained investment in effective intervention difficult. New Zealand urgently needs new public health legislation. The strategic approaches of both countries have failed to prioritise the broader determinants of health and their unequal distribution. This is in part because of lack of evidence of effective interventions, and in part because of concern that the health sector should not be held responsible for the policies and actions of the other sectors that, essentially, determine health.

While there has been investment in workforce development, this has been limited, especially for the indigenous workforces, as has investment in gathering the evidence needed to develop and sustain effective interventions, particularly in indigenous communities. Decision makers have failed to be convinced of the potential health benefits of significant investment in health promotion in the face of competing demands for acute care services and the lack of evidence of cost-effectiveness. While there have been partnership successes, getting health on the agenda of other sectors remains a significant challenge. Finally, while health promotion has had successes in improving overall health, the struggle for equity is a major challenge especially equity between the indigenous and non-indigenous populations.

There are many future challenges for health promotion in Australia and New Zealand. They include maintaining and strengthening systems that support health promotion. This will require powerful advocacy by the health promotion sector itself, and success in convincing societal decision makers about its achievements and future potential. Building capacity for health promotion in the personal healthcare sector remains a challenge, as does building strategic alliances with other sectors, and further developing ways of working to achieve shared benefits.

Another challenge is to find ways to strengthen participation in, and influence on, policy making and practice at the highest global levels, including involvement with global organisations (Labonte, 2003). While there are successes, such as participation in the development of the Framework

Convention on Tobacco Control (World Health Organisation, 2003), increasing globalisation means that the determinants of health needs, and their solutions, are increasingly coming from outside the two countries. Health promotion shares its values of equity and social justice with many other sectors and interest groups. Health promotion can join with them, not as leader but as a partner (for the need for partnership, see Part I, Chapters 4 and 5).

It is the issue of tackling health inequalities that poses one of the biggest challenges for both Australia and New Zealand. Above all, the health sectors need explicit political and policy commitment to the goal of reducing inequalities in health, especially for Māori and indigenous Australians, alongside the already established goal of improving the health of the population in general. However, there are grounds for optimism about the role of health promotion in this arena (Catford, 2002). New Zealand is making some progress with equity, in terms of Māori health promotion, and Australia is beginning the journey. In New Zealand ongoing commitment to, and honouring of, te Tiriti o Waitangi is required. 'By Māori for Māori' programmes need to be strengthened, and mainstream programmes must meet Māori needs. In Australia progress can occur only when there are genuine, respectful partnerships between the health sector and indigenous people whose knowledge, experience, culture and wisdom must lead the action (National Aboriginal Health Strategy Working Party, 1989).

Significant social and government commitment, combined with resources and resolve is still required. Analysis of the causes of inequalities, including the potential effects of racism in health, is also important (Jones, 2000). Health promoters have the ability to prioritise work with the least privileged in society and to measure success in achieving this in programme evaluation. The increasing range of available strategies and tools to tackle inequalities means it is possible to intervene at the policy, community and individual levels (Martin, 2000; Ministry of Health, 2002d; Simpson and Harris, 2003). The challenge will be met, in part, if the sector builds an equity approach into the everyday business of health promotion (Signal, 2002; NSW Department of Health, 2003).

Health promotion has contributed to the health development of the people of Australia and New Zealand. The challenges facing the health of the populations of both nations require strengthening of commitment to, and investment in, health promotion that assists individuals, communities and society as a whole to achieve health, wellbeing and equity.

References

Ajwani, S. and Blakely, T. (2003) *Decades of Disparity: Ethnic Mortality Trends in New Zealand 1980–99*. Wellington: Ministry of Health and University of Otago.

Applied Economics(2001) *Returns on Investment in Public Health: An Epidemiological and Economic Analysis*. Prepared for the Department of Health and Aged Care. Applied Economics. Sydney: Department of Health and Aged Care.

Ashton, T. (1999) The health reforms: to market and back? In Boston, J., Dalsiel, P. and St John, S. (eds) *Redesigning the Welfare State in New Zealand: Problems, Policies, Prospects*. Auckland: Oxford University Press.

Attwood, B. (2003) *Rights for Aborigines*. Crows Nest, Australia: Allen and Unwin.

Australian Health Ministers' Conference (2001) Department of Health and Ageing, Australian Government. http://www.health.gov.au/minconf.htm

Australian Institute of Health and Welfare (1999) *Development of National Public Health Indicators: Discussion Paper*. Canberra: Australian Institute of Health and Welfare.

Australian Institute of Health and Welfare (2002) *Australia's Health 2002*. Canberra: Australian Institute of Health and Welfare.

Australian Institute of Health and Welfare (2003) *Australia's Welfare 2003*. Canberra: Australian Institute of Health and Welfare.

Catford, J. (2002) Reducing health inequalities – time for optimism. *Health Promotion International*, **17**: 101–04.

Commonwealth Department of Health and Ageing (2000) *Health and Aged Care Portfolio Submission to the Commonwealth Grants Commission's Inquiry into Indigenous Funding*. Canberra: Commonwealth Department of Health and Ageing.

Commonwealth Department of Health and Ageing (2003) *The Public Health Education and Research Programme*. www.health.gov.au

Commonwealth Department of Human Services and Health (1994) *Better Health Outcomes for Australians*. Canberra: Australian Government Publishing Service.

Deeble, J. (1999) *Resource Allocation in Public Health: An Economic Approach*. A background discussion paper for the National Public Health Partnership. Victoria: National Public Health Partnership.

Devlin, N., Maynard, A. and Mays, N. (2001) New Zealand's Health Sector Reforms: Back to the Future? *British Medical Journal*, **322**: 1171–74.

Durie, M. (1998) *Whaiora: Māori health development* (2nd ed). Auckland: Oxford University Press.

Durie, M. (1999) Te Pae Mahutonga: a model for Māori health promotion. *Health Promotion Forum Newsletter*, **49**: 2–5.

Fear, H. and Barnett, P. (2003) Holding fast: the experience of collaboration in a competitive environment. *Health Promotion International*, **18**: 5–14.

Harris, E., Wise, M., Hawe, P., Finlay, P. and Nutbeam, D. (1995) *Working Together: Intersectoral Action for Health*. Canberra: Department of Human Services and Health.

Hawe, P. Wise, M. and Nutbeam, D. (2001) Policy- and system-level approaches to health promotion in Australia. *Health Education and Behavior*, **28**(3): 267–73.

Health Promotion Journal of Australia (1998) Issue devoted to aboriginal health *Health Promotion Journal of Australia*, **8**(1).

Health Promotion Forum of New Zealand (2000) *Ngā Kaiakatanga Hauora mō Aotearoa: Health Promotion Competencies for Aotearoa – New Zealand*. Auckland: Health Promotion Forum of New Zealand.

Health Targets and Implementation Committee (1988) *Health for all Australians*. Canberra: Australian Government Publishing Service.

Healthway (2002) About Healthway. www.healthway.wa.gov.au

Howden-Chapman, P. and Tobias, M. (eds) (2000) *Social Inequalities in Health: New Zealand 1999*. Wellington: Ministry of Health.

James. P. (2001) *The Puzzle, the Seed, the Voyage and the Guardian: Reflections On the Development of Health Promoting Schools in Aotearoa/New Zealand*. Auckland: Enigma.

Jones, C. (2000) Levels of racism: a theoretic framework and a gardener's tale. *American Journal of Public Health*, **90**: 1212–15.

Labonte, R. (2003) *Dying for Trade: Why Globalisation Can Be Bad For Our Health.* Toronto: The CSJ Foundation for Research and Education.

McQueen, D.V. (2001) Strengthening the evidence base for health promotion. *Health Promotion International,* **16**(3): 261–68.

Mahoney, M., Durham, G., Townsend, M., Reidpath, D., Wright, J. and Potter, J.L. (2002) *Health Impact Assessment: A Tool for Policy Development in Australia.* Report for Commonwealth Department for Health and Ageing. www.deakin.edu.au/hia, Melbourne: Deakin University.

Martin, H. (2000) *TUHA-NZ: a Treaty Understanding of Hauora in Aotearoa – New Zealand.* Auckland: Health Promotion Forum.

Mathers, C., Vos, T. and Stevenson, C. (1999) *The burden of disease and injury in Australia.* Canberra: Australian Institute of Health and Welfare.

Minister of Health (1989) *New Zealand Health Goals and Targets.* Wellington: Ministry of Health.

Minister of Health (2000) *The New Zealand Health Strategy.* Wellington: Ministry of Health.

Ministry of Health (1997) *Strengthening Public Health Action: A Strategic Direction to Improve, Promote and Protect Public Health.* Wellington: Ministry of Health.

Ministry of Health (1998) *Whaia Te Whanaungatanga: oranga whanau. The Wellbeing of Whanau.* Wellington: Ministry of Health.

Ministry of Health (2002a) Health Expenditure Trends in New Zealand 1980–2000. Wellington: Ministry of Health.

Ministry of Health (2002b) *He Korowai Oranga: Māori Health Strategy.* Wellington: Ministry of Health.

Ministry of Health (2002c) *Implementing the New Zealand Health Strategy 2002: The Minister of Health's Second Report on Progress on the New Zealand Health Strategy.* Wellington: Ministry of Health.

Ministry of Health (2002d) *Reducing Inequalities in Health.* Wellington: Ministry of Health.

Ministry of Health (2002e) *The New Zealand Health Monitor: A Ten-year Strategic Plan for a Coordinated National Population Survey Programme.* Wellington: Ministry of Health.

Ministry of Health (2003a) *Aukati Kai Paipa 2000: Evaluation of Culturally Appropriate Smoking Cessation Programme for Māori Women and their whānau.* Wellington: Ministry of Health.

Ministry of Health (2003b) *Pacific Health in New Zealand: Our Stories.* Wellington: Ministry of Health.

Ministry of Health, Public Health Consultancy and Te Rōpū Rangahau Hauora A Eru Pōmare (2002) *A Health Equity Assessment Tool.* Wellington: Ministry of Health, Public Health Consultancy and Te RōpūRangahau Hauora A Eru Pōmare.

Nathan, S., Rotem, A. and Ritchie, J. (2002) Closing the gap: building the capacity of nongovernment organisations as advocates for health equity. *Health Promotion International,* **17**(1): 69–78.

National Aboriginal and Torres Islander Nutrition Working Party (2000) *National Aboriginal and Torres Strait Islander Nutrition Strategy and Action Plan 2000–2010.* Canberra: Signal, National Public Health Partnership.

National Aboriginal and Torres Strait Islander Health Council. (2003) *National Strategy Framework for Aboriginal and Torres Islander Health* Canberra: National Aboriginal and Torres Strait Islander Health Council.

National Aboriginal Health Strategy Working Party (1989) *The National Aboriginal Health Strategy.* Canberra: The National Aboriginal Health Strategy.

National Health and Medical Research Council (1997a) *Case studies of Aboriginal and Torres Strait Islander health advancement.* Canberra: National Health and Medical Research Council.

National Health and Medical Research Council (1997b) *Promoting The Health of Australians: A Review of Infrastructure Support for National Health Advancement.* Canberra: National Health and Medical Research Council.

National Health and Medical Research Council (1997c) *Promoting the health of Australians: case studies of achievements in improving the health of the population.* Canberra: National Health and Medical Research Council.

National Health and Medical Research Council (2003) *Review of the implementation of the National Health and Medical Research Council's Strategic Plan 2000–2003.* Canberra: National Health and Medical Research Council.

National Health Performance Committee (NHPC) (2001) *National Health Performance Framework Report.* Brisbane: Queensland Health.

National Public Health Partnership(1999) *Guidelines for Improving National Strategy Development and Coordination.* Melbourne: National Public Health Partnership. www.nphp.gov.au

National Public Health Partnership (2003) *National Public Health Partnership Agenda 2002–2004.* Melbourne: National Public Health Partnership. www.nphp.gov.au

NSW Cabinet Office. *Families First.* www.parenting.nsw.gov.au/public/226_homepage/

NSW Public Health Bulletin (2003) *NSW Health Aboriginal Health Impact Statement and Guidelines. Incorporating Aboriginal Health Needs and Interests in Health Policies and Programmes.* Sydney: NSW Department of Health.

Northern Territory Health (2001) *The Bush Book.* Darwin, Australia: NT Health.

Nutbeam, D., Wise, M., Bauman, A., Harris, E. and Leeder S. (1993) *Goals and Targets for Australia's Health in the Year 2000 and Beyond.* Sydney: Department of Public Health and Community Medicine, University of Sydney.

Premier's Department, NSW (2000) Workforce Planning Issues http:/rrd.premiers.nsw.gov.au/rrd/public/2000/planning.html

Public Health Advisory Committee (2003) *A Guide to Health Impact Assessment: A Policy Tool for New Zealand.* Wellington: National Health Committee.

Ratima M. (2000) Tipu Ora – A Māori-centred approach to health promotion. *Health Promotion Forum of New Zealand Newsletter,* **52**: 2–3.

Ratima M. (2001) *Kia Uruuru Mai a Hauora Being Healthy, Being Māori: Conceptualising Māori Health Promotion.* Unpublished PhD thesis. Wellington: Department of Public Health, Wellington School of Medicine and Health Sciences.

Reid, P., Robson, B. and Jones, C.P. (2000). Disparities in health: common myths and uncommon truths. *Pacific Health Dialogue,* 7: 38–47.

Shilton, T., Howat, P., James, R. and Lower, T. (2001) Health promotion development and health promotion workforce competency in Australia. *Health Promotion Journal of Australia,* **11**: 117–23.

Signal, L. (1997) Partnerships for health promotion: reducing drug-related harm. *Promotion and Education,* **IV**(3): 43–45.

Signal, L. (2002) Tacking inequalities through health promotion action. *Health Promotion Forum of New Zealand Newsletter,* **56**: 10.

Signal, L. N., Martin, J., Rochford, T., Dew, K., Grant, M., Howden-Chapman, P. (2003) *Tackling Inequalities in Heart Health: A Review of the Health Services Work of the National Heart Foundation.* Wellington: Public Health Consultancy, Wellington School of Medicine and Health Sciences.

Simpson, S. and Harris, E. (2003) *NSW Health Impact Assessment Project, Phase 1 Report*. Sydney: Centre for Health Equity, Training Research and Evaluation, University of NSW.

Speller, V., Learmonth, A. and Harrison, D. (1997) The search for evidence of effective health promotion. *British Medical Journal*, **315**: 361–63.

Standing Committee on Aboriginal and Torres Strait Islander Health (2002) *Aboriginal and Torres Strait Islander Health Workforce National Strategic Framework*. Canberra: Australian Health Ministers' Advisory Council.

Trewin, D. and Madden, R. (2003) *The Health and Welfare of Australia's Aboriginal and Torres Strait Islander peoples*. Canberra: Australian Bureau of Statistics.

VicHealth (2002) About VicHealth. www.vichealth.vic.gov.au

Waa, A., Holibar, F. and Spinola, C. (1998) *Programme Evaluation: An Introductory Guide for Health Promotion*. Auckland: Alcohol and Public Health Research Unit.

Wehipeihana, N. and Burr, R. (2001) *Hikoi 2000 Evaluation Report*. Wellington: Hutt Valley District Health Board.

World Health Organisation (2000) *The World Health Report 2000. Health Systems: Improving Performance*. Geneva: World Health Organisation.

World Health Organisation (2003) *Updated Status of the WHO Framework Convention on Tobacco Control*. www.who.int/tobacco/fctc/signing_ceremony/co.

CHAPTER 18

Health Promotion in Canada: Back to the Past or Towards a Promising Future?

ANN PEDERSON, IRVING ROOTMAN AND MICHEL O'NEILL

In September 2003, the Canadian Dental Association held its first ever strategic forum as part of its annual general meeting. Speakers described the evolution of health promotion in Canada, possible strategies for promoting oral health and a proposed national oral health strategy (CDA, 2003). A few days later a critical article was posted on a national health promotion electronic discussion list in opposition to the then current federal government's healthy living strategy to reduce obesity, diabetes and heart disease through increased physical activity and better eating habits (originally authored by Finn, 2002). Echoing critiques from twenty years earlier, the author argued that this approach to promoting health blames the victim and fails to address the fundamental determinants of poor health. Two weeks later a call was made by the UN chief AIDS envoy, Canadian Stephen Lewis, for the federal government to rewrite or override its patent law to permit large-scale production of generic drugs to aid in the struggle against AIDS worldwide. His intervention made headlines in one of the national newspapers (see Nolen, 2003). These three examples, taken from within a period of one month, illustrate current health promotion activities in Canada and act as a reminder of its past whilst suggesting possible futures.

This chapter offers a critical reflection upon Canada's contribution to health promotion, making the distinction between health promotion as a bureaucratic entity or formal domain of study and practice, as opposed to health promotion as a process concerned with empowering people to take control of their own health (WHO, 1986). The former approach is evidenced by the institutionalisation of health promotion, such as the existence of government departments, research centres, training programmes and legislation (see Boyce, 2002). The latter approach encourages a broader critical gaze at public policies, health sector reform, partnerships and social capital. Taking both of these approaches into account it can be seen that Canada has had a mixed record when it comes to health promotion. Whilst it has offered much needed leadership both locally and abroad, and has introduced important innovations in thinking and practice, it has failed to make some of the critically needed changes in policy to ensure health for all. Consequently, the current situation shows some evidence of a reversion to the old discourse about lifestyles. At the same time there are promising new developments underway such as the introduction of anti-poverty legislation in Quebec (for further discussion of this and other dichotomies informing the process of health promotion, see Parts I and II, particularly Chapters 5, 12 and 19).

The history of health promotion in Canada

Details of the evolution of health promotion in Canada have been documented elsewhere (for example, Pederson et al., 1994; Health Canada, 1997; O'Neill et al., 2000). Here it is only possible to mention relevant highlights that contribute to the argument that Canada has played a significant role in health promotion in various ways, but that continued efforts are needed to optimise the potential for health and wellbeing of Canada's citizens.

Canada is routinely referred to as a world leader in health promotion (Green, 1994; Kickbusch, 1994; Raeburn, 1994) because of the release in 1974 of the seminal *A New Perspective on the Health of Canadians*, which became known informally by the name of the federal minister of health and welfare of the day, the Honourable Marc Lalonde (Lalonde, 1974). By introducing the health field concept (HFC), the Lalonde report put forward on behalf of the Canadian government the argument for taking not just healthcare, but all of the determinants of health into account. The HFC described health as arising from four equally important elements: human biology, healthcare organisation, lifestyle and the environment. Whilst the aim of the Lalonde report was to minimise the role of the healthcare system and enlarge the importance of the other three elements in an effort to restrain the increasing costs of Medicare, in practice, the lifestyle element became the major legacy of the report and inspired the creation of the federal health promotion directorate (Health Canada, 1997) and various provincial counterparts (see Pederson et al. 1994). An emphasis on the importance of lifestyle to health gave rise to criticism as well as support. Health activists, researchers and planners challenged what they argued was a simplistic understanding of the links between knowledge, attitude and behaviour underlying the health education and social marketing approaches arising from the health promotion strategy outlined in the Lalonde report (noteworthy critiques included Crawford, 1977; Brown and Margo, 1978; Labonte and Penfold, 1981; Hancock, 1986).

A decade after the Lalonde report, Canadians again achieved global influence when Health and Welfare Canada, now Health Canada, cosponsored the First International Conference on Health Promotion with the World Health Organisation Regional Office for Europe and the Canadian Public Health Association. Two noteworthy policy statements marked the conference, namely the *The Ottawa Charter for Health Promotion* (World Health

Organisation, 1986) and *Achieving Health for All: A Framework for Health Promotion* (Epp, 1986). The Ottawa Charter articulated a broad, structural view of health promotion that encompassed a wider array of strategies than were named in the Lalonde report, and *Achieving Health for All*, Canada's own statement on health promotion, echoed and complemented the tone and vision of the charter by embracing strategies such as coordinating healthy public policy, fostering public participation and strengthening community health services (see also Chapter 1 for a discussion of the impact of the Ottawa Charter).

The release of such documents at the national and international levels stimulated developments in the provinces and territories and contributed to significant growth in the supporting structures for health promotion practice in Canada. For example, both undergraduate and graduate level training programmes were created or expanded in the mid-1980s, research centres at universities were established, and research granting agencies at the federal level such as the National Health Research Development Program, the major funding agency for public health research at the time, sponsored strategic research initiatives concerned with health promotion. Two national health promotion surveys were conducted in 1985 (Rootman, 1989) and 1990 (Health Canada, 1993) and Canadian researchers were, and still are, among the international leaders in discussions of the evidence base for health promotion's effectiveness. Public health agencies and their professional associations, such as the Canadian Public Health Association, established positions for health promotion personnel. Initiatives such as the Healthy Communities project in English speaking Canada (Health Canada, 1997) and Le Réseau Villes et Villages en Santé (VVS, 2003) in Quebec found institutional and political support.

There is a division of responsibility between the federal and provincial governments in Canada with respect to health and healthcare. Provinces have actual responsibility for health and healthcare and the national government primarily plays a taxation and funding role. Fulfilling their healthcare responsibilities, various provincial governments established commissions and working groups to link health promotion, its messages about the determinants of health, and its proposed strategies, to the practical realities of delivering healthcare services. For example, during the 1980s, Ontario sponsored three separate processes in close succession, at different levels of political influence, each of which reported that the province should put greater resources into disease prevention and health promotion (see Evans, 1987; Podborski, 1987; Spasoff, 1987). Although they differed in emphasis, the reports shared a common view that health promotion efforts were needed to address health problems (Pederson, 1989).

Ontario also established an innovative health council that was chaired by the Premier and which undertook to generate a vision for health for the province and articulate health goals (Signal, 1993). Similar, but less extensive processes occurred in most of the other provinces in the country (see, for example, Alberta, 1989).

A review of the history of health promotion in Canada released in 1997 suggested that among the achievements of the Lalonde Report had been a broadening of the health discourse (see Health Canada, 1997). As noted, the health field concept opened up discussion about the relative contributions of the healthcare system, personal lifestyle, human biology and the environment to health status and disease outcomes. It was based on a critique of individualism, and the potentially victim-blaming nature of both health education and social marketing, that arose following the failure of early health behaviour strategies to make significant changes among population groups. Also noted above is the fact that a potentially radical view of health and health promotion occasionally found its way into public discourse. In time, however, this discourse was challenged by a competing view that arose not from social welfare activists, health educators and community developers but rather from epidemiologists, health economists and biostatisticians (see Kaufert, 1999). In a few short years, a focus on the prerequisites for health of the Ottawa Charter, those of peace, shelter, education, food, income, a stable ecosystem, sustainable resources, social justice and equity, was supplanted by discussions of the determinants of health. These were framed in terms of population health (Evans et al., 1994; Federal, Provincial and Territorial Advisory Committee on Population Health, 1994).

While the debate between health promotion and population health seemed innocuous to some, critics have suggested that the underlying premises and meaning of health promotion and population health are too different to be regarded as compatible (see Robertson, 1998; Raphael and Bryant, 2002). Others sought to combine what they perceived as the strengths of both approaches to develop comprehensive models and frameworks to improve health and guide action (Hamilton and Bhatti, 1996). Today, the discourse of population health remains visible in government documents and policy statements, whereas that of health promotion seldom appears or is medicalised (for example, the federal Women's Health Strategy speaks in terms of the determinants of health and population health but mentions health promotion in relation to cervical cancer screening. (See http://www.hc-sc.gc.ca/english/women/womenstrat.htm). The battle for discursive dominance reflects fundamental shifts in support for the vision and practice of health promotion in Canada. There is a return to language and programmes that reflect individual responsibility for health and illness and a weakening of the government role as provider of services and resources for health gain.

From an institutional perspective, health promotion appears to have been supplanted by other discourses and frameworks. Government departments at the local, provincial and national level established health promotion units in the late 1980s but dismantled them a decade later. To some extent, this pattern reflects the evolution of health promotion thinking and discourse, in addition to shifting political fortunes. It also conveys the challenge of maintaining an institutional presence in what has become a healthcare system driven by acute needs, technology and pharmaceutical developments.

The global contribution of Canada to health promotion

In spite of the vagaries of health promotion that have been noted above, Canada has made and continues to make a significant contribution to health promotion globally. This contribution has included ideas, leadership and resources. Moreover, Canada has benefited from developments and initiatives elsewhere. Hence, Canada's relationship to health promotion globally is perhaps best understood as a reciprocal one in which all parties benefit.

For example, the Lalonde report inspired action in many countries but also had an interesting bilateral influence on developments in Canada. The ideas conveyed in the report were quickly and enthusiastically adopted in other countries such as Sweden and the United States, but were reintroduced in Canada some years later and were significant as the rationale for the establishment of the Health Promotion Directorate, the first such national body responsible for health promotion. These exchanges between nations and international organisations were also the pattern for other ideas generated in Canada. For example, the concepts of healthy cities and healthy public policy were both born at a conference in Toronto in 1984, subsequently adopted by the European Office of WHO and imported back into Canada several years later when they seemed to have generated considerable momentum elsewhere. In other words, although Canada has contributed ideas to the international dialogue in health promotion, Canadians have also benefited from the positive receipt of these ideas and from the experiences of other countries in translating the ideas into practice.

Canada's leadership in the development of health promotion globally began even before health promotion emerged in the early 1970s. Prior to that, Canada was extremely active in the development of the major scientific and professional organisation in the field, the International Union for Health Education, with Michael Palko, one of the early presidents of the union, playing a leading role in the union and establishing a North American office in Canada. Subsequently, Lavada Pinder, a Director General of the Canadian Health Promotion Directorate, played a pivotal role in championing successfully the addition of health promotion to the name of the Union and in helping to expand its institutional and organisational membership base. More recently, Canada has helped to reinvigorate the North American region of the International Union for Health Promotion and Education (IUHPE) by providing leadership to develop a regional project on the effectiveness of health promotion, and over the years there has been a strong and steady presence of people from Canada and Quebec on the board of directors of the Union. Others, such as Ron Draper, the first director general of the health promotion directorate in Canada and Gerry Dafoe, the long standing executive director of the Canadian Public Health Association, made significant contributions to global leadership in health promotion though their work with the World Health Organisation, particularly through their organisation of the First International Conference on Health Promotion in Ottawa in 1986.

Again, although Canadians contributed leadership in these processes and to these organisations, Canada benefited from experiences gained in the international arena through importing ideas and models from international organisations. Perhaps the prime example of this influence is in fact the change in perspective about health promotion in Canada that resulted from the dialogue with WHO which led to the first international conference on health promotion, as evidenced by Canada's adoption of the language and vision of health promotion articulated by the WHO. A second example of such international influence is the establishment of national funding for healthy communities projects in Canada based on the experience of WHO EURO, despite the fact that the initial concept originated in Canada.

Canada has also participated in the global health promotion movement through the provision of human, technical and financial resources. These contributions have primarily been made through health promotion projects sponsored by the Canadian International Development Agency (CIDA) or the International Development Research Centre (IDRC). Here are a few examples among the dozens of such projects that occurred over the past decade, conducted in partnership with one or the other of the centres belonging to the Canadian Consortium of Health Promotion Research (CCHPR), a network of fifteen university-based units devoted to health promotion research and training (CCHPR, 2003).

One was a project carried out in Chile in the late 1990's that involved collaboration between the Centre for Health Promotion at the University of Toronto and the National Department of Health in Chile. This collaboration focused on the development of a national health promotion programme in Chile. Its successes included the establishment of not only a National Committee but also health promotion resource centres throughout the country as well as the training of health promotion practitioners (for further information the website can be explored at http://www.acdi-cida.gc.ca/cida_ ind.nsf/).

A second partnership in South America, coordinated by the Canadian Public Health Association, involved collaboration with the National School of Public Health in Brazil. In contrast to that of Chile, the initial focus of this project was local rather than national and involved strengthening the relationship between the National School and a local Favella in Rio de Janeiro, partly through a community health centre attached to the School. This enterprise is about to enter a second phase, after the successful completion of the first (see http://www.cpha.ca/english/intprog/brazil/about.htm).

The Canadian Society for International Health coordinated a third project, *Youth for Health*, in collaboration with the government of Ukraine, non governmental organisations and a national survey organisation. The project, which was conducted in Kyiv, produced a model for youth health promotion that is currently being tested and developed further in other Ukrainian communities in a second phase (see http://www.csih.org/what/yfh/ yfh1.html).

Partnering with, the Institut Africain de Gestion Urbaine (IAGU) based in Dakar, Senegal, the Quebec WHO Collaborating Centre for the Development of Healthy Cities and Towns, itself a joint venture between the Réseau Québécois des villes et villages en santé, the Groupe de recherche et d'intervention en promotion de la santé de l'Université Laval and the Institut national de santé publique du Québec, worked at the establishment and the evaluation of a network of healthy communities in six countries of sub-Saharan francophone countries in Africa (Simard et al., 1997).

A final example is the Training for Health Renewal Program (THRP), a partnership between the University of Saskatchewan health science faculty, the Prairie Region Health Promotion Research Centre and the Ministry of Health in Mozambique. THRP is involved in a systematic exploration of two related concepts, human-centred development as the ultimate goal of health work and new community health practice as a means through which health workers and communities take action to achieve human-centred development. The aim is to articulate the guiding principles for shaping curriculum and training initiatives in both countries (see http://www.usask.ca/healthsci/che/prhprc/thrp/thrp.html.).

As suggested by the aim of the Mozambique project, once again, Canada's contribution to global health promotion is a reciprocal one. This is also true for the other projects mentioned. In all cases, Canadian participants have benefited greatly from the experience of working with health promotion policy-makers and practitioners in other countries. Lessons have been learned about health promotion that often resulted in a rethinking and modification of their own practices in Canada. For example, at a workshop at the seventeenth World Conference on Health Promotion in Paris in 2001 that discussed three of the projects above, facilitators and barriers for projects of this kind were identified. It was found that many of the key ingredients for success had to do with the establishment and maintenance of respectful and strong interpersonal relations between delegates from the participating countries.

Examples of facilitating circumstances include a history of collaboration between the countries involved, time spent at the beginning to develop trust, vision, respect and understanding of the context, space devoted to building the team and a focus on ongoing close communication. Resources were also considered important, although there was a feeling that external resources should not be too large and that in-kind resources were as important as financial ones. Direct involvement of the funders was also thought to be important, especially with respect to evaluation. Barriers to success included changes in the political context such as those of government or changes in the physical environment. Others included unrealistic expectations of funding agencies, as when they failed to take context into account and cultural variations, including different concepts of time and language differences. Such facilitating circumstances and barriers are likely to apply to collaborations between countries with different income levels (for comparable discussions of collaborative community-based projects see Part II, Chapter 11).

As suggested by these four examples, Canada's global contribution to health promotion has been and continues to be primarily positive in nature.

Fundamentally, Canada is well regarded and is often perceived to be easier to work with than the former colonial powers by low and middle income countries, as the authors of this Chapter have been able to observe in their projects all over the world. However, the Canadian contribution to health promotion globally could be strengthened. Specifically, it could be more organised and visible. More resources could be applied. Perhaps most importantly, the Canadian government could do a better job of supporting the development of health promotion at home and in turning the rhetoric of health promotion into local and national action.

Lessons from the Canadian experience

Canada has played a prominent role in the evolution of health promotion in the past three decades and continues to play a role in its maturation. In the international arena, it has been shown how Canada, small in population but geographically vast, can nevertheless contribute to global health efforts. Canadians have learned from others, benefited from international collaboration, and have seen the value of academic practitioner partnerships in local and international initiatives. Canada's participation in international organisations has benefited not only those organisations but also Canadian institutions at various levels. Moreover, this exchange has given rise to an interesting process by which ideas developed in Canada sometimes find legitimacy elsewhere before they can be fully embraced at home.

Reflecting on developments in Canada itself, whilst health promotion has largely disappeared from government discourse (although it may be making a comeback in some places) it continues to influence disease prevention efforts, to inspire charitable and non governmental organisations, and to be influential in media campaigns and social marketing. Physical fitness and healthy lifestyles are back in vogue and the state has rediscovered its role in advocating a little ParticipACTION (the name of a well known government social marketing campaign promoting physical fitness). While Canada may be the home of the Health Field Concept, the Epp report and the Ottawa Charter, these documents seem to have ceased to inform the development of new ideas and they are no longer invoked in political addresses. The future of health promotion in Canada looks strangely like the past, exhorting individuals to take personal responsibility for their health in order to reduce healthcare expenditures.

Hence there are reasons for concern. Despite research that demonstrates the importance of social equity for health, Canada has witnessed a growing gap between the rich and poor in the past decade. For example, between 1989 and 2001, real family incomes for the bottom 20 per cent of family income earners in Canada dropped 6.8 per cent compared to an increase of 16.5 per cent for the top 20 per cent (Statistics Canada, 2003). The optimistic view that it would be possible to coordinate policy across sectors and generate health impact assessments has not been realised. There remain policy worlds that do not communicate, particularly between the economic and social sectors of government, despite groundbreaking events like the Quebec anti-poverty legislation (Noël, 2003). Health promotion has not been easy to integrate into a healthcare system dominated by acute needs and struggling to provide chronic care whilst budgets for health promotion and disease prevention efforts remain small. Finally, new threats to wellbeing arising from terrorism, ecological disasters and unforeseen bacterial and viral agents, including the SARS episode of 2003 that hit Canada very badly, have taken resources away from health promotion.

Despite these concerns, there remain reasons to be optimistic about Canada's possible future contributions to health promotion. Oral health, which was noted in the Lalonde report as a contributor to poor health in the 1970s, has not been a key dimension of health promotion campaigns in Canada for the past 30 years. It is, therefore, a momentous step to see the beginnings of a multi-stakeholder discussion of a national oral health strategy. It is also important to note that the Canadian Consortium for Health Promotion Research is still alive and well. Should Canada lead the globe in removing patent protections, that currently limit global access to generic anti-retrovirals by those suffering from HIV/AIDS, the country would again emerge as a world leader in health promotion, a reputation that it gained yet another time in recent years with the global fight against tobacco (for discussions of global AIDS and tobacco management strategies see Chapters 6, 8 and 9).

In the meantime, as Canadian researchers and practitioners tackle physical inactivity today, they are doing so with the benefit of 30 years of critical reflection, analysis and experience. Despite the reversion to outdated discourses, therefore, it is encouraging that health promoters in Canada have available to them the skills and expertise developed over many years, to support improvements in the health of Canadians and of many others around the globe in the early years of the twenty-first century.

References

Alberta Premier's Commission on Future Health Care for Albertans (1989) *The Rainbow Report: Our Vision for Health*. Edmonton: Queen's printer.
Boyce, W.F. (2002) Influence of health promotion bureaucracy on community participation: a Canadian case study. *Health Promotion International*, **17** (1): 61–68.
Brown, E.R. and Margo, G.E. (1978) Health education: can the reformers be reformed? *International Journal of Health Services*, **8**: 3–25.
Crawford, R. (1977) You are dangerous to your health: the politics of victim-blaming. *International Journal of Health Services*, **7**: 663–80.
Canadian Consortium of Health Promotion Research (2003) http://www.utoronto.ca/chp/chp/consort/index.htm
Canadian Dental Association (2003) *Strategic Forum*. 6 September. Ottawa: Westin Ottawa.

Epp, J. (1986) *Achieving Health for All: A Framework for Health Promotion*. Ottawa: Minister of Supply and Services, Canada.

Evans, J.R. (1987) *Toward a Shared Direction for Health in Ontario: Report of the Ontario Health Review Panel*. Toronto: Ontario Ministry of Health.

Evans, R., Barer, M. and Marmor, T. (eds) (1994) *Why are Some People Healthy and Others Not? The Determinants of the Health of Populations*. New York: Aldine De Gruyter.

Federal, Provincial and Territorial Advisory Committee on Population Health (1994) *Strategies for Population Health: Investing in the Health of Canadians*. Ottawa:Minister of Supply and Services.

Finn, E. (2002) Canada: World leader in health promotion? Available from CLICK4HP archives at :http://sundial.ccs.yorku.ca/cgi-bin/wa?A2=ind0309&L= click4hp&F=&S=&P=11048

Green, L.W. (1994) Canadian health promotion: an outsider's view from the inside. In Pederson, A., O'Neill, M. and Rootman, I. (eds) *Health Promotion in Canada: Provincial, National and International Perspectives*. Toronto: W. B. Saunders.

Hamilton, N. and Bhatti, T. (1996) *Population Health Promotion: An Integrated Model of Population Health and Health Promotion*. Ottawa: Health Canada.

Hancock, T. (1986) Lalonde and beyond: looking back at 'A new perspective on the health of Canadians.' *Health Promotion*, 1: 93–100.

Health Canada (1993) *Technical Report: 1990 National Health Promotion Survey*. Ottawa: Health Canada.

Health Canada (1997) *Health Promotion in Canada: A Case Study*. Ottawa: Minister of Public Works and Government Services.

Kaufert, P. (1999) The vanishing woman: gender and population health. In Pollard, T. and Hyatt, S. (eds) *Sex, Gender and Health*. Cambridge: Cambridge University Press.

Kickbusch, I. (1994) Introduction: tell me a story. In Pederson, A., O'Neill, M. and Rootman, I. (eds) *Health Promotion in Canada: Provincial, National and International Perspectives*. Toronto: W. B. Saunders.

Labonte, R. and Penfold, S. (1981) *Health Promotion Philosophy: From Victim-blaming to Social Responsibility*. A working paper printed by the Western Region Office, Health Promotion Directorate, Health and Welfare Canada.

Lalonde, M. (1974) *A New Perspective on the Health of Canadians*. Ottawa: Health and Welfare Canada.

Noël, A. (2003) *A Law Against Poverty: Quebec's New Approach to Combating Poverty and Exclusion*. Background paper, family network, Ottawa, Canadian Policy Research Networks, http://www.cprn.org.

Nolen, S. (2003) Spearhead AIDS fight, UN envoy tells Canada. *The Globe and Mail*, 25 September 2003: A1 & A20.

O'Neill, M., Pederson, A. and Rootman, I. (2000) Health Promotion in Canada: Declining or Transforming? *Health Promotion International*, 15 (2): 135–41,

Pederson, A. (1989) *The Development of Health Promotion in Ontario*. Toronto: University of Toronto, unpublished master's thesis.

Pederson, A., O'Neill, M. and Rootman, I. (eds) (1994) *Health Promotion in Canada: Provincial, National and International Perspectives*. Toronto: W. B. Saunders.

Podborski, S. (1987) *Health Promotion Matters in Ontario: A Report of the Minister's Advisory Group on Health Promotion*. Toronto: Ministry of Health.

Raeburn, J.M. (1994) The View from Down Under: The Impact of Canadian Health Promotion Development in New Zealand. In Pederson, A., O'Neill, M. and

Rootman, I. (eds) *Health Promotion in Canada: Provincial, National and International Perspectives.* Toronto: W. B. Saunders.

Raphael, D. and Bryant, T. (2002) The limitations of population health as a model for a new public health. *Health Promotion International,* **17** (2): 189–99.

Robertson, A. (1998) Critical reflections on the politics of need: implications for public health. *Social Science and Medicine,* **47** (10): 1419–30.

Rootman, I. Ed. (1989) *Health Promotion Survey Technical Report.* Ottawa: Health and Welfare Canada.

Signal, L.N. (1993) *The Politics of the New Public Health: A Case Study of the Ontario Premier's Council On Health Strategy.* Toronto: University of Toronto, unpublished doctoral thesis.

Simard, P., O'Neill, M., Diop, O. E., Ly, E. H., Diarra, D. and Badje, H. (1997) *Contraintes et opportunités pour la mise en oeuvre du mouvement Villes et villages en santé en Afrique francophone (rapport synthèse).* Québec et Dakar : GRIPSUL, IAGU et RQVVS.

Spasoff, R. (1987) *Health for all Ontario: Report of the Panel on Health Goals for Ontario.* Toronto: Ontario Ministry of Health.

Statistics Canada (2003) *Income in Canada.* Ottawa: CD ROM, Table T 802.

VVS (2003) Réseau québécois des villes et villages en santé. http://www.rqvvs.qc.ca

World Health Organisation (1986) Ottawa Charter for Health Promotion. *Health Promotion,* **1** (4): i–v.

CHAPTER 19

Health Promotion in the USA: Building a Science-based Health Promotion Policy

DEBRA LIGHTSEY, DAVID MCQUEEN AND LAURIE ANDERSON

Established goals and evidence are necessary, but not sufficient, to create health promoting policies in a large, federalised democracy. While some policies are undoubtedly created with a lack of scientific evidence, most have some support from sources considered scientific. The policy making realm invokes differing burdens of proof, depending on the controversies surrounding a policy and its support in the community. The United States has an unusual infrastructure for health promotion policy. Experts and constituents have developed national health promotion goals, backed by long-term data and broad capabilities to support health promotion. These have been made public in the document *Healthy People 2010* (US Department of Health and Human Services, 2000a). Through the *Guide to Community Preventive Health Services*, the US has developed a consensus-based process to determine when health promotion interventions have evidence of effectiveness (www.TheCommunityGuide.org).

This chapter examines the role of evidence in health promotion policy in the US, nesting proof in the larger context of policy making. This context includes not only that of proof, but also those of partners, politics and priorities. Each level of government whether federal, state or local, plays specific roles in all of these realms. These realms will be explored using the example of Clean Indoor Air policy in the state of Delaware.

Background

American health promotion has often been distinguished from its counterparts in Europe and Canada by its individualist orientation. This orientation reflects the origins of American health promotion in health education theory and practice and the seeming absence among American health promoters of the refinement of the Canadian and European efforts towards the Ottawa Charter goals, seen by many as the defining moment of health promotion in the West (for further discussion of the influence of the Ottawa Charter on global health promotion see Chapter 1).

Two distinct traditions emerged, separating the United States' developments from those of Europe and Canada: the European, framed by concerns with the social, economic and political roots of health, with a focus on the socio-political and the American, framed by the enlargement of the traditional scope of health education. The USA has had a strong focus on the individual and lifestyle approaches to health promotion and individualistic health promotion was seen as a core area for health educators. Since much of the underlying disciplinary base for theory and methods was found in educational psychology, there has been a strong concern with attitudes, opinions, beliefs and individual ways to change personal behaviours relating to health. Of course, these are general characterisations of a diverse field of practice and the spirit of the Ottawa Charter is to be found in much American health promotion practice, just as strong individual behavioural change approaches will be found in European approaches to health promotion. Nonetheless, the underlying differences between the two traditions remain to this day (for a comparable discussion of policy dichotomies, see Chapter 5 and, especially, Chapter 18).

Over the past three decades, health promotion in the US has grown into a large and diverse part of the American public health establishment operating at the local, state, regional, national and international levels. In the academic world health promotion is found as departments or components of departments of every school of public health as well as in many university-based settings. Similarly at the state and local levels there are departments of health promotion and many practitioners. At the federal level, one of the centres within the federal agency of the Department of Health and Human Services is named the National Center of Chronic Disease Prevention and Health Promotion (NCCDPHP). With such broad-based institutionalisation, the diversity of approaches to health promotion contained in it will reflect the diversity of approaches found elsewhere. Thus, the practice of health promotion within the US defies simple characterisation.

Despite its broad diversity of practice US health promotion is grounded in an effective, evidence-based approach to changing and improving the public's health. At every level health promotion practice demonstrates that the approaches taken are based on strong criteria of effectiveness. It reflects the tenet of public health that policies and the derived actions should be based on sound scientific principles. This means that there must be proof that involves data that can be collected routinely at the appropriate level and interpreted scientifically by all practitioners in the field. While this condition is considered necessary for health promotion policy enactment, it is rarely if ever sufficient.

Organised approaches to evidence-based policy for health promotion

One approach to creating an evidence-based policy is to create an institutional, structural response. This has been the case in the US. Briefly stated, the underlying principle is that evidence, however defined, is too complex an issue to be left simply for individuals to define. Evidence must be the product of the concerted effort of a number of experts in the field who define the parameters of what constitutes evidence. Methodology of how evidence is shown must be clearly stated and formalised. The opinions of scientists, academicians, practitioners, policymakers, public servants and the general public is integrated into an overall schema for assessing evidence. This process of consensus building through widespread engagement can be seen as a very American approach. It is, essentially, a tedious and laborious undertaking, involving time, effort and considerable cost. It is an approach befitting an economically highly developed, post-industrial society. It is the manifestation of a democratically fair solution to a complicated issue.

Policy making has its own institutional characteristics and is a complex endeavour for a country as diverse as the US. The making of policy and the institutional approach to evidence are intertwined since evidence, no matter how derived, is not the sole guiding component of policy making. While the focus is on the role of evidence and its importance in health promotion policy, it must be emphasised that many other factors play an important role in the making of policy.

Healthy People 2010: evidence and policy related through goals

In many instances, health promotion policy in the US is set institutionally by large consensus projects. This is most apparent in the successful efforts over 30 years to set national health goals. The goals are related to evidence in several ways, but most importantly they reflect the notion that the attainment of goals can be measured systematically overtime, proof that is linked to the development of scientifically based indicators that can be routinely monitored. This insistence that goals and their attainment must be measurable sets the US approach apart. Fortunately, with its highly developed public health infrastructure and sophisticated surveillance systems, the US is able to collect very accurate information on changes in health status and behaviour in the population.

The document *Healthy People 2010* is a salient example of a national effort to define goals. With its procedural openness, including the public availability of information and the attainability of documents, it is an exemplar of how health promotion ideas may be effectively integrated into a national approach to health promotion (for information and publications visit http://www.healthypeople.gov). In the development of each target area of *Healthy People 2010* the emphasis is on the quality of data to monitor the progress of the nation towards the target (for a comparison of this with other national and institutional attempts to set goals and monitor progress, see Part III, Chapter 14).

For example, smoking rates had been monitored over time and across states. As a result, the target setting method of *Healthy People 2010* could be based on evidence, as it is for other objectives that can be influenced in the short term, such as those related to physical activity, diet, smoking and alcohol-related motor vehicle deaths (US Department of Health and Human Services, 2000a). One challenge to this approach is that when sufficient evidence or measures do not yet exist issues may be left off the national agenda. For example, lack of reliable ethnic data makes establishing targets for some ethnic minorities impossible. Identifying these gaps can lead to new research and measurement. http://www.healthypeople.gov/Document/HTML/tracking/THP_PartA.htm

The Task Force on Community Preventive Services

In the United States, the Centers for Disease Control and Prevention (CDC) has taken the lead in assisting an independent non-federal US Task Force on Community Preventive Services to provide recommendations to the practitioners, policy makers and the public about the effectiveness of programmes to improve population health and maximise health promotion investments. Through systematic reviews of the intervention evaluation literature, the *Community Guide* summarises what is known about the effectiveness, economic efficiency and feasibility of health promotion programmes and policies. Evidence for monitoring national health indicators is provided by *Healthy People 2010* whilst evidence on the effectiveness of interventions to achieve these health goals is provided in the *Community Guide*.

The Task Force envisioned a *Community Guide* that would encompass *Healthy People 2010* priority areas; cover a broad scope of problem areas and related interventions; address risk behaviours that collectively have the largest impact on the health of the population; and consider major causes of poor health across the life span (Truman et al., 2000). For each interventions topic, such as those of nutrition, physical activity and tobacco use, a national body of experts is assembled to guide the review by reaching a consensus on critical determinants of population health that are amenable to intervention programmes. Their views are made explicit in the use of logic models, which describe phenomena that affect health, (see examples at: www.TheCommunityGuide.org) so the Task Force and the public can decide if fundamental determinants have been included.

Evidence of the effectiveness of programmes or policies that attempt to intervene on health determinants is collected and summarised in systematic reviews of the scientific literature. This process sheds light on where US investments in health promotion research and programme or policy evaluations have occurred, and where they have not. Where sufficient information exists, redundant investments to answer questions already known might be avoided.

Where no intervention research is evident, development and evaluation of potentially promising approaches can be considered. The Task Force's goal is to benefit from investments in intervention research already made in the public interest, translate these into effective public policy and programmes, and direct future research resources towards important unanswered questions.

The Task Force on Community Preventive Services makes recommendations based on the body of evidence that has accrued over time in the scientific literature. The work intends to define, categorise, summarise and rate the quality of evidence on the effectiveness of population-based interventions to impact on specific outcomes. The *Community Guide* will summarise what is known about the effectiveness and cost-effectiveness of population-based interventions for prevention and control, provide recommendations on these interventions and methods for their delivery based on the evidence, and identify a prevention research agenda. As reviews are completed they are made available on the Community Guide website (www.TheCommunityGuide.org) and published in the health promotion literature. Periodically reviews must be updated to include new intervention research and to take into account temporal changes in the sociocultural and environmental context in which these interventions occurred. For example, previously successful programmatic approaches to improve nutrition, physical activity, tobacco cessation and HIV/AIDS prevention may require different strategies to be effective in the present.

Recommendations in the *Community Guide* regarding the interventions are based on the strength of evidence of effectiveness, harms and generalisability. To categorise the strength of a body of evidence on the effectiveness of a specific intervention to impact on a given outcome, the Task Force considers the suitability of evaluation design to be able to attribute, with confidence, a change in an outcome caused by the given intervention; the quality of study execution and threats to validity; numbers of studies; consistency of findings; size of observed effects; and in rare circumstances expert opinion. The Task Force currently considers studies for which there are concurrent comparison groups and prospective measurements of exposure and outcome as most suitable, such as randomised or non-randomised clinical or community trials, multiple measurement pre- or post-designs with concurrent comparison groups, prospective cohort studies. All retrospective designs or multiple pre- or post-measurements without concurrent comparison groups, such as retrospective cohort studies and case control studies are rated as moderately suitable whilst designs with single pre- or post-measurements and no concurrent comparison group or exposure and outcomes measured in a single group at the same point in time such as the post only design are seen as least suitable (for greater detail on methods see www.TheCommunityGuide.org). The Task Force has noted that population-based prevention strategies frequently are multiple component and complex, and that randomised controlled trials may not be feasible or desirable to evaluate the effectiveness of community interventions.

Policy making in the US: proof, partners, politics and priorities

The implementation of policies, in the US, is made complex by the fact that not only does the federal government share power with states but also states share power with local government. The federal government's jurisdiction is limited, requiring that many policies be considered by 50 different units of government in 50 different states. The addition of local government intervention produces a vast array of policies across political jurisdictions, adopted at different times and for different reasons.

The factors that shape policy making process can be broadly categorised as the four Ps: proof from evidence that a policy is warranted; identifying partners who will champion the policy; politics, including the policy interests and electoral dynamics that characterise elected officials' decision making; and priorities, where the policy falls in the public's and policy makers' agenda.

This section will examine each of the four identified influences on health promotion policy, using the example of the enactment of state Clean Indoor Air restrictions in the state of Delaware. In 2002, Delaware became only the second state, after California, to enact a comprehensive clean indoor air law that covers almost all enclosed public places and workplaces, including restaurants and freestanding bars. Delaware also became the first state to repeal a state law pre-empting local government bodies from adopting smoking restrictions that are more stringent than state requirements, although this aspect of the 2002 law was overshadowed by its other provisions and drew little publicity and discussion. Pre-emption of local clean indoor air policy activity poses a major barrier to efforts to reduce second hand smoke exposure, and have been supported by the tobacco industry (Jacobson and Zapawa, 2001; Henson et al., 2002). A total of 22 states currently appear to have pre-emptive state laws in place.

Since Delaware adopted its law, four other states have enacted similarly comprehensive laws, including New York, Connecticut, Maine and Massachusetts. A number of states have also attempted to repeal pre-emption statutes, with some limited success. Delaware was also the first state to enact a comprehensive state law without previous experience with local clean indoor air ordinances.

Most tobacco control has been accomplished at the state and local levels (Jacobson and Zapawa, 2001). There is, however, a major federal role in supporting the proof, partners, politics and priorities needed to move tobacco control forward, as will be discussed below. The picture that emerges is of multilevel action, with different foci at each level. Progress is not linear, and one solution does not suit the whole nation. For that reason, evidence must take its place as only one of the drivers of health promotion policy.

Delaware is a small, mid-Atlantic state, comprising a population of less than 800,000 and an area of less than 2000 square miles bordered by the states of New Jersey, Pennsylvania and Maryland. It includes both urban and rural communities, as well as tourist attractions (see www.state.de.us/gic/facts/ history). Because of its size and location, it must compete with neighbouring states for business, including tourism and entertainment. Hence Delaware cultivates a corporate-friendly environment through its tax and incorporation policies, as well as a specialised judicial system for corporate law. More than 50 per cent of all US publicly traded companies and 58 per cent of the Fortune 500 companies are legally headquartered in Delaware (www.state.de.us/ corp), remarkable given its small size. The state is also home to several large legalised gambling venues that draw much of their business from neighbouring states where gambling is more limited.

Delaware's funding of tobacco prevention and control comes from a variety of sources. CDC funds Delaware's Tobacco Control Programme through its Office on Smoking and Health. Delaware also received tobacco control funds through the Robert Wood Johnson Foundation and from state funds, including tobacco settlement payments.

Proof

Although scientific evidence is the gold standard for which US public health professionals strive to inform public policy making, it is rare to find unanimity among researchers, and therefore policy makers are often called on to weigh the quality and veracity of evidence. Policy makers often need to act with incomplete or conflicting evidence. Public pressure to act, political opportunity, fiscal realities, strong ideologies and constituent interests all can drive this need.

That is not to say that it is wrong to act with less than solid proof because in a democracy, other truths hold equal or greater weight than science. There are many instances in which not acting is just as damaging or more so than acting without knowing all the consequences. This runs counter to the prevailing public health notion of a rational linear process of policy formulation from data collection to scientific consensus (Sommer, 2001). As a result, real world policy making can be anathema to those dedicated to the science of public health. If it is to contribute to public policy, public health science must strive not just for excellence, but also for relevance.

This relevance is never more important than when scientific proof is clear, and public health has clearly defined goals for action. Yet, health promotion interventions often face a higher burden of proof than more immediate forms of intervention (McGinnis, 2001; McGinnis et al., 2002). However, when conditions are right, proof can stimulate policy action.

In the case of second hand smoke, both the evidence for and the consensus on the goal were clear. In 1999, a summary of the components of comprehensive tobacco control programmes published by CDC's Office on Smoking and Health included eliminating non smokers' exposure to environmental tobacco smoke as one of four goals for such programmes (CDC, 1999). In 2000, *Healthy People 2010* included an objective calling on states to 'establish laws on smoke free indoor air that prohibit smoking or limit it to separately ventilated areas in public places and worksites.' A related objective also called for elimination of all state laws pre-empting local tobacco control actions (US Department of Health and Human Services, 2000b). Also that year, the Surgeon General recommended smoking bans as the most effective method for reducing second hand smoke exposure (US Department of Health and Human Services, 2000b). Finally, the Task Force on Community Preventive Services strongly recommended smoking bans and restrictions as effective interventions for reducing second hand smoke exposure in 2001 (CDC, 2000).

Using federal and other resources, and relying heavily on the national goals defined by CDC (CDC, 1999) as well by *Healthy People 2010*, Delaware's coalition formulated a state tobacco plan in January 2000. Given the broad national consensus it included clean indoor air as one of its goals (Delaware Division of Public Health, 2000). After funds became available from the 1998 Master Settlement Agreement between the tobacco industry and the states, the state conducted an Adult Tobacco Survey including measures of public support for clean indoor air policies.

Federal resources by way of CDC funds also allowed the state to track adult and youth tobacco use through the Behavioural Risk Factor Surveillance System, the Youth Risk Factor Surveillance System, and the Youth Tobacco Survey. These surveys provided state-specific evidence of the burden of tobacco use in the state.

Partners

Partnerships are widely recognised as necessary to implement effective public health interventions (see, for example, IOM, 2002; CDC mission statement at www.cdc.gov). Less often discussed is the role of partnerships in promoting sound health promotion policy (see Chapter 4 for further discussion of partnerships). While strong, science-based recommendations are a starting point, government agencies can only advocate policy change in the limited venue of their own administrations. For example, federal employees and many state employees are prohibited from activities considered to be lobbying. Similarly, federal funds cannot be used to lobbying for specific legislation. Government representatives are often permitted to pursue the policies of the elected and appointed leaders of the administration, so working to place health promotion policy on administration legislative and regulatory agendas is an important lever in policy change. However, legislatively initiated policy is more plentiful, and therefore often a preferred method for those seeking change.

Non governmental organisations play a key role in the policy making process. Their agendas are not always identical to those government scientists may view as being empirically justified, but they are often in the best position to propose policy options to the full spectrum of decision makers. They also, importantly, are constituents of government agencies, and must therefore play a role in developing plans, goals, science and programmes.

At the federal level, executive branch agencies develop relationships through the creation of mechanisms such as advisory groups, joint projects, conferences and professional affiliations. In the case of tobacco, CDC maintains a number of partnerships with national organisations, from the disease-specific, such as the American Cancer Society, the American Lung Association, and the American Heart Association to those that focus exclusively on tobacco issues, including Americans for Non-smokers' Rights, the Campaign for Tobacco Free Kids, the American Medical Association's Smokeless States Initiative, the Advocacy Institute, and the American Legacy Foundation. Others represent state and local tobacco control programmes such as the Association of State and Territorial Health Officials or focus on specific population groups, such as Tribal Support Networks. Many of these national groups have state and local affiliates whom, given their national organisation's relationships and their roles in each jurisdiction, are also likely to engage with their state tobacco control programmes.

Delaware funded by the Robert Wood Johnson Foundation and CDC, supports the IMPACT Coalition, comprising more than 35 organisations representing healthcare institutions, youth groups, local communities, educational organisations, grassroots networks and state agencies (see www.state.de.us/dhss/dph/shatitis.htm). These partners implement programmes and are able to present policy options to legislators and administrators. The collaboration created by the coalition also serves policy purposes, achieving consensus on policy goals and providing a forum for coordination. While no federal or state funds can support lobbying activities, the unified message helped these organisations to work bring a concerted effort to bear using less restricted resources.

The systematic building of constituencies through this coalition enabled the state to pursue the goals identified through federal and state consensus processes. Federal and private support, then, created conditions that gave rise to an active policy force for tobacco control, laying the groundwork for the Clean Indoor Air reforms that would follow.

Politics

Although political forces are difficult to quantify, actions taken by policy makers must take into account the opinions of supporters and constituents. This is assured by the two-year election cycles for lower house members in most legislative bodies. Politicians are driven by the need to be responsive to voters and contributors whilst the influence on policy makers by constituents is an essential feature of democracy.

In 2000, as the Delaware health and social services agency developed its legislative agenda to propose to the incoming Governor, the IMPACT partners asked the public health division to make clean indoor air a priority. The division presented this proposal to the Cabinet Secretary's office. Since the Cabinet Secretary did not wish to propose that the newly elected Governor take on a potentially controversial subject that was not in her election platform, it was suggested that IMPACT might be more effective in working directly with legislators to propose the legislation. It was acknowledged that the administration would be under more pressure than recognised advocacy groups to draft a moderate bill (Silverman and Gatto, 2003).

Members of the coalition drafted legislation that would have been the strongest in the country. It proposed to outlaw smoking in any enclosed area to which the general public was invited, as well as outdoor areas within 20 feet of an entrance or exit to such an area (141st DE General Assembly, Senate Bill 99). This included stand-alone bars, some private clubs, and all gambling establishments.

While in many states and localities the tobacco industry organised opposition to smoking bans through restaurant associations and smokers rights groups, no such activity took place in Delaware until after the passage of the Bill. However, a number of business interests did push for changes in the proposed law. A total of 28 amendments were offered during the two years of debate on the bill. Most sought exemptions for a particular type of establishment from the ban, with the gambling establishments most widely expected to succeed. In addition to gaming facilities, exemptions were sought for: tobacco retailers; fire, rescue or ambulance company facilities when used for fundraising purposes; fraternal organisations; stand-alone bars (known in Delaware as taverns and taprooms); restaurants; brew pubs; hotel and motel bars and lobbies; small, seasonal hotels and motels; and hotels affiliated with gaming facilities. Other amendments sought to remove the requirement that smokers be at least 20 feet from an exit or entrance, restore the pre-emption clause or delay the effective date for specific types of businesses.

While these amendments demonstrated a large group of opponents, no organised opposition emerged. Most groups expressed concern about the law's economic impacts, given the ease of crossing into other states for entertainment and tourism. Given that all offered the same evidence and rationale, to decide which businesses to exempt proved to be a near-impossible task for legislators.

Tobacco control advocates relied on published peer-reviewed scientific studies that challenged claims about economic harm from smoking bans (Glantz and Charlesworth, 1999). They relied on overwhelming evidence that these policies are effective in reducing second hand smoke exposure, and a national consensus that this exposure is a serious health threat that should be addressed. These groups stood together, while the opposition never came together. After two years of debate, the measure passed with only two changes to its broad prohibitions: the outdoor ban applying to areas within 20 feet of smoke free facilities was eliminated, and fundraisers by fire, rescue and ambulance companies were exempted.

The IMPACT coalition's ability to present a cogent and unified message in the face of relative chaos in the opposition led legislators to pass a controversial bill overwhelmingly. By gaining the Governor's support, the coalition strengthened its position during the second year of the debate.

Politicians were also moved by the supportive editorials in the state's largest daily newspaper, the *Wilmington News Journal* (Wilmington News Journal, 2001). The tobacco control programme's long-standing efforts at public education contributed to strong public support for the law. The state's use of CDC's model Adult Tobacco Survey, supported by tobacco settlement dollars appropriated by the state, was able to document that 87 per cent of residents thought people should be protected from second hand smoke, and showed that people would be more likely to patronise venues if they were smoke free (Ratledge, 2002).

Priorities

A fundamental challenge facing health promotion policy in the US is its relative priority when compared to medical treatment. For whereas public investment in the former seems to require evidence that future savings will offset the cost of the investment, no such demands are made of the latter (McGinnis et al., 2002). Policy makers must balance health needs against a wide array of public needs for policy and resources.

In Delaware the state agency, in consultation with the Governor's staff, did not request resources to implement new smoking restrictions. This was a crucial decision, because it limited debate to the policy issues in the committees responsible for health, rather than involving, in addition, those responsible for budgets. The lack of budgetary implications meant that this law did not need to be a budget priority, but did need to be a political priority.

In addition to becoming the number one priority for the non governmental members of the IMPACT coalition, the bill became a priority for its lead sponsors as well as for the Governor. Because of the fragmentation of opposition, no priorities were set among those groups opposed, and the clear priorities of colleagues and constituents prevailed. However, the state could not have set these priorities alone. The federal identification of goals and evidence, coupled with the federal investment in tobacco control programme infrastructure and interventions, provided the basis for this remarkable change in policy. The ability to document the problem and gauge public readiness for action was also bolstered by federal assistance, both technical and financial.

This chapter has focused on the underpinnings of US government health promotion policy. While others have discussed the federal role as limited in clean indoor air restrictions (Jacobson and Zapawa, 2001), the example explored here makes it clear that while this role is indirect, it is not trivial. The federal role in providing scientific evidence, programme infrastructure, and programme funds and technical support makes a significant contribution to development of policy at state level. States are able to better read their partners and politics, and help set public priorities, than those at national level. But by providing the context and the tools the stage is set.

The title of this chapter focuses on evidence-based policy. While evidence is desirable and should be the underpinning of sound policy, factors of partnership, politics and priorities are at least equally influential in sharing most policy debates. Public health practitioners and researchers must acknowledge this reality and attend to these other realms, without compromising the goal of policies with proof. While some may believe that a more technocratic approach is preferable, democracy demands complex dynamics, of which proof is just one element.

Also instructive is the use of an environmental approach to reduce exposure to second hand smoke in the US. While the traditional focus on the individual and lifestyle approaches to health promotion still dominates health promotion policy in the US, the evidence base and consensus process have yielded societal action on a number of factors that are beyond individual choice. In addition to second hand smoke, government has acted to employ evidence-based policy interventions recommended by *The Community Guide* in several other areas, including motor vehicle safety, water fluoridation, tobacco price increases, and school policy changes. (See www.thecommunityguide.org). These approaches result in much discussion and occasional controversy about the appropriate role of government versus individual choice in promoting health. Nonetheless, the US continues to favour the role of individual choice in decisions regarding health, while recognising that in some areas of health concerns environmental and public policy approaches are the most proven methods for improving the health of the public.

References

Centers for Disease Control and Prevention (1999) *Best Practices for Comprehensive Tobacco Control Programs.* Atlanta GA: US Department of Health and Human Services.

Centers for Disease Control and Prevention. (2000) *Effectiveness of Smoking Bans and Restriction to Reduce Exposure to Environmental Tobacco Smoke (ETS). MMWR Recommendations and Reports, 49(RR-12).* Atlanta GA: US Department of Health and Human Services,

Delaware Division of Public Health (2000) *A Plan for A Tobacco-free Delaware.* Delaware Health and Social Services, http://www.state.de.us/dhss/dph/plan.htm

Glantz, S.A. and Charlesworth, A. (1999) Tourism and hotel revenues before and after passage of smoke-free restaurant ordinances. *Journal of the American Medical Association,* **281**(20): 1911–18.

Henson, R., Medina, L., St Clair, S., Blanke, D., Downs, L. and Jordan, J. (2002) Clean indoor air. Where, why and how. *Journal of Law, Medicine & Ethics,* **30**(3 suppl.): 75–82.

Institute of Medicine (2002) *The Future of the Public's Health in the 21st Century.* Washington DC: National Academy of Sciences.

Jacobson, P.D. and Zapawa, L.M. (2001) Clean indoor air restrictions: Progress and promise. In Rabin, R.L. and Sugarman, S.D. (eds) *Regulating Tobacco.* Oxford, UK: Oxford University Press.

McGinnis, J. (2001) Does proof matter? Why strong evidence sometimes yields weak action. *American Journal of Health Promotion,* **15**(5): 391–96.

McGinnis, J.M., Williams-Russo, P. and Knickman, J.R. (2002) The case for more active policy attention to health promotion. *Health Affairs*, **20**(2): 78–93.

Ratledge, E.C. (2002) *Tobacco Attitudes and Media Survey.* University of Delaware Center for Applied Demography & Survey Research.

Silverman, P. and Gatto, F. (2003), Delaware Division of Public Health. Telephone interview conducted on 1 December 2003 by the author.

Sommer, A. (2001) How public health policy is created: Scientific process and political reality. *American Journal of Epidemiology*, **154**:12 (suppl.): S4–S6.

Truman, B.I., Smith-Akin, C.K., Hinman, A.R., Gebbie, K.M., Brownson, R., Novick, L.F., Lawrence, R.S., Pappaioanou, M., Fielding, J., Evans, C.A. Jr., Guerra, F.A., Vogel-Taylor, M., Mahan, C.S., Fullilove, M., Zaza, S. (2000) Developing the guide to community preventive services: Overview and rationale. *American Journal of Preventive Medicine*, **18**:1(suppl. 1): 18–26.

US Department of Health and Human Services (2000a) *Healthy People 2010*, 2nd ed. Washington DC: US Government Printing Office.

US Department of Health and Human Services (2000b) *Reducing Tobacco Use: A Report of the Surgeon General.* Atlanta, GA: US Department of Health and Human Services.

Wilmington News Journal. (2001) *Banning all Smoking in Indoor Public Places Would be Smart Move.* (Editorial) 22 April.

WHO, EURO (1984) *Health Promotion: A Discussion Document on the Concepts and Principles.* Copenhagen: WHO.

WHO, EURO (1998) *Health Promotion Evaluation: Recommendations to Policymakers.* Copenhagen: WHO.

World Health Assembly (1998) *Resolution WHA 51.12 on Health Promotion.* Agenda Item 20, 16 May 1998. Geneva: WHO.

Author Index

Subject Index